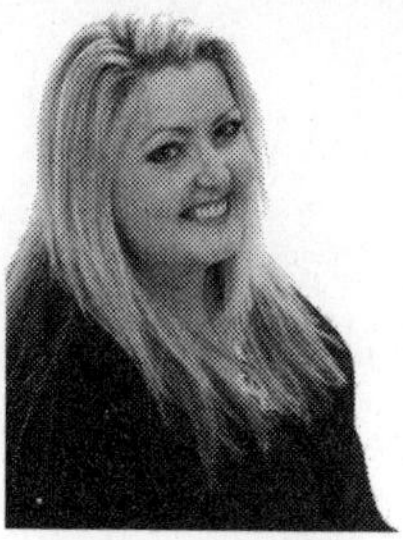

Sheyne Rowley has worked extensively with children and their families for nearly 20 years – the first ten years as a childcare worker and teacher in schools, kindergartens, daycare centres and the home environment, both in Australia and abroad; the last nine years with distressed families, dealing specifically with what appears to be unsolvable cases of significant sleep dysfunction in children aged up to six years. Her unique strategies have seen parents from across the globe contact her to enlist her help in resolving their child's sleep-time issues, which she can do in as little time as three days.

Sheyne's remarkable success rate has seen her secure regular appearances on Channel 7's *Sunrise* since March 2003, where she is known as 'The Australian Baby Whisperer', as well as appearances on Channel 9's *Mornings with Kerri-Anne* and the ABC's *7.30 Report*. In 2008, she was delighted to speak in Parliament House at the launch of PACAN (Parliamentarians Against Childhood Abuse and Neglect). Sheyne is also a popular choice as ambassador for many peak bodies.

Sheyne released her first book *Dream Baby Guide* in 2009 to glowing reviews and it rushed off the bookshop shelves. She was thrilled to see families implement her techniques and achieve amazing results. A whole new dimension to her work began as parents supported each other using this new wisdom.

In 2012, Sheyne welcomed her first precious daughter into the world. She continued working part-time with families, while adjusting to a very challenging motherhood journey herself.

In 2014, she was to face one of the greatest trials of her life as she supported her 24-month-old daughter through life-saving cancer treatment.

To this day, Sheyne believes that the reason she was able to identify and alert the medical teams to her daughter's condition at an early stage, and help her through that treatment so successfully was because of her natural parenting style. That style is the Dream Baby approach.

Sheyne decided it was essential that she release a new and easy-to-follow book that focuses on a healthy, respectful style of parenting, promoting natural sleep.

Dream Baby Guide: Sleep

The essential guide to sleep management in babies

Sheyne Rowley

ARENA
ALLEN&UNWIN

This book is intended as a source of information, not a medical reference book. While every care has been taken in compiling the information contained herein neither the author nor the publishers can be held responsible for any adverse reactions to the suggestions offered. The reader is advised to consult with a medical health professional for any concerns they may have before they embark on any of the suggestions contained herein.

First published in 2015

Arena Books, an imprint of
Allen & Unwin
83 Alexander Street
Crows Nest NSW 2065
Australia
Phone: (61 2) 8425 0100
Email: info@allenandunwin.com
Web: www.allenandunwin.com

Cataloguing-in-Publication details are available
from the National Library of Australia
www.trove.nla.gov.au

ISBN 978 1 74237 588 5

Index by Puddingburn
Set in 11.25/13.6 pt Bembo by Bookhouse, Sydney
Printed and bound in Australia by Griffin Press

10 9 8 7 6 5 4 3 2 1

FSC www.fsc.org MIX Paper from responsible sources FSC® C009448

The paper in this book is FSC® certified.
FSC® promotes environmentally responsible,
socially beneficial and economically viable
management of the world's forests.

For my Dasha Sofia, my extraordinary,
brave, loving and funny little miracle.
You are my reason for being.

Contents

Preface

I'd like to introduce myself. First and foremost I am a mother. An extremely attached, attentive and aware mother of an extraordinary little three-year-old girl. My career has spanned a wonderful 25 years. The skills I have learned and developed over this time, and spent over two decades implementing in other families' homes to help restore their balance, harmony, sanity, marriages and sleep, are the very same skills that saved my own precious daughter's life.

I always wondered why I was The Australian Baby Whisperer, and it wasn't to save everyone else's families: it was to save my own. I have just been fortunate enough to help others along the way. To each of those families, I am eternally grateful. To all those readers new to the *Dream Baby Guide*, you will enjoy a deep understanding and connection to your precious baby that few truly have the chance to enjoy.

I believe in the Dream Baby Philosophy because it has not only helped the thousands of families I have worked with, but my own daughter too.

What is a dream baby?

A dream baby is a baby who has a balanced life, whose individual sleep needs and nutritional needs are met on a daily basis, who feels emotionally settled and is able to cope with the general flow of his day. A dream baby feels safe and comfortable in his environment, and has the emotional skills to enjoy both playing by himself and interacting with others. Most importantly, a dream baby can be heard and believes his needs can be met, and can understand and predict what his carers are asking him to do. A dream baby has parents who understand his needs and, based on their own wisdom, can help him achieve happy days based on that wisdom.

Sleep and behaviour are intimately connected to the way you communicate and interact with your child during the day. They depend on a mixture of skills developed and emotional trust acquired through a respectful flow of communication, play styles implemented, emotional securities fostered, nutritional needs being met and predictable routines. Without a daytime balance, there is no easy path to peaceful sleep. With a daytime balance, sleep just happens.

It's been six years since I released the *Dream Baby Guide*. In the first year of release I quickly learned that my readers were smart, thorough, had a good memory for important information, wanted to do things the right way, but needed to get their lessons fast. When I first wrote the book I was so concerned about the children that I gave extremely detailed and quite repetitive information. I've learned a lot since then . . . I became a mother. I now know that for all my worry about those precious babies I was offering advice for, the parents were more worried than I could ever be, so a concise, easy-to-follow guide was needed.

Then something extraordinary happened, a critical observation. As I worked within the *Dream Baby Guide* philosophy with my own daughter, as is my natural parenting style, my baby was able to achieve in every area of development, but still unable to sustain sleep comfortably, a significant issue. By understanding my daughter's capabilities, I was able to see her limitations clearly and one hurdle was too high to jump, therefore I never, ever left her to cry. I did as I advise everyone else to do in the book. I tried to find the reason she kept waking, so I could heal that first, fix that, during her daytime – through her diet – her body. What I found was utterly horrifying, but detected so early that it increased her survival rate from 40 per cent to 97 per cent. My daughter had a tumour in her spine and chest cavity. She was diagnosed with cancer at just 24 months of age. That early diagnosis led to a much better prognosis.

I am beyond grateful and without words to adequately express my relief when I say that my daughter has completed treatment, which was extremely successful, and while she still lives with cancer, it is stable and there is a 97 per cent chance of things remaining that way for the rest of her life.

What this meant to me as a philosopher, an author and a mother was so important that I went about updating this book immediately. It's critical for parents to be able to equip their children with the skills and balances in life that they need, so that the common causes of tears at sleep time and behavioural disruptions during the day are erased, making it very easy to see the areas of true challenge for your child. While cancer is rare, with only one in every 260 children diagnosed, my point is that if you can know your child well enough to be able to spot something hidden and sinister like cancer, then the philosophy in this book is a must in every home to identify common issues such as allergies, adenoids, learning difficulties, and hearing and sight issues.

Enjoy reading, and, most importantly, enjoy getting to know your baby so well that achieving peaceful nights and happy days becomes easy.

Sheyne Rowley,
May 2015

PART 1

GETTING STARTED

1

The Dream Baby approach

If you've been struggling with disrupted nights and exhausting days, you'll probably find it hard to believe that using my Dream Baby approach to help your baby or toddler sleep well may be the most fulfilling journey you embark on during the first precious years of your child's life. Why? Because my approach involves getting to know your baby and learning about all the things that make her tick. It involves empowering your child to cope with change and separation independently, a gift she will carry with her for life. And, just as importantly, it will help *you* develop a confident style of parenting so the challenges you face as a carer are exciting rather than frightening, and the experience is more joyful than frustrating.

My approach is not about trying to fix sleep alone. In fact I challenge many of the old ways of thinking about sleep – those stock-standard 'solutions' such as routine management or control crying, that tend to be carried out in isolation of the daytime environment. Instead, I'll show you how every aspect of a child's day impacts on her sleep. I'll show you how an imbalance at sleep time is a direct reflection of an imbalance somewhere else during the day and I'll show you how to identify where that imbalance may be so you can correct it, thus correcting your sleep issue.

This book is *not* a bits-and-pieces manual, where you flip to a page for quick answers regarding your particular problem. To find out why, please read this first chapter from beginning to end because I set out an overview of my highly successful Dream Baby approach. It's a completely holistic philosophy – an all-encompassing approach to parenting that looks at sleep as just one (if very important) element of your and your child's life.

In fact, the Dream Baby approach is about establishing a strong family philosophy. Through happy, healthy days, you can equip your child with the emotional tools to sleep well during peaceful nights and ensure your entire family's emotional wellbeing.

Is the Dream Baby approach suitable for any age?

The Dream Baby approach is a complete parenting philosophy you can utilise from when your child is just six months old and throughout her early years (and even beyond). The importance of balanced communication and a confident style of parenting during the first three or four years of a child's life is often underestimated. However, it is during these years that parents should be laying the foundations for a firm, trustworthy and loving parenting approach within their family because this, in turn, will influence the entire future for your child and family in an extremely constructive and positive way.

Whatever your child's age, it's never too late to start, though you'll need to begin at the basics set down here for six-month-old children. On the upside, your child will learn the skills more quickly the older she is. What doesn't change is the method, which is the same whether she's six months or 24 months old: a consistent approach where she can look to you for clear guidance, and you can help her develop the communication skills she needs to live happily through day and night.

Looking in the right place

After working with babies and toddlers for more than 20 years, during ten of which I've regularly presented on television, I've received tens of thousands of letters and emails asking for help.

In most of the emails and letters I receive, the primary reason given for a child's sleep problems is a medical condition that might have occurred during the child's first few weeks of life, or be from an illness three months prior. It might be an ongoing difficulty with reflux, or something simple such as teething.

It appears that parents tend to first look for a medical reason.

But after more than 20 years working with parents and children to solve sleep-time issues, I can say categorically that medical problems are generally not the cause of sleep disruption. In fact, in all my years of caring for children, I can count on one hand how many times sleep disruption was the result of a medical problem. Only once in my career has profoundly disturbed sleep been due to a serious illness.

While there is no denying that reflux, irritated airways and general illness and discomfort can contribute to sleep difficulties, these problems are all usually quite manageable. Nevertheless, many parents will highlight these issues and tell me all the things they've done to correct them.

Few parents say, 'I can't lie my baby down to change her nappy because she's impossible to manage', or 'I can't put my baby down to play or she cries', or 'My baby won't let me feed her', or 'My baby won't sit in the high chair/car seat/pram/bath'. Ironically, however, it's these sorts of behaviours I look for first to get a clearer and more balanced picture of issues that might be affecting a child's sleep-time, and they are almost always the real causes of sleep-time disruption.

The six keys to your dream baby

So what aspects of a child's day are likely to affect the way she sleeps? The answer to this question forms the bones of my approach and each point will be dealt with individually in the chapters that follow. In simple terms, I help parents address the following aspects of their and their child's life:

1. Sleep requirements, routines and associations.
2. Communication.
3. Play and developing independence.
4. Nutrition.
5. Environment.
6. Interpreting your child's cries.

In the spirit of my all-encompassing approach, none of these elements can be addressed in isolation from the others. So while my approach may require a little bit of extra work for you to begin with, just like a good investment, your effort will repay you handsomely down the track.

1. Sleep requirements, routines and associations

Not every child requires the same amount of sleep, and yet much of the literature and sleep programs available prescribe just one sleep routine per age group.

My experience is that children tend to fall into two main groups with regard to sleep: those with a low to average sleep requirement; and those with an average to high sleep requirement.

You can't ask your child to go to sleep at a certain time or stay asleep for a particular length of time without knowing how much sleep she's capable of taking or when it's appropriate for her to sleep. So the first step in addressing sleep issues is to assess just how much sleep your child requires.

Once you've determined how much sleep she needs (and it's not that hard to do!), you're in a better position to adopt an appropriate daily routine to suit her and develop a consistent sleep-time settling, resettling and waking routine.

The other element of routine is sleep associations: that is, the set of predictable conditions your child associates with falling asleep, stirring during sleep, or waking. Sleep associations can be either 'parent governed' – those provided by a carer, such as patting or rocking – or 'independent' sleep associations that a child can do by themselves. The predictability and consistency of your child's sleep associations can affect her ability to sleep peacefully.

2. Communication

I'm often asked to nominate the most important element of my approach when addressing sleep-disruption in small children. I think many people expect me to answer 'routine', but in fact about 85 per cent of my childcare philosophy concerns communication. This is because to correct any typical sleep-time problems, we need to be able to communicate clearly with our children, to ask them to look to us for guidance and to co-operate with us when we put them to bed. If your child is to sleep through the night or for a significant period of time during the day, she must be able to allow you to put her into bed and leave her in the conditions she'll encounter several times throughout any sleep period, which in most cases is tucked in her soft, warm bed in her own room without you there.

In fact, good communication will help you create a balanced and harmonious environment for every member of your family, day and night, week after week. It will enable you to have true and lasting understanding and co-operation in your home. And when there is stability and harmony in the family home, the natural bonuses are children who have deep, healthy, restorative sleep, are not fussy at meal times and can happily explore and play and therefore learn and grow. So by the time your child has reached 18 months of age, if you've communicated well with her from an early age, other people may be surprised at how amazing the bond is between you, and how easy you make parenting look!

Communication is the backbone of my approach to sleep repair and I can't emphasise enough how important communication is for you, your baby and your whole family!

3. Play and developing independence

Play is one of the most important elements of a child's life. Through play, children have fun while learning vital skills. Among many things, play teaches children independence, something that is necessary if they are to learn to fall asleep without direct parental assistance.

And yet, in many of the homes I visit, babies struggle when put down for just a moment, and quickly become stressed if their mum or dad stands up and walks one or two metres away, even to grab a glass of water. For many of the families I work with, the root of their babies' sleep-time and daytime behavioural issues is anchored in their children having difficulty feeling safe in their own space, an issue that needs to be worked through on a daily basis.

Children deserve the opportunity to discover the joy of a quiet play with their toys, to be able to feel comfortable and safe playing alone without feeling anxious. In the long term, learning to play independently equips children with the tools required to navigate their world. In the short term, independent play will help them settle and resettle independently.

Role play is another form of play we can engage in with our children to teach them vital skills that will help them manage their days and nights without anxiety.

In the chapters on play we will explore the importance of role play in helping children to settle and sleep.

4. Nutrition

Nutrition and sleep go hand in hand: food provides fuel and the capacity to sleep; and sleep provides fuel and the capacity to eat.

Balancing food with sleep can be tricky, especially since food may take the place of lost sleep, or affect a child's ability to sleep. To help our children sleep we need to understand the impact on their sleep of low iron and poor meal-time behaviour, and vice versa. That is, good diet and good sleep work together, as do positive meal times and good sleep.

5. Environment

Environmental elements such as light, noise, movement, comfort, temperature and comfort items like cuddly toys or dummies can impact upon a baby's ability to sleep. Most unsettled babies respond very quickly to some environmental help, whether it's reducing light or noise, or wrapping them for comfort and security.

This book contains detailed information on ways to ensure your child's sleeping environment is conducive to great sleep.

6. Interpreting your child's cries

There's a lot of debate about control crying and all hybrids of it, and I don't believe they are good strategies. Sadly, the result of the debate around control crying can be that parents are left with nowhere else to turn other than to eliminate all crying and fully assist a child to sleep. Both of these methods are extreme approaches at opposite ends of the same spectrum, and both create their own version of learnt helplessness in a child.

The approach I advocate is about balance. If crying is a child's only way of communicating, it's important we learn how to understand her and communicate with her. My sleep repair approach advocates a balanced strategy where all your child's needs are met well before you even embark on independent sleep. This means that by the time you start to show your child how to sleep, environmental factors, healthy, balanced communication, the vital skill set and an appropriate routine are already in place.

Babies don't like change. Anything slightly new will evoke a reaction and a need to ask you if she is okay and if this is normal, healthy and safe. A balanced approach is essential in your answers to those questions. This, combined with understanding how your child's body falls asleep, stays asleep, how often she can wake, and how long it could take for her to be able to fall asleep again, will give you the tools you need to help your child sleep independently and well.

How to use this book

This book is divided into three parts.

Part 1, Getting Started, includes this current overview of my philosophy and approach. It also includes a chapter on how and why we sleep, determining how much sleep your child needs and common causes of sleep disruption.

Part 2, Establishing A Balanced Family Philosophy, covers other issues most sleep problems can be traced to and which therefore need to be addressed if a child's sleep is to be repaired. They are:

- communication
- developing independence and play
- nutrition
- environment.

Part 3, Sleeping Well For Peaceful Nights, is devoted to sleep repair. I've put this section last because I don't believe there is any point trying to repair sleep until all the causes of your baby's sleep disruption have been identified and addressed during the day first.

Creating your Dream Baby Profile

Before embarking on any kind of sleep repair the first step is to read through Parts 1 and 2 of this book and draw up a profile of your child and family. This will give you a snapshot of where you are now, so you can see what areas need repairing.

Your Dream Baby Profile will help you understand the *causes* of any sleep-time or behavioural issues so you can repair those to correct sleep rather than putting a Band-Aid on the symptoms. This usually takes a good week of work. It's important to review The Checklist on page 346.

Each section of the Dream Baby Profile corresponds to a chapter in the first two parts of this book. When you've finished reading the first two parts of this book and have completed your Dream Baby Profile you can create your own personal plan for your child and family.

A blank Dream Baby Profile is on page 11–12. You can either fill it in there, or photocopy it.

Making a plan and putting it into action

When you've drawn up your Dream Baby Profile you can devise a sleep repair program based on your child's unique requirements. Following the successful implementation of this program (and you'll be surprised how easy it is once you know what you need to do!) your baby should be able to:

- go to sleep all by herself every time without tears after a gentle snuggle and a song, and a loving tuck-in and good night
- sleep right through the night for 11 to 12 hours without the need for feeds or intervention (unless there is a diagnosed medical reason for night feeds)
- eat well throughout the day
- play happily with or without you
- cope with you putting her down on the floor or in the cot, and even stepping out of the room, without stress
- sleep a minimum of two and a half to four hours during the day, with at least one of those sleeps being one and a half to two hours in length, if not two sleeps of that length
- be co-operative at the end of the day from 5 to 7 p.m., albeit tired and ready for a full night's sleep, but not miserably unhappy and unsettled.

Now if you're thinking, 'I've tried everything, I've been to sleep school and had people come into my house and nothing's worked so how could this work?' rest assured. Many families have sought the help of countless services both public and private – but appear to have achieved only inconsistent, if any, results. If you've tried but failed to repair your sleep issues in the past, don't fret or feel despondent. This program has so much more to offer than you will have been exposed to.

So be excited because you're about to become a baby whisperer!

About the Dream Baby Profile

This will help you develop your personal program, which is broken down into two parts.

The first part is your homework, where you start to work on the skills and changes required to equip your little one with all the skills, environmental and emotional comforts they need to be naturally confident to sleep without stress. Combine your personal Dream Baby Profile with The Checklist on page 346.

The second part will be where you implement your new daily routine, including your settling techniques with the new environmental factors to restore harmony into your house. For this you will refer to the final support document called 'Before you start' on page 351.

My Dream Baby Profile

Sleep, routines and role play

1. What is your child's average sleep requirement? ____________
2. Which routine suits their sleep requirement? ____________
3. Choose a settling routine (see pages 324–31) ____________
4. Choose a resettling routine (see pages 331–33) ____________
5. Date you will start settling/resettling role play ____________
6. Date you will start waking routine (see pages 333–35, start one week before sleep repair) ____________

Communication

Lines of communication (percentage of time):

Child-governed line ____________ %

Parent-governed line ____________ %

Negotiated ____________ %

Date you will implement the flow of communication (see pages 428–29) ____________

List the other specific communications you are going to work on, e.g. nappy-changing: ____________

Play and independence

1. Can your child play happily both independently and dependently in their play and sleep environments? Yes / No

   List the date when you will:

   1a. Start play stations and play strategies ____________

   1b. Start playtime in the cot ____________

   1c. Introduce a short-term absence cue ____________

2. Emotional toolkit input: can they cope with simple emotions like frustration with toys? Yes / No

   Do they have patience waiting for meals, nappy changes, baths and outings? Yes / No

   List the date when you will:

   2a. Introduce playtime in the high chair ____________

   2b. Start playtime sitting in the bath ____________

   2c. Begin the nappy change communication strategy ____________

Nutrition

1. Do I need to introduce more meat? Yes / No
2. Am I offering too much (TM) or too little (TL)

Milk?	TM / TL
Water?	TM / TL
Fruit?	TM / TL
Vegetables?	TM / TL

3. List the date you will start a new meal plan (see Chapter 9) ____________
4. List the date you will start a new feeding technique (see Chapter 9) ____________

Environment

Give yourself a week to incorporate these changes while you do your homework.

Changes required:

1. Light:

   External? Yes / No

   List the date you will put up a block-out clock ____________

   Internal? Yes / No

   List the date all lights will be covered or removed by ____________

2. Noise

   Do I need to introduce white noise? Yes / No

   If yes, list the date ____________

3. Temperature

   List the changes you need to make ____________

   Date you will have the changes ready ____________

4. Movement

   Do you need a wrap? Yes / No

   Do you need a Safe T Sleep? Yes / No

   List the date you will start practicing on a doll ____________

Please note: do not use any of the movement environmental aids until you start your daily routine and new settling/resettling routine, or you will taint your child's defined expectations.

Will you keep or remove comfort items? Yes / No

2

Sleep: Understanding the basics

Before we begin exploring the triggers of sleep disruption and building a strategy to solve them, I'd like to briefly take you through the very basics of how sleep works.

There are three areas this book will touch on in resolving your sleep-time issues: the first is the biology, then the psychology and finally the physiology. In essence, this is the body, the mind and the environment.

Take the time to read through this brief insight into sleep basics.

What is sleep?

Sleep is a state of unconsciousness during which most voluntary muscles are inactive and the brain is relatively more responsive to internal rather than external stimuli. Scientists believe that, during sleep, the body repairs itself and the brain processes memory and the activities of the day. In children, there is strong evidence that sleep is vital for both growth and successful brain development.

Based on the above information, it's pretty obvious that sleep is vitally important to growing bodies.

The stages of sleep

Scientists who study sleep have identified two kinds of sleep: REM (rapid eye movement) and non-REM (NREM) sleep.

Non-REM sleep is divided up into three (or sometimes four) stages. Each of the four stages of sleep is characterised by differing brain waves and other physical characteristics. The different stages are:

1. Stage N1 – I call this surface sleep
2. Stage N2 – I call this power sleep
3. Stage N3 – I call this healthy sleep
4. Stage 4, REM – I call this dreamy sleep.

People transition through the various stages several times during the night.

Stage N1: surface sleep

Surface sleep is a transitional stage between:

- wakefulness and sleep
- sleep and wakefulness
- sleep, stirring and sleep.

During this transitional stage short dream snippets may occur, usually involving recall memory and featuring images from the day. Brainwave tests show that the brain's electrical activity slows, moving from alpha waves to theta waves. The sleeper may experience sudden muscle contractions which give them a jolt. This sleep lasts for between three and eight minutes.

Stage N2: power sleep

In stage 2, your child is fully asleep and is well on his way to deeper stages of sleep. This occurs about five to ten minutes into a sleep cycle and is characterised by slower breathing and a drop in heart rate. Once he's at Stage 2, he's likely to stay asleep for a prolonged period. If you're holding him, this is when he becomes limp and heavy in your arms and you're safe to move him because he's less likely to stir.

Stage N3: healthy sleep

After around 20 to 30 minutes in the first two stages of sleep, the body drops into an even deeper stage of sleep that I call 'healthy sleep'. During this stage the body maintains and restores itself: it grows and heals. This is when growth hormone secretions are at their highest.

When a child first goes to bed at night, this stage of sleep is at its longest but the length of this stage gradually shortens as the night progresses. This appears to be why the first sleep of the night is always the best.

This is the deepest level of sleep and it is when the brain emits its slowest waves – theta and delta waves.

Stage 4, REM: dreamy sleep

During the REM dreamy sleep stage the brain becomes active. The heart rate increases and the eyes flutter. It is believed that during this stage the brain is as active, if not more so, than when your child is awake. Imagine that . . . sleep being an exhausting task. In stark contrast to the fluctuations in body metabolism, which is also at its highest levels, muscle activity is almost non-existent, and the body is virtually in a paralysed state.

For children aged six months to two years, around 30 per cent of their sleep is REM sleep; for adults it's around 20 per cent.

The function of REM sleep is not yet fully understood but research has linked it with the inner workings of the brain, in contrast to healthy sleep, which is linked with body repair. So while healthy sleep still functions to replenish the brain, there is speculation that information learnt during the day may be processed by our brains during REM sleep. Other brain functions may also be mediated during REM sleep, such as problem solving, memory consolidation and creativity.

How the sleep cycle works

Adults and children move through the stages of sleep several times during the night. Each sleep cycle may last around 40 to 45 minutes in total but can be as short as 20 and, more commonly, 30 minutes.

So while your child's sleep has a beginning and an end, it also has several peaks and troughs as he moves back and forth through the different stages. The most important windows for you to remember are: settling at 7 p.m., and partial wakings (three-eight minutes) between 10-11 p.m., 2 a.m. and 4-5 a.m.

How much sleep your child needs

Every child requires a certain amount of sleep during a 24-hour period, but every child's sleep requirement is different. An average baby between six and 12 months of age will have a daily sleep requirement of between 13 and 17 hours. A baby or toddler between 12 and 24 months of age will have an average daily sleep requirement of between 13 and 16 hours.

Knowing your child's average daily sleep requirement will help you work out their day sleep routines so their night sleeps are unaffected and remain steady. If your child's 24-hour sleep intake, averaged over a week, is:

- 8 to 14½ hours, they have a low sleep requirement (LSR)
- 14½ to 15½ hours, they have an average sleep requirement (ASR)
- 15½ to 16½ hours, they have a high sleep requirement (HSR).

You can break your child's sleep requirement into two distinct portions of the 24-hour cycle:

- day – 7 a.m. to 7 p.m.
- night – 7 p.m. to 7 a.m.

I've divided the day at 7 a.m. and 7 p.m. because nature is your home environment's alarm clock – sunlight, birds chirping or squawking, traffic rumbling, increased room temperature and the house creaking into life as people get up and get ready for the day ahead will, on average, occur around 7 a.m. for most of the year. Therefore, you will need to put your child to bed by 7 p.m. the night before to ensure he gets his night sleep quota of 11–11½ hours.

Establishing a healthy night-time body clock, or 'circadian rhythm', is achieved in the first five years of life. Therefore, a 7 a.m. rising time should be put in place early so your child's energy peaks between the hours of 9 a.m. and 5 p.m.

At the end of this chapter is a sleep diary, where you can record your child's sleep patterns to determine his current average sleep requirement.

Sleep associations

Children learn a set of predictable conditions called sleep associations, which they use to manage the transitions between wakefulness and sleep and vice versa, or between the stages of sleep. Children rely on these sleep associations to help them go to sleep and wake up. They also rely on these same sleep associations when they stir during sleep as they transition from one sleep stage to another.

During all sleep cycles children become semi-conscious for brief periods, during which they become slightly aware of their surroundings. They stir, make sure the environment is the same as when they first fell asleep and their associations are still available. If nothing has changed, they'll go back to sleep without help. If, however, the associations they went to sleep with *have* changed, they'll need to recreate those conditions before they feel comfortable enough to go back to sleep.

How well your child sleeps can depend on how predictable and consistent these transitions involving sleep associations are.

There are two kinds of sleep associations:

1. Carer-dependent – sleep associations provided by a carer.
2. Independent – sleep associations children can do by themselves.

The importance of transitions

To help your child sleep well, you need to be aware of how and when your child transitions from one stage to the next.

There are three transitions that especially affect a child's sleep:

- Settling.
- Resettling.
- Waking.

Each transition is interlinked and it is the continuity between all three that results in good sleep.

Settling

Settling is the process of *going to sleep* from a state of wakefulness or moving from consciousness to stage N1 or surface sleep. The settling conditions you provide for your child will have an impact on his ability to resettle during a sleep session.

Resettling

Resettling is the process of *going back to sleep* from stage N1 or surface sleep. Surface-sleep windows last around three to eight minutes. While a child may be partially aware of his surroundings, he won't be fully conscious of them.

Waking

Waking is the process of coming to a full state of consciousness from a state of sleep. The waking conditions you provide for your child can have an impact on his ability to resettle through a sleep session elsewhere in the day.

Carer-dependent sleep associations

Typical sleep associations involving a carer's intervention include such things as:

- feeding
- patting
- rocking
- motion (such as that provided by a pram or car)
- lying in your bed

- sleeping in your arms or upright against your shoulder
- lying on the couch next to you
- you putting a dummy in his mouth.

In this situation, a child associates these events (rocking, patting, holding) with sleep. If the sleep associations required by your child to go to sleep involve your intervention, it's likely he'll need you to recreate those associations in order to go back to sleep again. This can happen over and over during each sleep session throughout night and day sleeps.

The effect of dependent sleep associations

A young child knows nothing about the concept of sleep or of time passing. So when he falls asleep after feeling the sensation of being tired and then wakes up some time later, he not only doesn't know he's been asleep, he doesn't know that time has passed. It seems so obvious when you think about it, but it's something adults tend to forget.

He only has associations with the sensations leading up to being asleep. These associations are his personal coping strategies for when he feels tired. A child develops these associations by looking to his carers for guidance about what to do when he starts to feel tired. These coping strategies are either a learnt *dependent* pattern of association, such as patting, breastfeeding, or sucking a dummy, for example, or a learnt *independent* pattern of association, such as sucking a thumb, playing with the tag on his teddy or tugging on his ear.

So when a child opens his eyes after being asleep, if he still feels the sensation of being tired, he expects everything to be the same as when he first had that tired feeling. Even after hours have passed, he will expect to still have his usual sleep associations available to him and to be in the same place he was in when he went to sleep. If those associations have changed after he's gone to sleep – for example, his breastfeed has ended, or he's no longer in your arms – he may become startled or cry for assistance.

If this happened with you and your child, the trust he has in you when he feels tired is compromised and he may associate the feeling of being tired with you disappearing without his knowledge. This is likely to result in him fighting sleep.

Secondly, you are sending negative messages to your child about his cot. If you never put him in the cot while he's awake, or you never leave him in the cot awake, or you take him out of the cot when he wakes in the night, or you stay with him until he's asleep again, you're sending him the following message: you should *not* be in your cot when you are awake, and you should not be in your cot alone.

Doing this repeatedly teaches him that his cot is not a safe place to be and that being tired is not a safe feeling to have. Of course, this is simply not true if he's in a house where he's loved, his room is safe and his cot is warm and comfortable. Hence, it's very important to be mindful not to burden your child with this concern.

Independent sleep associations

Independent sleep associations might include:

- feeling snug in a wrap
- feeling warm and comfortable in the cot
- a teddy
- a darkened room
- thumb sucking, hair twirling.

The effect of independent sleep associations

If children originally go to sleep in their cot, in a dark room, without anyone there, then once they've been taught to self-resettle they will feel comfortable to look around briefly before drifting off back to sleep in the middle of the night.

Common causes of sleep disruption

Babies can and do have the ability to sleep, even if they are struggling because of a lack of sleep. The key is identifying the cause of their disrupted sleep.

There are two major causes of sleep disruption:

1. Classic routine and association issues.
2. Significant communication and behavioural difficulties, particularly in the area of emotional security.

Classic routine and association issues

The first group of children, which the traditional sleep repair services are designed to help, are those with routine and sleep association problems. Often the problems these children have are due to them requiring less sleep than they're being asked to take, and/or they have sleep associations that are dependent on their carers rather than things the children can do independently. Unfortunately, as mentioned earlier, many services assume all babies require the same amount of sleep, whereas in fact some babies require less, and some require more. My approach starts with determining just how much sleep *your* baby requires.

Communication and behavioural difficulties

The second group of children requiring sleep repair include those with significant communication or behavioural difficulties. However, most sleep repair services focus on the first group, so what happens to these children? Despite them often having loving, intelligent, attentive parents, their problems tend to be treated using the same strategies designed for the first group. This can actually exacerbate rather than alleviate symptoms of daytime and sleep-time disruption. There appears to be a lack of understanding or assessment process to identify or help the children and families that fall into this second group and this is why I have been run off my feet for years working with them.

I call this second group 'special care' families, and they need to establish a parental philosophy in order to facilitate daytime harmony, which ultimately establishes sleep. In other words, these children just need a little extra guidance from their parents during the day.

In order to repair these cases of sleep dysfunction, a daytime management and communication plan needs to be implemented. For these children, sleep cannot be repaired in isolation from the rest of their daytime activities because their sleep problem mirrors communication and emotional security imbalances during the day.

The skills required to help children fall asleep peacefully in their cots and beds and then sleep well at night are the very same life skills they need to develop to equip them with a strong and dependable personal 'emotional tool kit' during the day. This kit will allow them to grow up feeling comfortable in their own skin, to feel respected and autonomous, to be respectful and reliant on wisdom, to be flexible, and to make wise choices based on learnt wisdom. In my opinion, they will also be less likely to struggle emotionally in early childhood and adolescence.

My program offers a balanced and gentle approach to all children needing sleep repair, and is therefore extremely effective and respectful for both groups.

Effects of sleep disruption for children in group two

Without help, research has proven that the short-term effects of communication and behavioural difficulties are:

- early childhood health problems
- parental mental and physical health problems

- disrupted cognitive development
- ADHD (attention deficit hyperactivity disorder)
- obesity in children
- school-bullying and confidence issues.

So a sleep problem for group two can be much more significant than simply the loss of sleep in early childhood. It's interesting that the long-term effects listed above are more prevalent in males than females and a large proportion of my client base are male children under five years of age. That said, I have my fair share of little girls, but I find boys are quite sensitive and need lots of clear guidance, predictability and reassurance.

Put simply, a solid parenting philosophy being established initially will not only facilitate the pathway to healthy sleep before problems begin, but also to healthy communication and emotional development for our children today, tomorrow, next year and for the next decade.

Homework

1. Questions

Answer the questions below:

- Do you understand the cycle of the four stages of sleep? If not, reread pages 14–15.
- Do you understand how your child transitions between awake and asleep? If not, reread page 17.
- Do you understand what a sleep association is and the difference between dependent and independent sleep associations? If not, reread pages 17–19.

2. Information for section 1 of your Dream Baby Profile

Keep a sleep diary of your child's sleeping pattern for seven consecutive days, in order to assess your baby's average sleep requirement, routines and sleep associations. An example of part of a sleep diary is below.

Example of part of a sleep diary

Sleep diary for Lily

Day 1: 5/1/2013

Time	Awake/Asleep	Waking or settling routine
6.34 a.m.	Awake	
9.30	Asleep	

10.00	Awake	
2.47 p.m.	Asleep	
3.17	Awake	
7.15	Asleep	
11.30	Awake	
2 a.m.	Asleep	
4.00	Awake	
4.07	Asleep	
7.15	Awake	

Total daytime sleep = 1 hour
Total night-time sleep = 9 hours, 23 minutes
Total 24-hour sleep = 10 hours, 23 minutes

Day 2: 6/1//2013

Time	Awake/Asleep	Waking or settling routine
7.15 a.m.	Awake	
10.12	Asleep	
12.22 p.m.	Awake	
3.54	Asleep	
4.25	Awake	
7.15	Asleep	
10.54	Awake	
11.05	Asleep	
7.15 a.m.	Awake	

Total daytime sleep = 2 hours, 41 minutes
Total night-time sleep = 11 hours, 49 minutes
Total 24-hour sleep = 14 hours, 30 minutes

Day 3: 7/1/2013
Total daytime sleep = 2 hours, 21 minutes
Total night-time sleep = 9 hours, 37 minutes
Total 24-hour sleep = 11 hours, 58 minutes

Day 4: 8/1/2013
Total daytime sleep = 58 minutes
Total night-time sleep = 10 hours, 45 minutes
Total 24-hour sleep = 11 hours, 43 minutes

Day 5: 9/1/2013
Total daytime sleep = 2 hours, 5 minutes
Total night-time sleep = 9 hours, 40 minutes
Total 24-hour sleep = 11 hours, 45 minutes

Day 6: 10/1/2013
Total daytime sleep = 1 hour, 42 minutes
Total night-time sleep = 11 hours, 7 minutes
Total 24-hour sleep = 12 hours, 49 minutes

Day 7: 11/1/2013
Total daytime sleep = 2 hours, 6 minutes
Total night-time sleep = 11 hours, 14 minutes
Total 24-hour sleep = 13 hours, 20 minutes

To find your child's average sleep requirement add the total hours slept per day together and divide by the number of days. For example, based on the sleep diary above:

Day 1: 10 hours, 29 minutes
Day 2: 14 hours, 30 minutes
Day 3: 11 hours, 58 minutes
Day 4: 11 hours, 43 minutes
Day 5: 11 hours, 45 minutes
Day 6: 12 hours, 49 minutes
Day 7: 13 hours, 20 minutes
TOTAL: 86 hours, 26 minutes = 12 hours, 21 minutes

On your Dream Baby Profile, write in your child's average sleep requirement and whether they are a low-, average- or high-sleep requirement baby. Also briefly summarise their routines and sleep associations.

PART 2

ESTABLISHING A BALANCED FAMILY PHILOSOPHY

3

Communication: Achieving a balance

As I mentioned in Chapter 1, communication makes up around 85 per cent of my approach to addressing sleep-disruption in small children. Above all else, communication is my 'magic wand' to empower children with a strong and dependable emotional tool kit during the day, which in turn helps babies settle and resettle independently. With clear communication parents and carers can ask babies to look to them for guidance and to co-operate when they put them to bed. And taking the time to establish a clear and predictable style of communication with babies is much more valuable than just establishing good sleep patterns.

By addressing the reasons for a child being uncomfortable with sleep-time guidance during the daytime communications streams first – like when you ask them to lie down for a nappy change, sit in the pram or high chair for a meal, or play independently on the floor while you leave the room to grab the washing basket, go to the toilet or dress yourself quickly – we are able to work through the feelings associated with the tasks of listening, waiting and being in their own space without you in sight, to ensure the emotions and experiences of going to bed are familiar, normal and manageable for them.

Sleep-time disruptions are usually a direct reflection of some form of imbalance during the day, be it routine or meal-time problems. In my experience, these imbalances are most often caused by imbalanced or unclear communication.

The three lines of communication

A child's life is full of new and challenging things. One of the most caring things you can do for your child as she learns and grows during her early years is to be a loving tour guide, sharing your wisdom and providing guidance when required.

Being your child's tour guide on the journey of life during these early years will involve three lines of communication:

1. Child-governed.
2. Parent-governed.
3. Negotiated.

Let's look at each communication line individually.

1. Child-governed line of communication

This is where your child makes a request and the parent happily obliges. The child governs the outcome of the situation. In some situations, this is a healthy line of communication and is useful for learning communication skills and independence. To be balanced, however, a child-governed line of communication should constitute only about one-third of a child's waking day from six months of age to five years.

A child-governed line of communication can be used in situations such as playtime, requests for cuddles, ends of meals, etc. The list is endless.

2. Parent-governed line of communication

A parent-governed line of communication is where a parent makes a request and the child obliges. This is healthy and useful for helping a child learn communication skills, social skills and for developing the child's emotional tool kit.

Parent-governed communication is most valuable during times of transition in a child's day, such as nappy change, meals and sleep times, plus health and safety issues and regular daily events.

3. Negotiated communication

This is a mutually agreed line of communication where the outcome of a situation is negotiated by the parent and the child. It is the last communication line to be introduced, and should only come into play after a child is around 12 months old. You need to establish clear child- and parent-governed lines of communication before introducing a healthy balance of negotiated opportunities. A negotiated outcome should constitute one-third of a toddler's waking hours from 12 to 15 months onwards. This line should never replace a parent-governed line, but rather be additional to it.

Times that negotiated communication can be used include playtime activities, simple choices like which food they want at meal times or which t-shirt that day, choices of location for outings, etc.

These three lines of communication can be used with children when they reach four to six months of age and all the way through to school and beyond. Ultimately, they should be used equally throughout a day.

Finding the balance

Communication is a two-way process, and requires parents and children to listen as well as be heard. Parents whose communication works only one way, and who are overly controlling, leave their children damaged or ill-prepared to cope with the complexities of adult life.

Controlling children produce controlled, ineffective parents. This can become a perpetual cycle in some families and be extremely destructive.

Just as damaging is the equally extreme approach that gives a growing child who is new to the world nearly 100 per cent control. This can result in children who disregard authority, are inflexible, unable to accept guidance, and controlling of those around them.

In addition to these inflexible qualities you also risk overburdening your child. Children are developing autonomy in early childhood but if they are forced to make decisions that only lead them to poor outcomes they develop what's known as 'shame or doubt' in themselves.

Often, when I visit distressed parents and babies in their home, I find parents desperately trying to help their upset babies by listening intently to everything the baby is telling them. They provide all the feeds the baby demands, they pace with them for as long as they ask, and pick them up every time they request it. This, these parents believe, means they are *hearing* what their baby is trying to tell them. After all, babies know when they're hungry, have a full nappy, are feeling a little sore in the tummy, or simply want to be fed to feel happy even when they aren't hungry.

When parents have addressed all of their child's demands and the child is still upset, they begin to look for medical reasons for the tears. Surely if they have done everything the child has asked, shouldn't the child be happy?

Well, doing everything a baby demands does not equal a happy baby. While listening to your baby is extremely important, and something most parents are good at, it is not a balanced approach on its own. You can't always look to a baby for guidance about how to make her happy because she doesn't always know what she needs. If you let a baby guide you, she might want to stay up all night, but that certainly isn't what she needs and it won't ultimately make her happy.

Babies are impulsive and do not understand consequences. So a baby may refuse solids and opt for what she knows – breast or bottle milk – but her hunger during the middle of the night and her grumpy moods indicate drinking just milk is insufficient. You know she needs solids and it's up to you to guide her.

I'll give you an example from an adult's perspective. Imagine I've just entered a distressed family's home. I observe the scene. The baby is upset, the parents are looking desperately to their baby for guidance to make her feel better but they are getting nowhere. I always ask the same thing: 'Okay, you've called me in as an authority on this situation. What exactly do you want from me?'

The parents almost always look at me desperately, often on the verge of tears: 'We have never done this before. We desperately need help, we don't know what to do. Can you please just tell us or show us what to do?'

Since I do have experience in the area of making babies happy, imagine if I didn't share it? How much confidence would parents have in me if I spent our entire day together asking them what I should do to improve the situation they are in, or looking to them for guidance? They would lose faith in me altogether, they would become upset, and they would probably get frustrated or angry with me.

Well, bingo! This is *exactly* what babies are saying to a parent when they are upset: 'Help me feel better, Mum and Dad. Tell me what to do. I just don't know.'

We need to aim for a balance with babies and children, in which they are respected and able to make decisions and control certain aspects of their day, however during the times when a child is transitioning from one daily routine to another, a parent must govern events and outcomes via clear communication. During these times, parents need to make executive decisions for their baby that the parents *know* will improve the situation so their baby can feel happy in the long run. They will have taught their child what to do so they feel a level of control and personal direction, yet established the original routine based on their experience and wisdom. The key to achieving this balance during these times is clear communication.

So while it's important that about a third of your communication throughout the day be child-governed, many events occur each and every day during which you need to guide your child. This is because she is simply too little to appropriately run these events without your guidance. For example, it is crucial when you are asking your baby to lie down to have her nappy changed, or to lie down and go to sleep, that the communication line is parent-governed. At these times you need to be a loving guide and teacher, because you know that meeting your child's every demand is not meeting her long-term needs or in her best interests.

How balanced communication helps repair sleep

Ideally, while babies are still young and at home, their parents should be the ones to teach them what it's like to be guided, to have to wait, to sometimes have to do things differently, or to just trust others. To never provide those opportunities through loving and patient guidance at home means parents leave these important life lessons to others who won't know their child as well as them, or not have as much time or patience to gently help their child through this time as they would.

We need to be able to ask children to look to us for guidance, and for them to co-operate when we put them to bed in order to correct any typical sleep-time problems. They are learning to trust the emotions they're feeling when we're guiding them, and learning that those emotions are safe. If they are to sleep through the night or for a significant period of time during the day, they have to be able to let their parents put them into bed and leave them in the conditions they'll encounter multiple times throughout any sleep period, which is generally being tucked into their soft, warm bed in their own little room, and without their parent in the room.

So when someone asks me, 'When is my baby going to learn how to sleep?' my answer is, 'When you teach them!' You must be able to guide your child, and in order to guide her you must be able to communicate clearly with her.

It's not difficult to establish simple, easy-to-understand and trustworthy lines of communication to convey your wishes and intentions. While it requires a deliberate effort on your part, the rewards outweigh any effort you put in. You'll see your child confidently pick up these skills as you promote happy playing, no-fuss eating and sleeping and a predictable flow to the day. With clear and balanced communication, you and your baby will be able to relax and get the most out of the first two years of her life. You'll have the confidence that your child has had the right balance of food, sleep and stimulation during the day to encourage a full, undisturbed night sleep and your child will feel empowered, with an understanding of each situation via clear communication and familiarity.

Trust yourself

Your baby only knows what she's experienced. If you've taught her to feed, be patted or lie on your shoulder while you pace with her, then that is all she knows. At this early age she doesn't have the logic to think of a better way. As the adult and guide, you do, and you need to help her by showing her how to do things better.

As well as showing your child a better way, you need to take the burden off her. When I walk into a house and spend time with a new family with very little experience of parenting, I take the burden off them immediately. I say, 'Look to me for guidance. I will show you a better way.' And each time the parents or the baby does something that will make their or their baby's life stressful, I correct them by showing them a new and better way. Sometimes that brings tears, sometimes not, but once the new way has been learnt, there will be no more tears in that area.

When there are tears from a child or parent, I remain confident because I have more experience than them, so I understand more about particular scenarios.

Similarly, as a parent, you need to trust yourself. You know much better than your child what she needs, as opposed to what she wants. You also know that you love your baby and would never make a decision regarding her from a place other than love. Build your confidence on that platform and you can help her be happy.

Without a doubt the ability to understand and subsequently communicate with your baby on a deep and intimate level are achievable goals for *any* parent. All the families I have worked with over the past 15 years, regardless of the severity of the disruption they were experiencing, have been able to quickly learn effective communication skills to understand their babies or toddlers and to restore harmony to their home in as little as two to five days. The challenge after that lies only in maintaining a confident style of parenting and communication.

Once you've embarked on your new confident communication approach, you will need to give yourselves and your child a good three to four weeks to feel absolutely comfortable with it. The bulk of the learning will happen for you within a five-day period, but learning to be consistent parents will take you far longer. Go easy on yourself and don't get frustrated.

As time progresses, your child settles down and relaxes as she learns you're predictable and trustworthy, and you feel more equipped to guide her. You'll have developed her self-esteem through positive communication and predictable, simple-to-understand language. You'll continue to work through areas your child finds difficult so you can help her achieve a sense of confidence in all areas of her life. You'll also encourage positive communication from her through consistent role modelling of excellent communication. Your baby's sense of her routine will allow you to guide her without tears and stress. Her every basic need will have been met.

When there is imbalanced communication

When I work with babies I often find their parents are very good at listening to their children's governing lines of communication, and are happy to oblige their baby's every whim, but are not so good at the parent-governed line of communication.

Can you imagine how uncomfortable you'd feel if you stayed at a friend's house and weren't told where you'd be sleeping or what was planned for the day and night? You'd probably feel unable to relax because of the need to watch your hosts to work out what was going on, what was expected of you and when. This is how babies and toddlers feel every day if no one keeps them informed about what's going on, when and how!

If your child is having difficulties during the day, you need to look closely at your parent-governed line of communication. If you're not communicating clearly with your child, she may feel vulnerable, and may struggle against your guidance (or anyone else's, for that matter).

If your communication is lacking in the area of the parent-governed line, your baby may not cope well during periods of transition from one part of the day to the next. Signs of a weak parent-governed line of communication include:

- Nappy changing time: the child tries to roll over and crawl away. Many parents without a governing line in place feel the need to do away with the change table altogether by around eight to ten months for safety reasons.
- Getting dressed: the child arches her back, flails around and gets very upset until she's picked up or stood up.
- Getting into the high chair: the child becomes stiff, arches backwards and tries to kick off the seat so you can't sit her down.
- Staying in the high chair: she screams and throws things off the table and insists on getting out within three to eight minutes (her attention span), whether she's eaten enough or not. She often won't let you put a bib on her.
- Eating: she shakes her head, waves her hands, pulls the spoon out of your hand, covers her mouth with her forearm, or puts her mouth on the tray or back of the seat, all while pulling cute 'you can't feed me!' faces.

- Getting into the car seat: she goes stiff and slides out of the seat towards the floor as you try to put her in a sitting position so you can do up the buckle.
- Getting into the pram: she becomes stiff as in the high chair scenario, and often gets very, very cross at you (even at eight months).
- Staying in the pram: she insists on being carried, and if you don't pick her up quickly she squirms out of the buckles and tries to stand up. If she's unable to stand, she cries and turns to you, gesturing to be picked up.
- Constantly demanding to be picked up: she crawls over to you and tries to stand up, often tries to squish between you and the kitchen bench, pushing you out of her way and crying until she falls over, and becomes upset.
- Playing with things you don't want her to, such as the TV, so you're always having to move her away or put items out of her reach: parents who haven't set up expectations for their baby by the time they're crawling typically find it difficult to set boundaries around these sorts of items.
- Not playing independently: she demands your constant attention and clings to you when you attempt to sit her on the floor. These babies may still squirm down and venture off to play on their own terms, but that is a child-governed line and is very different to when you ask them to play.
- Sitting on your lap: she's unable to stay seated and focus on a task.
- Can't drift off to sleep or go back to sleep: she becomes upset when you attempt to leave her in her cot, which results in you having to assist her to sleep. The assistance often includes milk feeds, nursing, rocking, patting, shushing, lying next to her, holding firmly, etc.

Toddlers aged between 12 and 15 months who are experiencing difficulties with communication and guidance may also have problems, such as:

- not coming inside after playing outdoors
- not packing away toys and books or other play things
- not holding your hand when you're out and about
- pinching or scratching or smacking others when they feel cross
- not listening and paying attention (they have learnt that when someone speaks, it generally means they can continue with what they're doing, so they tune out)
- not letting parents watch their television shows.

These are just some examples of the more typical daytime problems that arise from an underdeveloped parent-governed line of communication. They indicate that the child is feeling overburdened with running the day.

Poor communication styles

When I work with carers who are having difficulties at sleep time or with daytime behaviour I find they tend to have one of four kinds of communication styles.

1. Basic communication with no definition

These carers talk clearly about upcoming events, and state a clear expectation of behaviour, but fail to follow through and define the statement. For example, they may say, 'Nearly time for a nappy change, Charlotte.' They follow this with, 'Time for a nappy change, lie down.' At this point they place the child on the change table. The child immediately rolls over and spends the next few minutes trying to crawl away, then crying each time she is laid down again. This behaviour indicates the statement by the parent, 'Lie down', has not been defined, and Charlotte hasn't been shown what it means to not try to get up. Charlotte thinks 'lie down' means 'roll over' because that is what she's allowed to do each time that statement is made.

2. Delayed communication

These parents do not talk clearly about upcoming events or state expectations. This may be because they do not think their baby will be able to understand them, so they don't tend to use language consistently until their baby starts to talk to them. These parents generally feel they have never been much for talking. Occasionally they say they feel like they're being fake or insincere when they talk to their baby. So while they think through everything clearly in their own mind, they rarely share the information with their child. They will, however, say indirect general statements such as 'Come on, let's go!'

3. Nervous and uncertain communication

These are the parents who either make everything a question automatically, without even thinking about it, or make it a question because they've predicted their child will get upset at the statement and impending transition. Good examples of this are: 'Are you ready to lie down for nappy change?' 'Do you want some lunch?' 'Do you want to have a bath?' or 'Do you want to have a sleep?'

There's nothing wrong with asking questions. In fact, for at least one-third of a baby or toddler's waking day parents can ask questions as part of a child-governed or negotiated line of communication. However, at particular points during the day when children need their parents' guidance, such as eating, nappy change, bath, going to sleep and so on, parents should refrain from asking questions.

Often, when I ask these parents to make a clear statement, they attempt to do so but use an upward inflection, which makes the statement sound uncertain or like a question.

If you know your child needs a nappy change, for example, guide her confidently by saying in an appropriate way: 'It's time to have your nappy changed.'

4. Confusing communication

While some people are talkers and naturally use a forewarning stream of language, they are not necessarily routine with their style of communication. For example, they may say 'Time to change your nappy' one day, then 'Come on, let's get rid of that poo' the next, followed by 'Let's get you some new pants, Mr Stinky Bum!' the day after. Using different language each time makes it that much more difficult for a child to learn and understand what is being said. Therefore, it may take much longer for the child to understand and be relaxed with their parent guiding their day.

What's your communication style?

Keep a diary for a day recording how you communicate with your child.

1. Lines of communication

   What percentage of your daily communication was child-governed? ______________ %

   What percentage of your daily communication was parent-governed? ______________ %

   What percentage of your daily communication was negotiated? ______________ %

2. What kind of communicator are you?

4

Communication: Developing your parent-governed line

Many people think that successful communication with a baby or toddler is challenging, even impossible. However, it's not at all challenging to communicate with a child using a parent-governed line of communication if you can identify:

- Why: understand your own motivation for wanting to develop a strong parent-governed line of communication
- When: identify the appropriate times to use your parent-governed line
- How: use predictable and consistent language and gestures in a set pattern.

Why: your motivation for wanting balanced communication

Children only know what they've been taught. Luckily, it's your choice what you teach your child. You can teach him how to deal with normal daily life scenarios in a way that will empower him with the emotional tools he needs to cope in the future. Or you can teach him to simply avoid any situation that will evoke emotions.

Teaching your child how to deal with normal healthy emotions he experiences and empowering him with solutions, without fearing you may lose his friendship or people may judge you, is parenting from a place of love and confidence because you're taking your child's overall needs into consideration and setting appropriate boundaries based on those needs, even if he doesn't always agree with you.

This is in stark contrast to parenting from a place of fear or pride, where you're concerned you're 'being mean' or 'breaking your child's spirit' or '[insert latest buzz term here]' by asking your baby to lie down for a nappy change or teaching him to listen or co-operate occasionally through the day.

No parents want to hold their children back or limit their ability to explore and feel safe by not exposing them to the normal life conditions they'll encounter when they interact with someone outside their house, or outside the protective arms of their parents. So, for example, while children may want to touch hot oven doors, parents teach them these are no-touch zones because it's obviously dangerous for them. This is safe, loving guidance and not emotionally damaging. Nor are clear, safe and loving boundaries set around basic listening and co-operation.

When you see or meet other children, the things that might make you think 'I don't want my child to behave like that.' would be a child screaming and demanding things, refusing to listen, crying or being aggressive with other children, etc.

Then there are the children who make you think, 'What a beautiful child. I'd love my child to be content and happy like that.' Those children usually have bright personalities, may be a bit cheeky but accept guidance from their parents, play happily, engage in interactions with those around them, are verbally engaging and show clear socialising patterns. They're also the children who'll go to sleep for their parents when they're tired, eat reasonably when they're hungry and accept a simple 'not now' or 'no' from a well-meaning parent. These children will possess their skills and confidence as a result of clear communication, guidance and boundaries.

Being confident enough to provide clear guidance based on your desires for your family – even if that guidance causes a few minor dramas initially – will set you apart from someone providing no guidance or blindly following an ideology.

What motivates you to provide clear guidance at certain times of the day via parent-governed communication is your desire to have a positive relationship with your child so he can be the happy, well-adjusted child you want to raise.

When: events and routines using parent-governed communication

Babies transition several times a day. Some of the major transitions they experience are regular events such as meal times, nappy changes and bedtime. Babies feel most vulnerable during these transitions for a couple of reasons. Firstly, they are impulsive and see no reason to move from one activity to another. Secondly, they are intelligent and like to follow patterns – like most humans they develop habits.

If you don't tell your child what to expect before and during periods of change, everything may suddenly become chaotic for him – he may feel unsafe, resulting in tears or clingy and demanding behaviour. By being demanding, a baby is trying to restore a sense of control and predictability to his day, no matter how inappropriate his behaviour may be in order to achieve it.

Most of the tears I encounter in babies and toddlers – apart from those caused by basic needs like hunger, tiredness and the need for comfort – occur during transitional episodes of the day when parents try to guide the event without adequate communication. The children's tears result from feeling out of control which makes them feel uncomfortable, angry or frustrated.

Tears during transitions only occur when the transitions are parent guided; never when the baby requests a transition himself, such as when he squirms in your arms to be put down on the floor to play. Clearly he's aware of the change about to occur when he guides it, it's when you instigate a change without adequate communication in place, or for the first time, that he will become unsettled.

As parents, we need to create predictability using clear parent-governed communication around routine daily events. These are times when you create a set of conditions that your baby or toddler can predict, and ultimately feel in control of because he knows what to expect. Some examples of event routines would be:

- changing his nappy
- getting dressed
- eating a meal
- getting ready for sleep
- playing independently
- having a bath

- getting in the pram/car/high chair
- coming inside from outside.

Once your child has had the opportunity to practise routine events with you guiding him and has learnt to be comfortable with not controlling certain aspects of his day, he will be empowered with all the information he needs to recognise what is required of him at sleep time.

How: the seven steps of clear communication

The key to communicating clearly with a child is consistency and predictability. When you communicate with him in a consistent and predictable way during routine events during the day, you engender trust in him and significantly reduce or eliminate tears when teaching him a new routine around sleeping, eating or playing.

The aim is to use repetitious language and gestures, or 'cues', to guide your child from one part of the day to the next. The familiarity of these cues enables him to feel safe: though you make the decisions about key areas of his day based on your wisdom and a desire to meet his best long-term needs, he feels in control.

Your primary intention when communicating with children under two should be *being understood*. This means you need to be totally accountable for what you say and for the clarity you give to each statement.

You should create a flow of communication that's easy to use and simple to understand, a way of saying: 'Here we are now', 'This is where we're going next', and, 'This is my expectation of your behaviour'. When you reach the next location you begin again: 'So here we are now', 'This is where you're going next', and 'These are my expectations of your behaviour'.

I call this 'laying a path in words' and it contains the following seven steps:

1. Pre-empting.
2. Forewarning.
3. Stating event and expectations.
4. Defining your statement.
5. Praising.
6. Following through.
7. Completion.

Now, let's look at these seven steps of the flow of communication in more detail.

1. Pre-empting

This is where you state the task your child is involved with now, and what he can expect to happen next. Your pre-emptive dialogue contains three stages:

1. State the current event the child is involved in: 'Lachlan can help Daddy feed the puppy dog.'
2. State the upcoming event and your expectations of his behaviour: 'Then it's time for a bath. *Nearly time* to sit down and wait for Daddy.'
3. Finish on a positive by redirecting his attention back to what he was engaged with: 'Now, where's that puppy's food?'

The final stage will enable you to prepare him for the next event, and quickly get him back into the current enjoyable task to avoid tears and tantrums so that by the time you mention the event again it won't be a big surprise and will be unlikely to trigger as strong a reaction as if it was simply sprung on him.

To use a pre-emptive line of communication is considerate because it empowers your child with an understanding of what's going to happen in his day before it unfolds. This prevents tears or inappropriate behaviour because he doesn't feel unsettled or frightened by any unexpected changes in his daily routine.

What we are aiming to do by pre-empting is to reduce the amount of time you have to spend either correcting inappropriate behaviour or dealing with it. This is a win–win situation because you are able to structure the day based on your baby's true needs, and he will still feel in control of his day because you've made it predictable for him. This is the key to a content and happy baby or toddler.

By using your pre-emptive language consistently and making it a simple part of your communication style, you create harmony. You also teach your child to be open, expressive and respectful of your desire to be involved in his plans for the day. This style of communication will follow him throughout his life.

2. Forewarning

Forewarning is where you transition your child smoothly from one event to another with alert of upcoming changes. This ensures he has time to prepare and knows where he's moving to next, so he feels in control of it.

Get into the habit of articulating your plans two to five minutes in advance of each transition of the day. Just like pre-empting, state the current event, state the upcoming event and your expectations of his behaviour, and finish on a positive by giving him something to look forward to so you encourage him to co-operate. For example, if you plan to pack away his toys and sit him down for lunch, say 'Last one, then it's time to pack away toys so we can sit down for lunch. Blocks in the box. Yummy chicken and vegies and your favourite Wiggles spoon.'

3. Stating event and expectation

As opposed to the 'nearly time to' of the pre-emptive step, this portion of the flow indicates it's now 'time to' transition into your next event. This is where your child may resist you a little, but with lots of forewarning you can help him understand what 'it's time to' actually means. You take him to his, say, high chair and pat the seat, saying: 'It's time to sit down and wait for Mummy.'

Be careful about how you manage this stage. If you say to a child, 'Sit down and wait', ensure he understands the meaning of the statement by always getting him to sit down for you. This is a clear parent-governed statement and is not up for negotiation, so don't taint or confuse it by saying 'Would you like to sit down and wait?' or implying by your actions 'When I say it's time to sit down, it means sit down . . . but if you cry, arch your back or hit me, you don't have to sit', otherwise you'll encourage tears every time you ask him to do anything. This is why you need to define your statement.

4. Defining your statement

Defining your statement is the difference between being a good communicator and someone who makes little sense to your baby. Being aware of what you've said to him and considerate enough to show him what that statement means is far easier than dealing with the fallout when he can't listen to you because you make no sense to him. Be aware of what your style of communication is teaching him.

If you say to your child something like, 'No touching Daddy's computer', then pick him up and move him somewhere new, he either gets upset because he wasn't finished playing with it, or he heads straight back to continue playing with it. This is when many parents get frustrated and think their baby is not listening to them. In fact, you haven't taught him what your original statement meant. Taking him away from an object does not teach him what 'no touch' means and will not prevent the same scenario playing out again, particularly if he's taken a shine to the colourful buttons on the computer that everyone else seems to be allowed to play with.

Try to see it from your baby's perspective. Imagine sitting on the lounge relaxing and flicking through a magazine, and your partner saying, '*Ne lisez pas ce livre*'. When you look at him he just looks back at you with raised eyebrows then turns away. You have no idea what he just said but given he's looked away you figure it mustn't be important, so you carry on relaxing and reading. Then he comes over to you and repeats, '*Ne lisez pas ce livre*', before taking you to the kitchen to look at the coffee machine and press all the buttons for you. After a while you finish looking at it and automatically go back to what you were doing before, which was relaxing with your magazine. Your partner sighs and comes over again and repeats, '*Ne lisez pas ce livre*', before taking you to see the new alarm clock in the bedroom.

Each time you finished looking at what your partner was showing you, you simply went back to doing what you were enjoying. The statement '*Ne lisez pas ce livre*' had no meaning to you because each time he said it he took you to see something different. By then you stopped listening to him; it was just easier to look out for where he was going to take you next, or if he was going to take you somewhere new.

To show you what the statement '*Ne lisez pas ce livre*' means I'm going to define it in a way that will teach you what its true definition is. Imagine sitting on the lounge relaxing and flicking through a magazine and your partner says to you, '*Ne lisez pas ce livre*'. When you look at him he comes over to you and taps the magazine, shakes his head and repeats, '*Ne lisez pas ce livre*'. He takes the magazine out of your hand and places it on the coffee table repeating, '*Ne lisez pas ce livre*'. You look at him then reach out to pick up the magazine again but he waves his hand in front of the magazine and repeats, '*Ne lisez pas ce livre*'. Each time you reach for the magazine he blocks your hand or waves over the magazine and repeats, '*Ne lisez pas ce livre*' as he shakes his head. He then hands you the remote to the television and says '*Vous pouvez regarder la télévision*'. He gives you a hug, points to the magazine and shakes his head again and says '*Ne lisez pas ce livre*', then points to the television and smiles, repeating, '*Vous pouvez regarder la télévision.*'

It's clear that he doesn't want you to read the magazine and would like you to watch the television instead. His actions and persistence of communication and intervention define his statements for you. This is exactly how children learn. You must speak and define the statement by physically encouraging your child to stop touching the computer until he understands what 'No touching Daddy's computer' means.

The other mistake people make in defining a statement is to give it an incorrect meaning, and then get upset with their child for doing what they've been taught the statement means. For example when a mother says, 'Lie down while Mummy changes your nappy', then allows the baby to roll over and get up on his knees, she teaches him that 'Lie down while Mummy changes your nappy' means 'Roll over and get on your knees'. Similarly if a parent asks a child to 'Sit down for morning tea', then allows him to stand up and walk away with the food in his hand, it teaches him 'Sit down for morning tea' means 'Stand up and wander around with your food'!

Children don't do these things because they're deliberately ignoring the instruction. They are actually doing what they think they've been told to do.

One of the most unfair and confusing things you can do is teach your child to not listen to your statement or to think it means something else, and then get upset with him for doing what you've taught him. This is why I'm against smacking children. As well as not believing in enforcing co-operation through fear, it's easy to confuse a child by making him believe that smacking him means you're blaming him for the problem that has arisen, and this is almost never the case.

No matter what parenting style you adopt, the vital skills around defining a statement are the most basic and courteous language tools you can employ to ensure you're acting as a loving teacher for your child to learn from.

5. Praising

Always praise your child when he responds to your parent-governed line appropriately. Be sure you use a very specific type of praise such as 'That was beautiful listening to Mumma, thank you for standing up and walking to Mumma for shoes on'. Use body language, such as turning sideways, looking preoccupied with another task, avoiding eye contact and ignoring obvious protests or undesirable behaviour when he is resisting your governing line.

6. Following through

Once you've defined your statement, follow through for as long as it takes to ensure your baby understands the definition fully. This doesn't mean harping on about it for hours; but following through with words and actions until he acknowledges what you've said or stops trying to do anything other than what you're defining.

The way an eight to ten month old will acknowledge your request is by getting cross or upset at being prevented from doing his chosen thing. This is different to him not understanding you are requesting something of him. When he doesn't understand what you're asking of him, he just repeats the same action regardless of your intervention. It's when he stops and looks at you and gets cross or upset that he's identified that you are intervening. At this point, acknowledge this and say 'Good listening', then repeat your statement: 'No touch the power point', before moving him away to a new activity.

In an older baby you need to seek recognition from him that you've asked him not to touch the object, or not to do anything other than what you've stated. In crawlers, this often comes in the form of stopping the action of trying to touch an object, sitting on his bottom and looking at you and the object and then you again. He may hold his hand out without touching, in which case say, 'That's right, good listening. Mummy said no touch' in a calm, patient manner. You can then clap, or kiss him or just smile warmly, then move him on to a new activity.

If you've asked your baby to lie down to have his nappy changed, follow through and prevent him from doing anything but remain lying down until he stops resisting. Offer distractions and stay calm while following through with your definition. Only once he's understood and accepted the request should you carry on and complete the nappy change. If he starts to resist again, stop changing the nappy and manage his behaviour.

The reluctance of a strong-willed child should not cause you to rush to finish the task at hand. If you rush in response to your baby's temper you teach him to be stroppy at you to make you hurry up. Carry on with your task, activity or request consistently and patiently until you come to the natural end and then move to the next step of your communication.

Asking your child to listen doesn't mean you should be aggressive, impatient or bossy in your tone. Be both patient and compassionate: 'Mummy knows it's hard to lie down and wait. I know you feel a little bit cross', but remain consistent with the definition of the statement 'Lie down and wait'. Remain warm and friendly even when he gets cross the first time you ask something of him.

By the time your baby is around 15 months, his ability to understand and learn is amazing and you will only need to define a basic boundary and follow through a couple of times before he understands the boundary from that point on. By the time your baby is close to 18 months of age, he will be able to learn to happily accept a new boundary with a simple clear request, often without challenging you if you use clear pre-emptive and forewarning language and role play.

7. Completion

If you want your child to look to you for guidance, you need to be trustworthy and reliable. This means being consistent, which is where the completion of the flow of communication is vital. If you do every single step in the flow of communication correctly but then forget to wrap up the event with a line of parent-governed communication you're being inconsistent with the message you are delivering.

Here's an example. At sleep time, you ask your baby to go to sleep, define that statement and, after a grumble or a big protest, he goes to sleep. Then he wakes during the night and cries. You once again ask him to go to sleep and you follow through. Then, in the morning, when he wakes and cries you think to yourself, 'Great, he's had enough sleep', so you walk in and pick him up. Your baby doesn't know 7 a.m. from 2 a.m. so you've been inconsistent by allowing him to govern communication at 7 a.m. but not at 2 a.m. This will confuse him regarding whether he needs to cry to ask you to pick him up because you did in the morning, which teaches him to always cry just to see what will happen.

When you establish a parent-governed line around all sleep times, you teach your baby that when he wakes up he can have a chat or a play and can trust that you will come in to him in due course and get him up. As a result he won't feel the need to cry out.

Example of routine communication: nappy change

1. **Pre-empting**: 'Charlie, Mummy is just getting dressed but *soon* it will be time for nappy change. *Nearly time* to lie down and wait for Mummy.'
2. **Forewarning**: 'Last one, Charlie, then it's time for nappy change. *Nearly time* to lie down, wait for Mummy.'
3. **Stating event and expectations**: '*It's time* to change your nappy. Let's go.' Charlie looks up and you say 'Up up' and he raises his arms. You carry him if he's still a crawler or say 'Let's go' and gesture for him to follow you. He grabs a toy and runs towards the room where the change table is and stands waiting for you. Pat the table and say, 'Lie down. Wait for Mummy.' You lie him on the change table and say 'Lie down. Wait for Mummy' again. He lies down and babbles, chats or sings along with you while you change his nappy. As the nappy change draws to a close, you play a little game or do a little nursery rhyme, much to his delight.

4. **Defining your statement**: If he moves to roll over or stand up, make the wait sign (see page 58) with your hand and say 'Wait'. Remember, 'Lie down. Wait for Mummy' means 'Don't try to reposition'.
5. **Praising**: If he's lying happily and doesn't look like he's going to challenge you, praise him: 'Good lying down, Charlie'; 'Good waiting for Mummy, Charlie'.
6. **Following through**: To manage behaviour use your cues: 'Lie down', 'Wait', 'Legs down', 'Hand out. Mummy do it!' Add nursery rhymes, small toys and songs to hold their attention.
7. **Completion**: At the end of the nappy change, when *you* are ready, get your baby up with the up cue (see page 59) or use the wait game. Give him a cuddle and kiss, then leave the room with a little ritual that could be closing the door or turning off the light or putting the nappy into the bin together and washing hands.

Tips on how to communicate clearly with your child

How you use a parent-governed line of communication with your child will impact on how he perceives your guidance, and the guidance of others. You'll achieve the best results by being confident, respectful, encouraging and appreciative.

Use confident statements, not questions

Use your parent-governed line of communication with confidence so your child trusts your ability to guide him. Avoid making a statement sound like a question, and be aware that when establishing your parent-governed line of communication, it's not only sentence structures involving words like 'can I', 'should we', 'could you' that can change a statement to a question. Sometimes all you need to do is change the pitch or inflection of your voice at the end of a sentence.

For example, say 'Lie down and wait for Daddy' out loud as if talking to your child. Now say it again but lift the inflection at the end of the statement. Now say it again but drop the inflection at the end of the statement. Which inflection did you naturally use when you first said the statement? If you dropped the inflection, then it was a confident statement. If you lifted the inflection, it was a question.

I believe in respectful communication, so if you ask a question with words like 'should we', 'could we', or use an upward inflection at the end of a statement, expect to receive an answer, which you will need to respect if you're to establish a respectful two-way open language stream within your house.

If you catch yourself turning a statement into a question, quickly correct yourself by repeating the statement with a downward inflection if your child hasn't already responded with a cry, a head shake or 'No!' If he's answered, try again a few minutes later, starting with your forewarning step with a statement like 'Okay bubba, last time and then it's time to ______!' with a downward inflection.

Stay confident and follow through as usual with your parent-governed line of communication by defining that statement.

The first stage in teaching yourself to make confident statements is hearing yourself when you use an inappropriate inflection or sentence structure when you're trying to guide your child with a parent-governed line of communication. The second stage is hearing it then quickly correcting it. The final stage is thinking it, correcting it in your head, and then saying it correctly first-off. It takes about five days to correct the habit of a previously automatic inflection and sentence structure.

Be consistent

Communicating in a consistent way can be difficult for even the most experienced parent. Being consistent is much easier when you're not busy or preoccupied – that is, when you aren't on the phone, at the shops, at a friend's house, having friends over, in a rush, busy cooking, cleaning or talking with your partner. The problem is, many babies find inconsistency or unpredictability unsettling.

To be consistent and predictable, always deliver your statements in a clear and consistent way, defining them as statements. Remain aware of your child and his needs and actions, and be consistent with your language, expectations, definition and follow through, regardless of anything else that is happening.

Being consistent means your baby learns to listen to you, and learns to follow through when you talk and ask respectfully. However, this is a two-way street, so when your baby asks you to listen to him, be attentive to his needs and don't put him off for a hundred other chores or the moment the phone rings.

Ensure that both you and your partner are on the same page by discussing a general plan on how you think things should be done in your house, establishing boundaries or house rules, and agreeing on how you'll both manage certain parts of the day in a consistent, predictable way.

If you are inconsistent, by the time your baby is around two years old he will have learnt to only listen to you when you repeat yourself. This will also mean that on a social level he'll have learnt to not listen properly to people when they ask respectfully the first time, but to wait until they get frustrated with him.

Be polite, gentle and loving

Some parents believe guiding a child involves frowning and growling. Others veer towards being apologetic and overly concerned. My advice is to guide your child in a way that is compassionate and understanding by using loving, happy, upbeat tones and having confidence in fulfilling your loving duty towards your child. This tone should remain as you define your statements and requests, even if your child is a little unhappy with your consistent guidance on your first few attempts.

Ask politely and be upbeat, while remaining confident in your right as a parent to make requests or guide your child. If your child gets very stroppy about you governing certain times of the day, help him feel more comfortable with this healthy balanced line of communication by adopting a confident, matter-of-fact and respectful tone.

Be reassuring

It's important to be reassuring and understanding with your child if he's uncertain about a new routine so he learns to cope with the situation. Reassure your child with cheerful confidence and smiles to help him avoid or recover from tears and fears quickly. Express your reassurance not only with words but with a sense of humour, the tone of your voice and your body language.

Remember, your language has the power to change situations from negative to positive. If your child is having difficulty in an aspect of his day be encouraging, with comments like, 'Let's go and see your beautiful room. Where's that big blue car on your sheets?' and remain confident as you enter his room. Continue this even if he cries. You need to guide his impression of his room, his cot and his entire sleep environment with happy, confident tones and persistence.

Be enthusiastic

Try hard not to ever lose your sense of humour, your enjoyment of watching your baby's clever way of working out how the world works, your love of life and your desire to be the best possible parent or carer you could ever possibly be.

I've sometimes sat with parents who are crying and saying the most untrue and unkind things about themselves in front of their wide-eyed children. By feeling worthless and allowing a negative inner dialogue to affect your self-esteem around your child, you bully yourself into a place of no confidence. Your child will be unable to relax if you appear upset, as he will read this as potentially dangerous to him and will need to cling to you and try to govern the day to create predictability to calm himself.

When you're communicating with your child, be enthusiastic. Try to (or appear to) enjoy most aspects of the day, have a sense of humour about most events, and only become more serious when you need to define a statement and help him learn a new cue or routine he's struggling with. This may sound difficult for mothers struggling with postnatal depression, or fathers concerned about their partner and baby, but it's really important to appear happy, confident and full of love and enthusiasm while you're with your baby – even if you have to fake it at first.

Use humour

Babies over ten months respond very positively to humour. Used effectively, humour can also defuse potentially stressful situations with toddlers so that they laugh – rather than cry – at things that are a little overwhelming. For example, with a toddler who is easily embarrassed, it's lovely to help them giggle at some of the things that may happen by sharing the experience and the response with them.

Take every opportunity to make your child laugh. A tickle at a random time of the day will make him giggle and he'll look forward to your next interaction.

Use body language

As well as words, children under two will try to read your body language, which consists of both eye contact and the actions of your full body. It's important, therefore, that your verbal language matches your body language. When you ask a baby to trust you so he can relax and allow you to govern him through certain parts of his day, your body language needs to be relaxed and confident.

I see parents trying to use a parent-governed line of communication while, for example, asking their baby to wait in a high chair. When the baby gets cross or demands to be picked up, the parent will say, 'Wait' at the same time as putting their hands under the baby's arms and leaning in to cuddle him, or they'll try to do things extra quickly and pick the child up without defining the request. If you've started a routine event using parent-governed communication and your child, whether eight or 18 months of age, is having a hard time learning to allow you to govern the end point of the event they used to be in charge of, your body language *must* remain consistent with your verbal language.

On top of this, if you're asking him to switch his attention from visual cues (where the baby feels he needs to watch your actions to predict your movements) to verbal cues, try to keep your movements to a minimum. Moving around a lot won't encourage him to relax while he gets used to being a separate entity from you, particularly if he's immobile. For example, if you're just starting him on independent play, it's important to stay in one particular area. Walking in and out of the room may make him nervous and feel that he needs to watch you all the time. This will obviously discourage play and the child won't enjoy that most basic of early childhood desires and needs, which is to explore and challenge their environment.

This doesn't mean you need to stay still, it just means you should plan to work in one area or room of the house at a time. Tidy the kitchen, prepare the food for the day, gather any clutter into a basket on the bench ready to put away later. If you move around the kitchen bench to the other side, your baby may interpret your body language to mean you're going to leave the room, and cry and ask to go with you. After working through one room, use clear language as you transition to the next room, so he learns to trust you to always tell him when you plan to move from one room to another, rather than him having to try and read your body language and guess your actions.

If your actions are predictable your baby can trust that you won't disappear – or reappear – without telling him, which means he can focus on his toys.

Use eye contact

From birth, a baby's gaze drifts towards the human face, so eye contact is a great way to get his attention, or ensure he has yours. When you want to make sure your baby has heard you, or you want to let him know you've heard him, use eye contact.

Very occasionally, when you're using your governing line of communication and your child's behaviour indicates he's not going to co-operate, staring at him may suggest you're open to negotiation or are looking to him for guidance. Avoid eye contact that will encourage loud crying or tantrums, which is his way of telling you what to do. Instead, state your intention then carry on with your chores or task.

If your baby is very upset and needs a little reassurance, then make eye contact and repeat your request confidently, for example, 'It's okay, bubby. Mummy just needs you to wait. I know you feel cross, but you're okay.' Remember, however, that your motivation when you reassure him is *not* to fix it but to just let him know you can hear him; you know he's upset but you are confident the feeling he has is a safe and normal feeling and your request remains.

Avoiding eye contact should be used only very occasionally and only when you have a very cross child screaming and arching to be picked up out of the high chair, pram, cot, or wherever. It is not a daily strategy, or something to be done for prolonged periods of time. It's designed to help a child who thinks he needs to scream or tantrum as a form of communication to learn a new way of communicating.

Stay positive to build their self-esteem through language

Each child is a clean slate, and you play a vital role in shaping your child's self-esteem and self-image, so the way you communicate with him is key. Be mindful of what you're telling him directly or indirectly. For example, if he shudders when he tastes a super sweet pineapple for the first time, say something like: 'Oh, sweet new taste. Look, Mummy try it too! Nice and sweet', rather than 'Oh, you don't like that', or 'You don't want that?'

When you make statements such as 'He doesn't seem to like ______', 'He only drinks ______', 'He hates having a bath', 'He gets upset when he sees Grandma', 'Dogs frighten him', 'He doesn't like sharing his toys', you're building your child's image of himself and the world around him, so make sure your statements build your child's positive image of himself and the world around him.

Examples of positive language include, 'Charlie did good listening for Daddy today, Mummy', 'Charlie did good lying down and waiting for Daddy when I changed his nappy! Yeah!' Positive language should be used even if it has been a challenging first day with your new cues. We want to tell our children they are good sleepers, they love their cot/room, they're good eaters, they love vegetables, like water, like to play with their toy, love bath time, are happy, good listeners, a good friend, funny, love to be active, are good at sitting and waiting – the list goes on and on.

Destructive communication and behaviour

I often encounter destructive communication and behaviour, and am never shy about pointing it out to parents because a child's entire life journey can be damaged if he forms opinions about the world around him based on a set of negative untruths or manipulative innuendoes intended for someone else in a moment of anger.

Every child should grow up free from the burden of your relationship's highs and lows, the emotional insecurity of an adult, or a negative view of the world.

The following is a list of destructive communication styles that will negatively impact on a child's relationship with his carers, siblings and others.

Competitive parenting: children as pawns

Parents competing for their children's affections with subtle verbal inputs can destroy the relationship between the child and the other parent. This often occurs when one parent is upset with the other and says things like:

- 'Naughty Daddy should be home now!'
- 'Mummy doesn't like bathing you, does she?'
- 'Daddy doesn't want to play with you. He'd rather watch the television.'
- 'We don't want Mummy to help us, anyway, do we?'

Undermining the other parent can happen in non-verbal ways too, for example when one parent always takes over when the child demands it, not allowing their spouse and the baby the chance to find their own way and thereby limiting the relationship potential between the two of them. One person will rarely be able to do things just like the other. Give your partner and child the time to find their own way together without coming in and 'rescuing the baby'. Undermining your partner is destructive because it can make the child think the parent isn't up to the task and it can make the parent attempting the task question their parenting skills. This can impact on the time and interaction the parent and child have, risking their bond.

Undermining yourself or others

- 'I'm a terrible mummy.'
- 'Naughty Mummy.'
- 'I'm sorry, I'm a bad dad, mate.'
- 'Is Mummy so terrible that you don't want to ______?'
- 'Do you hate being with your dad so much that you ______?'
- 'Daddy can't do it.'
- 'We don't like Granny coming over, do we?'

Bickering with your child like a sibling

The 'yes', 'no', 'yes', 'no', argument is a tormenting and toxic communication style. You are the adult. State the answer. Do not bicker with your child.

Negative input about their sibling relationship
The lines go something like:

- 'Stop annoying your brother.'
- 'Why can't you play together?'
- 'You're so rough with your brother.'
- 'He doesn't want to play with you.'
- 'You two are a nightmare together.'

Teaching your child with an-eye-for-an-eye
- 'They bite you. You bite them back.'
- 'They hit. You hit back.'

Trying to teach empathy through guilt
Trying to teach empathy through guilt might occur when a parent goes to play with their child and the child pushes the parent away because he's playing on his own or with someone else. The child doesn't do this to be mean: it's just that sometimes he's busy and not yet at the stage of co-operative playing. Often in the child's mind the arrival of an adult mid-game can represent the end of a play session, which may not be what he wants if he's very absorbed in his activity. This apparent rejection can feel a little hurtful for mums, though it more often happens to dads. Because the parent feels hurt, the next time the child comes to play with them, the parent pushes him away so he can feel how hurt the parent felt.

Be aware that the child will not link the two situations and this won't teach him empathy at all. You actually *will* hurt him because he's only a child and he'll wonder why you're behaving like this. He's then more likely to role play that behaviour back to you because he's learning how to interact socially with others, and you will have started a vicious cycle of negative interactions.

Teasing, mocking or laughing at your child when he is angry
Never tease, mock or laugh at a child when he is angry. While you may find his displays of emotions or even his triggers entirely adorable, these emotions are overwhelming for a tiny person. If you don't show an understanding of that to your child by responding appropriately, he will be left feeling he has no emotional support or safety nets.

Wanting to be wanted
Wanting to be wanted creates a pattern of dependency in order that a parent can feel important to or needed by a child. One of the saddest

things I've seen in early childhood education was a parent who hovered and said goodbye as many times as it took for their child to cry before the parent felt satisfied and could leave.

This stems from a need for validation that the parent is loved, which is an unfair burden to put on a child. It's not a child's responsibility to love you, it's your responsibility to love him. A parent needing tears to feel important to their child is a toxic form of parenting which stems from low confidence in their parenting ability. Parents are the most important people in the world to their children and have an absolutely irreplaceable role in their children's lives. You will never ever need to question this fact!

Make the time to make it work

Between six and 12 months, babies need a lot of repetitive communication in order to understand statements, which means staying with them, repeating statements and being patient. When you're teaching a child of this age not to touch the oven door, for example, make sure you don't have lots of other distractions, and don't get frustrated about the time it takes to teach the baby to understand that 'no touch' means 'no touch'. It may take a few consistent statements and definitions for him to learn the message and each session will require your full attention and patience.

By 12 to 15 months, you'll still need to be repetitive and follow through, but the process will be much faster, so you won't need to allocate as much time to teaching him something new.

From 15 months to two years, if you're having trouble establishing your parent-governed line of communication, you need to make sure you're prepared because you will encounter far more behaviourally motivated resistance from your baby. You'll need to stay calm, compassionate and ultra-confident while still appearing to have plenty of time to achieve the stated request and outcome. Remember that it is tricky for the child. Empathy is your key here.

Manage your child with the same amount of spirit and determination that he possesses, but always stay on his side and be empathetic while you follow through. If he's bold and confident, parent him with the same boldness and confidence. If he's overly bossy and entirely inflexible, however, be strong, clear and absolutely consistent, without going into battle with him.

Allow the time to set your child up and equip him for coping in the big wide world so he can happily and confidently engage with his peers and carers. By allowing him to throw a tantrum or scream when faced with an event not governed by him you're leaving him ill prepared to cope outside the home when dealing with others. If you don't take the time to teach your child to co-operate and be flexible, his friends and teachers at kindergarten will, which might come as a big shock to him!

5

Communication: Cues and routines

Cues to create patterns of routine communication

Within a normal day or week certain events recur multiple times. These include nappy changing, getting dressed, sitting in the high chair or car seat, having a bath and sleep time. As discussed in the previous chapter these events are often the transitional triggers that cause tears for your child and stress for you.

By making these events predictable and consistent for your child, you build her trust. You then have a manageable set of conditions to deal with each time you encounter a routine situation. It also ensures your baby feels completely in control of the event because she can pre-empt and therefore feel she owns each step, even when Mum, Dad, big sister or Granny changes her nappy.

The wait game

When I need to guide children into, through and out of an event routine like a nappy change, or getting dressed, or getting out of the pram, I use a fun game to help them learn to look to me for guidance so they know they don't need to cry to be picked up. I call this strategy 'the wait game'.

The wait game is a valuable tool that not only gives you practice at governing the outcome of a situation, but also ensures your baby or toddler understands it is normal and fun. The wait game incorporates a simple sign-language cue, which is very convenient when you're out with your child or she's focused on making a racket and can't hear you. A quick flash of this simple visual sign will enable her to understand your request. The game is conducted in response to certain behaviours and needs to be incorporated at the end of all parent-governed times of the day.

Making the wait sign

The sign I use in the wait game is an L-shape made with my thumb and first finger. To do this, start with a closed fist, and angle your hand so your bent-over fingers are facing towards your child. Open your fore-finger and thumb to make an L-shape so your child can see it briefly, then withdraw your hand as you close it to a fist again. This is designed to be a brief flash that just catches her gaze without irritating her, or stopping her from doing what she's doing.

Your child won't necessarily look at your hand. This doesn't mean she didn't register the sign. In fact, whether she appears to register it or not, she quickly learns its meaning.

When you're first playing the wait game, you may choose to offer the sign when your child starts a particular behaviour you want to correct, and again after you've re-positioned her correctly. After the first few days of playing the game you can start to rely more heavily on the word 'wait', and only offer the sign at the end of a request when she's in the correct position.

How to play

The wait game is a simple verbal and visual cue that can be incorporated into most parent-governed events of the day. It should be played in a fun way based on anticipation and excitement about what's going to happen at the end of the game, which is generally a snuggle or tickle. Play it while introducing and following through on your expectations of your child's behaviour. For example, when she's in the high chair and you've wiped her face and hands and removed the tray, quickly flash the sign and, with a big smile and maybe a giggle, say 'Waaaaaiiiiiiit! Wait.' In this way she starts to associate that request with fun feelings she can enjoy.

While you're asking your child to wait, undo her buckles. Remind her again to wait for you, so she is not governing when you pick her up. You are teaching her to feel comfortable with you governing the outcome of the event.

If your child raises her arms or leans forward in a gesture to say 'pick me up', define your statement by showing her what 'wait' means. So take her hands and put them down in her lap while saying, 'Hands in lap, wait for Daddy', or gently push her back into a safe sitting position, saying, 'Sit back. Wait for Daddy.'

Continue to make her wait until she's sitting as you would like. This may cause tears if she becomes annoyed or feels uncomfortable with you being in charge. However, as with most things in early childhood, practice makes perfect.

Your child will need to progress through the ladder of learning (see pages 70–72) and you'll need to be patient and confident until she starts to recognise and enjoy the process. Once she's sitting with her arms down and waiting for your guidance, you can use your up cue (see below). When you've picked her up, raise her in the air and say, 'Good waiting, darling,' then blow raspberries on her cheek and have a bit of baby fun.

This way, when you are in the supermarket and she gets stroppy about waiting in the checkout queue or demands to reach some sparkling lolly wrappers, you can flash her a smile and your wait sign without even opening your mouth, and she will sit back, put her hands in her lap and look at you with a big smile.

The wait game gives you the chance to change the mood, and offers a valuable break to hand your child a toy to distract her.

If your baby is aged six to ten months, play the wait game in a fun and consistent way. If you've followed all the basic instructions and your baby is struggling to calm down, try to distract her with a toy. The moment she calms down or is distracted, use your up cue and pick her up.

The up cue

The up cue is a very simple way of helping your baby learn to rely on your verbal communication rather than what she can see. You walk past your baby a hundred times a day and if she has to look at you to see whether you're going to pick her up or not every single time she'll become distracted from her toys over and over, becoming unsettled and eventually upset. Because she can't predict what you'll do in this situation, she may become uninterested in, or unable to focus on, play, and want to be carried around all day. However, if you use a verbal cue such as 'Up, up' each time you plan to pick her up, she will be able to play, knowing she doesn't need to anticipate you picking her up unless you say, 'Up, up.'

When you use the up cue and say 'Up, up', you are not *asking* your baby if she wants to get up, so don't wait for your baby to lean forward and gesture up. The up cue is a parent-governed line of communication designed to tell your baby that you – not her tears or tantrums – govern when she will be picked up. So say 'Up, up', then happily and confidently pick your baby up without asking permission.

Responding to their requests

From the earliest age, babies are able to clearly communicate with their parents. And for most parents understanding what their baby is saying or asking for – whether it be needing a nappy change, hunger or tiredness – comes naturally. However, things can become complicated when parents have to decide whether what their child is asking for is something the parent would prefer she didn't have. This is often where parents doubt their ability to understand their child.

It's usually in the 12- to 24-month age group that things can get a little tricky if the baby doesn't like the way things are happening. At this age children are still learning to live with their emotions, so guiding them can become difficult. Therefore if clear and honest lines of communication haven't already been introduced, it's important to introduce them quickly.

Once your child is good at telling you what she'd like, or where she'd like you to take her, there'll be times when you'll have to deal with her wanting things she can't or shouldn't have. When this happens, assess the situation from an adult perspective, even if your child is turning bright pink with fury. It's when you fail to assess her true needs and confidently assert your right as a parent to guide things that the situation can go pear shaped. Instead, your child, who has very little life experience and no way of consciously resolving a situation, is burdened with telling you how to do things. This sort of situation can result in a baby having a mother breastfeed her from 2 a.m. until 5 a.m. as a means of going back to sleep, or a toddler insisting on going to bed at 11 p.m. and getting up at 4 a.m., ready to start the day.

Distraction isn't always the answer – sometimes 'no' is the answer

The first strategy I find most people use if they don't just buckle and give in immediately to their baby's demands (which can be healthy and natural on some occasions) is the good old distraction technique. While distraction can be a good strategy and has its place in a balanced parenting approach, it should never be used as the only way to deal with a baby asking for something, or doing something you don't want her to do. Using only distraction can result in a baby throwing a tantrum out of frustration because she thinks she hasn't been heard or understood.

Often it is more honest, after showing her that you've heard and understood her, to simply say 'no'. Parents often give in to their child if they have to acknowledge what the child wants, even when the parents really don't want the child to have what she's demanding. Many only give in because they're nervous of saying 'no', yet saying 'no' and explaining why is good when it comes to establishing boundaries. In fact not saying 'no' can be confusing and tormenting.

Say 'no' to impractical requests

It's important to lay appropriate foundations for play and behaviour during the day. Sometimes that means saying 'no', especially when a child's request is impractical or unachievable. For example, if she can't yet walk and you give in to her desire for you to hold her hand and walk with her all day, you're telling her she can't do anything without you. This example can be applied to many different scenarios.

Don't repeat their request as a question

Another common strategy that parents use when answering a child's question is to repeat the question back to her. This also lands her in hot water:

> Child: 'Biscuit!'
> Parent: 'You want a biscuit?'
> Child: 'Yes.'
> Parent: 'No biscuit now. It's dinner time.'

Broken down, the parent here is asking, 'Would you like a biscuit?' The child responds 'Yes', but is then told, 'Well you can't have one'. This is very confusing! Remember: ask a question, expect an answer and respect the answer! Don't repeat a request as if it is a question! It's an example of turning a parent-governed line of communication into a question, which creates a child-governed line of communication, and ultimately the child's answer is not respected.

Don't use 'later'

A further common mistake is when parents try to be less direct:

> Child: 'Biscuit?'
> Parent: 'You can have a biscuit later.'
> Child: 'Biscuit!'
> Parent: 'Soon you can have the biscuit.'

The child continues to ask for a biscuit and eventually, frustrated at not receiving one, drops to the floor in a tantrum. What's happened is that the parent has answered the child with what appeared to be a 'yes', but wasn't. A young child doesn't understand the concept of 'later', which could be in a second or hours. All that's heard is a positive response, what sounds like the child might get to have a biscuit.

Until your child is five years of age, you need to be more specific and give her daily routine landmarks to predict what 'later' is so you don't leave her hanging. A more honest and fair answer is a clearly stated, 'No biscuits now. All gone, bye biscuits.' This doesn't mean you can't offer her a biscuit later. It just means you answer her clearly and don't lead her to believe you might give her the biscuit soon.

Pre-empt possible problems with clear communication

Pre-empt any possible problem areas within the flow of your child's day. If you know she may ask for a biscuit when she smells food cooking, tell her what she can expect before you start to cook and tell her your expectations of her behaviour and what she can expect of you: 'Mummy is going to cook your dinner now, yummy chops and mashed potato. Nearly time to sit down at the table for your chops and vegies. No biscuit, all gone biscuits, yummy chops with dippy sauce.'

The ability to say 'No _____, now, my darling. It's time for _____' is a vitally important line of communication for parents because babies need simple, clear acknowledgement and answers.

Use specific language and specific praise

I often hear parents with a child 12 months to two years old using very broad terms when it comes to communicating with or praising their baby. It's important to be extremely specific and break down your language when it comes to showing your expectations and appreciation of specific events. 'Good listening' is a very specific term for praising purposes, as are 'Good eating', 'Good sitting' and 'Good waiting for Mummy'.

It's equally important to be conscious of how empty a statement to your baby can be. For example, saying 'Please be good for Mummy' doesn't give any definition of what 'good' is. Some other common examples of empty statements include 'Eat nicely', 'Behave', 'Be nice' and 'Play nicely'. All of them are far too broad for your average under-two year old to understand.

You need to describe each of the above more clearly to a baby or toddler. So, for example, 'Eat nicely' needs to be broken down into understandable tasks such as: 'Pick up your spoon. Scoop it up, in your mouth! Good eating with your spoon!' or 'Cup on tray! Good listening, Bella. Look [point], cup on tray. Yeah!' and clap.

'Behave' would need to be broken down into understandable tasks such as, 'Good sitting, bubba.' 'Be nice' could be broken down into understandable tasks such as 'No hitting. Be soft to Daddy', as you encourage baby to stroke Daddy's face with her hand. 'Nice being soft, bubby. Oh, soft.'

'Pack away, please' could be broken down into 'Time to pack away. Joshua, pick up the block [point to the block], in the bucket, ta for the bucket, letting go of the block! Good packing away, Joshua. Good putting the block in the bucket! Pick up more blocks, in the bucket, let go.'

Each one of these specific styles of communication requires you define your statements the first few times. So you need to physically help your child until you can see she understands what the terms mean.

Whether you start using this style of communication at ten months or 18 months of age, your child will still need to go through the same learning process. They cannot skip a step simply because they are older or have an advanced understanding of language. You will need to start from scratch no matter what age your baby is, and once this style of communication is achieved, you'll need to remain consistent to avoid slipping back.

Separation anxiety

It's important to understand separation anxiety and the role your communication plays in developing and maintaining trust. Because, of course, separation is a major concern for your baby when she's learning to go to sleep independently. If you cannot leave a room during the day when she's playing happily, you can't expect her to cope with you leaving her in her dark room when she's worn out and tired.

Until the age of around four to six months, your baby is generally quite content to be left in the care of others, but as she grows she starts to develop a sense of 'object permanence'. This is where she learns that things and people continue to exist even when they are out of sight. Once she develops an understanding that she can call out to you from a neighbouring room, and you occasionally return at her insistence, she begins to look for a more permanent pattern during these events. The problem starts when she can't find a predictable pattern within these absences. In fact, the patterns are so varied that there are some days you do not return for hours, while on other occasions you return within minutes.

To make matters worse, she spends a little time gazing lovingly at her best friend (Mum or Dad) before happily starting her play, but when she looks up to watch you again you've suddenly disappeared and she can't see you anywhere in the room. You are now being inconsistent for her.

This is where a child might feel more comfortable guiding you rather than being in a situation where she can't predict what you will do. Focusing on play becomes difficult because she starts to be more focused on where you are, and as a result play becomes a challenging task. It's simply easier for her to ask to be taken everywhere with you, comfortably perched on your hip so she can predict what you'll do rather than risk feeling vulnerable and unsure of her environment. Unpredictability around your movements and absences triggers anxiety in your baby as she loses trust around you staying in the room or leaving and coming back. Her response is to try and avoid such a situation from repeating itself.

Absence cues

Separation anxiety varies from child to child, based mainly on the consistency of the communication provided by parents. Some children still experience stress around a carer leaving their line of sight well into their second year.

This is a normal and healthy stage of development but knowing a baby is upset and calling to them can be difficult for parents, whether they're running to the bathroom for 30 seconds or leaving their child in the care of someone else for the day. As babies have no concept of time, it's hard to explain to them the difference between going to the bathroom and going to work for the day. Parents need to look at ways of being honest, and creating some kind of predictability for their child to trust. This is where language cues and the associations developed around those cues become very valuable tools. By implementing the following short- and long-term absence cues, and then working through the emotions that occur around those events, you can develop trust with your baby in as little as one to three weeks.

I often see parents, with only love and the best of intentions, being their child's complete emotional solution throughout the day, only to expect their child to be totally self-soothing at night. This is an unrealistic expectation to place on any child.

Instead, we need to help our children learn to relax when we leave their line of sight during play or other 'alert' times of the day, so they're able to relax when we leave them at sleep time. The idea is to give children the chance to learn, via brief intervals with lots of positive reinforcement, how to cope with the sensations they feel when we leave the room during the day. This allows them to build confidence around the event long before they experience it at sleep time, so they can relax into their new settling routine without the stress of separation anxiety.

Short-term absence cue

The way to do this is to consistently use short-term absence cues each time you leave your child's line of sight, such as, 'I'll be back.' And every time you return, always say 'I'm back'. The first time you use the cue, make your absence short. Each time thereafter, gradually leave for longer and longer periods. Always say 'I'll be back' when you leave her line of sight, and always say 'I'm back' when you return.

Consistently informing your child of your movements is courteous and enables her to relax and do what all babies love to do: explore, play and learn, rather than feel the need to watch your every move.

Avoid ever saying the cue from another room or you'll encourage your baby to focus on listening for you all the time. This defeats the purpose because the conditions she encounters when she's going to sleep shouldn't involve her listening for you through the door, or thinking she can call out to you all night and you will respond each time.

What to do if your baby cries

The worst thing you can do if your baby cries when you leave the room is rush back in to fix her distress. Instead, assess the situation from an adult's perspective. A parent going to the bathroom under predictable conditions is definitely *not* something their child needs rescuing from and not the message you want to deliver to your baby. It would be debilitating for a child to think she is not okay or cannot calm down until you've held her and fixed things each time you re-enter the room. This is not teaching a baby appropriate coping strategies to normal emotions.

Sometimes you will carry on with your chores and reassure her by saying, 'You're okay, Bubby', then redirect her focus, 'Where's your car?' If, however, your baby has found this a difficult task, sit down casually beside her, and without fixing it for her (by picking her up, patting, rocking, etc.), show her how to calm down through play. If you maintain an attitude that everything is okay and that despite her tears she's okay, she'll be able to assess that she's okay.

Long-term absence cue (saying goodbye)

When you are absent for what feels like an eternity and your child frets, she will fret each and every time you leave her line of sight throughout the day. This is where the bulk of the stress around separation anxiety arises. If you plan to be away for a long period of time, such as when you go to work, to the gym for a few hours, or to the hairdressers, it's very important to say a proper goodbye.

Many people think babies under 12 months are too young to understand or be bothered by you leaving. However, if you don't pre-warn your baby when you're leaving for a substantial period of time, she will develop negative associations with you leaving the room, and will end up crying every time you leave her line of sight, even when you quickly go to get something in the other room. This pattern of behaviour will impact significantly on your ability to settle her at sleep time.

The trick is to create a predictable goodbye routine, because repetitious patterns produce the most laughs and the most relaxed demeanour in babies. An example of this is when you take your child to her grandparents' house, and Grandpa always takes her to look at the same rose bush, turn on the same tap, and Grandma always sings the same nursery rhyme. Very quickly your baby learns to expect and enjoy this pattern of events.

So, for example, if you're going to work, take the time to allow her to walk you to the door or car and to kiss and cuddle you goodbye. Wave to her and, importantly, involve her in the final part of the routine so she completes the farewell process herself. This could be something as simple as closing the car door or the garage door with you. By creating a predictable end to the goodbye routine and involving your child in it you are giving her a routine to look forward to as well as a sense of control over something she may find difficult so she can move on.

Even if saying goodbye results in a few tears, it's still important to allow her to feel the emotions tied up in someone she loves leaving her for a long period of time. This ensures she doesn't lose trust in you. It's obvious there will come a time when she is very sad to say goodbye for an extended period of time but it's okay for her to feel those emotions. These are normal feelings to have and nothing to shelter her from. It's so much more important to be honest with your baby and let her feel a little sad for a few moments than allow her to lose faith in you.

Developing trust during separation

The first rule in developing trust with your baby around separation anxiety is to be honest. Try to *never* walk out of a room without saying goodbye or 'I'll be back'. Imagine how frantic you'd feel if you looked up and your baby was gone, and you called out and heard nothing, then went looking and found nothing. Obviously, our fear as adults would be justified but for a baby it feels the same way when she looks up from what she's been doing, and you're gone. So she calls out, and nothing, so she looks for you and finds you've disappeared. This is very frightening for a baby.

Having worked in childcare centres for years, one of the worst things I dealt with was when parents snuck off without saying goodbye to their babies because they didn't want them to cry. What they didn't realise was that when their children looked up and around, then looked for them and couldn't find them, they got upset anyway. And worse, not just a little upset as they would have if their parents had said goodbye, but extremely upset and in some cases frantic. The most difficult thing for these children was the confusion that followed. They'd continue to cry and look for their parents for at least an hour and in some cases the better part of the day, whereas children whose parents were honest and said goodbye usually cried for between 30 seconds and five minutes and could then carry on with their day.

The children whose well-meaning but misguided parents snuck off without saying goodbye would turn up at childcare the next day clinging desperately to their parents' legs, feeling uncertain about the environment because it was associated with uncomfortable feelings from their previous visit. This same situation happens in the home environment when parents or others the baby loves and trusts aren't honest about leaving. Parents are not doing their baby or toddler any favours by being dishonest and not telling them when they leave, be it for a short or long time.

Positive feedback

Be your child's emotional safety net. When you tell her you plan on leaving her line of sight for a short period of time, your intention is to verbally assure her she can carry on playing, trusting that if you leave the room for a short period of time you will let her know, and tell her when you return so she can carry on playing undisturbed. This means she doesn't need to stop playing when you have to leave the room for a moment because her need to watch you to predict your movements is negated by your verbal cue and the events that always follow your actions. Instead she can know your movements and the outcome of them without even looking.

When you use your short-term absence cue, say it casually without trying to take her attention off what she is doing. Initially, while she's learning to trust that this new cue means you always come back within a short period of time, she will look up, and perhaps cry, but over time as she starts to trust this cue her need to look up will diminish and she will continue to play. This is your ultimate goal, so the way you say 'I'll be back' casually, without even looking at her, tells her you are very relaxed and not concerned for her, and this fills her with a sense of security.

And remember what I said about eye contact. Engaging your baby in eye contact can suggest you're about to talk to or play with her, so to make eye contact as you say your short-term absence cue then leave the room is a confusing message. The short-term absence cue should be said casually as you confidently walk out of the room regardless of her reaction. Spend a brief period out of the room and then re-enter confidently and say hello in a happy tone with a smile, regardless of her reaction. Your response to her reaction when you return to the room is what tells her if she is okay or not.

Remember how children react when they fall over and look to their parent to assess if they are hurt or not, and the parent's reaction ultimately determines if they start to cry or dust themselves off and carry on happily. It's the same in all situations where children feel uncomfortable. Don't make her think that you leaving the room is a bad thing by being frightened or overly reactive to her reactions.

If your baby is mobile and she follows you as you leave the room, allow her to follow you, even if she crawls or walks after you crying. This tells her you are not concerned, she is not in any danger, and she can feel comfortable in expressing the way your movements make her feel without being given the wrong messages about those feelings. Unless she hurts herself, don't vary your action from your original plan on these chores or toileting journeys. You should still close the bathroom door and walk back into the original living area that you left once you've completed your chores and say, 'I'm back'. Even if this means walking right past her on your way back. It's perfectly normal for a child to want to be near you, and if she can move it is fine for her to follow you, but don't teach her she needs to be carried when you're walking around the house because it is unnecessary and limits her opportunities to explore her environment.

Don't taint your cues

The golden rule of all communication is consistency. If you want your child to trust you, be predictable and consistent 100 per cent of the time. So always use your short- and long-term absence cues, always be reassuring in your response to her reactions and consistent in the messages you deliver when she expresses her emotions. Never adopt an 'I'm too tired to do this today' attitude.

It's normal to get tired and not have as much enthusiasm and energy every day of the week, so it's best not to push the envelope for yourself or your baby on these days. Therefore, if you don't feel you have the energy, simply carry on with your day and don't ask anything particularly challenging of your baby.

To taint a cue could mean you change the definition of, say, 'I'll be back' and the associated expectations your baby has of your behaviour around that event. This would mean you were unpredictable and therefore untrustworthy, and this will result in clingy behaviour in your child.

You can teach a baby very quickly to cry to get you to come back in the room, rather than play and wait for you. And you do not want to teach her that because you're not going to be able to maintain this, and it is a destructive strategy to use around your baby's sleep time.

Triggers for episodes of anxiety

Now that you understand the root cause of some basic separation anxiety in the home environment, it's important to understand the things that may disrupt the carefully balanced conditions of trust within your new language framework. If lack of trust is the cause of the tears, and communication to create predictability in her environment is the solution, anything that disturbs this predictability could easily disrupt the flow and trigger episodes of anxiety in your baby again.

On days when it's clearly not working, your ability to guide your baby with strong, clear, parent-governed lines of communication is one of the most reassuring tactics you can adopt to re-establish trust, along with your pre-emptive and forewarning cues. You'll soon see it is a quick and helpful strategy to help her settle down quickly and trust your guidance again. When she's feeling anxious, allow her to govern fewer areas of the day, depending on how unsettled she is. She's simply unsure of your predictability again, and you need to quickly establish her trust.

Some of the triggers could be things like a sudden change in the environment like the arrival of a new sibling, a sibling going to school after being home for the weekend, a change in carer for the day, a sneaky exit by you, someone being unwell, tradespeople in the house, Daddy arriving home from work, or going to a family barbecue where she's been passed around a lot. And obviously the big triggers might include a hospital stay, a holiday, or moving house.

During these times remain consistent, retain the ability to guide your baby or toddler, and follow your flow of communication by laying a path in words for each transition of the day until she calms down. The more you learn to understand your child the better equipped you are to be consistent.

6

Communication: The ladder of learning

The ladder of learning and what to expect

Whether you are a child or an adult, it takes time to learn a new skill, and learning a new style of communication or a new routine is no different. Fortunately, babies learn at an amazing pace, so you can be certain that, given the opportunity, your baby will thrive under your loving and consistent guidance. That said, all children, whatever their age, will need to climb a ladder of learning with a particular new skill or routine. So don't put off teaching a baby the process, or skip any of the steps. Once each step has been learnt and effective communication has been achieved, you can enjoy your happy and content baby and maintain your positive communication by being consistent.

The rungs of the ladder

Your primary goal when communicating with a child under two is to simply be understood. A child of six months is obviously going to have a different level of comprehension compared to an 18 month old, but the ability to understand a simple request during the normal flow of a routine is an equally complicated task for both age groups if effective balanced communication streams haven't been introduced.

The bottom rung of the ladder

The bottom rung of the ladder is where a child-governed line is the main form of communication. Let's take nappy changing as an example. Features of this rung might be that when you try to lie your child down to change his nappy he rolls over, refuses to stay in one spot, becomes emotionally overwhelmed, cries or does anything other than what you want him to do to ensure changing his nappy is a pleasant experience.

Achieving the transition from bottom rung to top rung does not happen without your child having to go through a natural learning process. Remember to be realistic and fair with him. It might take a day, or sometimes two or three days, for him to become familiar enough with a new flow of events that he feels he can truly relax and trust that the process is predictable and, therefore, safe.

The rungs in between

On the second rung of the ladder, your child is unfamiliar with the new routine and fights, but you remain consistent and confident, even if it feels a bit uncomfortable. Keep your eye on the top rung for motivation.

By the third rung your child will be familiar with the routine but may need repetition and consistency to trust the process and relax. You may still experience some resistance but as you repeat your cues and remain confident he settles quickly.

On the fourth rung your child is familiar with the routine and trusts your consistency. In the nappy changing example, he will start to relax and play with his toy. Towards the end of the event he will become a little unsettled as he tries to pre-empt the end. You need to stay calm, maintain a steady pace, and complete the event appropriately.

At the fifth rung your child manages the new routine through predictability. If he isn't mobile, when it's time for nappy changing, he'll look towards his room, gesture to lie down, look for his toy in its usual location and play happily until the nappy change is complete. If he's mobile, he may crawl or walk to his room and follow the above-mentioned actions of a non-mobile baby.

The top rung of the ladder

The pinnacle is when an appropriate parent-governed line of communication is in place and your child is empowered with the flow of events and feels in control of the routine because he can pre-empt the sequence of events you've taught him. For example, you lie him down to change his nappy, and he lies still, happily playing with a toy while you change the nappy, blow some raspberries on his tummy and so on. You clap your hands and say 'Up, up' and he waits for you to pick him up. You have a cuddle and thank him for lying still during his nappy change and turn out the light together on your way out the door.

How you may feel during your child's climb

Teaching a child something new is a thrill to me because I know how well it will turn out. I use these strategies all the time because they work! Hence, when a parent tells me it all seems too hard, and their baby gets cross, I say: 'I know how this story ends. This first rung of the ladder is like reading the first chapter of a book. Once you get past it, the rest of the story just flows and is easy.'

I completely understand that parents of children still on that first rung don't know how it ends, and out of fear they may fail to progress any further. Even though the bottom rung of the ladder is climbed relatively quickly, many parents find it virtually impossible to see past this brief period when their baby or toddler is crying or having a tantrum about the new and unfamiliar conditions. Some parents assume their baby is feeling fear, pain or neglect. In reality, most children are just uncomfortable with the unpredictability of the event, and in an effort to stop feeling this way they try to go back to their old set of conditions (no matter how inappropriate they were). When the old conditions are not reinstated, a child may become frustrated, angry and upset at his lack of control.

When this happens, remember to assess things from an adult's perspective:

- Where is he?
- Who is looking after him?
- What am I asking of him?

If you're teaching him to lie down for a nappy change, sit and wait in his high chair until a meal is finished, sit on your lap for a story, lie down in his cot, in a house where he's loved, and you're creating a new, improved way of doing things, the answers to these three questions are: 'At home', 'Me or my partner, so no one better' and 'To change his nappy'. This is all reasonable and nothing to feel anxious about. You were the one who taught him to do something in a certain way in the first place, and you are now simply teaching him something new once again.

Be patient and fair and don't expect your child to get things immediately. Give him a day or three to be fair. When he cries, put your needs and feelings aside and stay calm and confident so he is reassured. If he thinks the new routine makes you uncomfortable he won't relax and the process will become drawn out. If you remain steadfast and see things through, you'll be amazed at how quickly your under-two year old learns to listen, understand and master a new skill.

When your child resists guidance

It's natural and normal for your child to resist guidance when you first implement a parent-governed line of communication. He needs to climb several rungs before you achieve this type of communication consistently. Once this is in place and you and your child have become confident with that balanced flow, you can incorporate your third line of communication – negotiation – and you'll have a parent- and child-governed home. This change is challenging for your child, and may be met with a little or, in the case of a few toddlers, a lot of resistance.

When a child struggles with being guided I may spend up to three weeks guiding him by using my language cues even when things are going well. This gives the child the opportunity to feel comfortable and get used to being guided at both happy and challenging times, which creates more positive associations with guidance. Once the resistance stops, I slowly reintroduce choices. If your child copes well with a more open style of communication (negotiation) by happily accepting the responsibility of making some choices without trying to govern all areas of the day again, it's fine to continue guiding him and gradually offering more choices. Don't confuse him by letting him believe you're looking to him for guidance again or he may feel the need to create a trustworthy predictable day again by governing it himself through inappropriate behaviour. Retain a confident parental guiding role in your child's life.

Whether the resistance from your child is driven by a strong character or a naturally assertive or even bossy nature, or because he's feeling uncomfortable with a new or foreign set of conditions, your response should always be the same. It is perfectly natural for him to feel the whole range of normal, healthy human emotions. There's nothing normal or healthy about a child only ever feeling happy. Your child also has a right to express the way he feels when he experiences those emotions. He's new to this world and, even for an adult, feelings of frustration, unfamiliarity or anger can be overwhelming and need to be vented. Your child's daily moods and reactions to certain events are not directly proportionate to your parenting ability.

If you don't allow him to express his normal emotions you risk creating a culture in your family where your child cannot be honest about the way he's feeling because he fears it may upset you. Never discourage a child from feeling or openly expressing his emotions. Never avoid a normal situation because it may evoke emotions. It is your response to your child's expression of emotions that tells him if he's still safe under those circumstances, despite his feelings at that time.

It's very important that your child be able to rely on you to be the solid ground on which he can stand when he feels uncertain and uncomfortable in a particular situation. Imagine how he feels when you've asked him to sit in his high chair, and you're following through and defining that statement for the first time in his life. He'll be unsure and may become very upset at the unpredictability of the situation. Then imagine how he might feel when you smile, stroke his hair and say in a confident and loving voice 'It's okay, bubba, it's just time to sit down, you're okay!' then carry on with your chores until he settles down.

While your child may still feel cross or upset about the situation, you have told him by your actions and language that you're not concerned for him. Since he determines whether he's at risk based on your response to his reaction, he can feel cross or upset about the situation without feeling as though he's in harm's way. An example of this is when you see a child running at the park, and then suddenly falling over. If he hasn't seriously hurt himself, he looks for his parent immediately and more often than not, a parent will react in one of two ways: 'Awwwww, ouch' with a look of concern, extended arms and words, the v-shaped eyebrows and a contorted mouth; or 'Oops, over he goes, you're okay little guy, up you get.'

If the parent looks or sounds concerned, the child drops his little head and starts to cry immediately. He will often need a cuddle of reassurance before he is better and off he goes again. If the parent looks more confident, the child will often get up, rub his smarting hands or knees and carry on, safe in the knowledge that his mum and dad don't think he's at risk.

This is an important example because when you're helping your child work his way through a new process, which will often only take a day or so to learn, he *will* express himself if he's not pleased about the change, and he'll look to you to gauge if he's okay or not in this new situation. Your role as a parent is to assess the situation from an adult's perspective. If you assess a situation from your child's perspective, meaning you react by becoming upset too, you will mislead him and deliver the wrong message about this new routine and basic request to your child.

If you've assessed that your child is safe, loved, and only feeling uncomfortable about learning something new, you need to let him know that he's safe and not at risk by being confident and reassuring. He is permitted to get upset, and even allowed to have a full-scale tantrum if he feels totally overwhelmed, but you shouldn't burst into tears and get angry alongside him. The important thing to be conscious of is your response, and the message it conveys to your child. You can empathise confidently without looking guilty or concerned that your child is upset. If you need to practise this, do so while you're having a shower, or driving in the car alone (if that ever happens). Put yourself in the situation and verbally practise responding in an empathetic but confident and reassuring way.

Always follow your flow of communication, and remember that it only takes one or two positive, confident sessions to teach your baby something basic and new like nappy changing without tears or tantrums. Once you've established the language cue around that event you can forewarn him of your expectations and his response to the situation will become positive and a reflection of your response.

Responding to their resistance

Right from the time when their baby is six months old, I encourage parents to be mindful about what their actions teach their baby. All parents need to be cautious about giving currency to inappropriate behaviour, like back arching, screaming or hitting out, or undesirable communication, such as screaming and tantrums. If you carry on with your request and ignore these behaviours (by cleaning the table while you wait for him to calm down, or adjusting your shirt while he vents) without making eye contact or changing your actions, he quickly learns that you only respond to his calmer behaviours, and he'll only be picked up when he's *not* screaming, hitting or back arching. This results in your baby finding a more positive way of asking to be picked up without screaming or crying to get your assistance.

To respond with communication or body language to inappropriate or undesirable patterns of behaviour teaches your child to continue to do them in order to make you listen to him. When he goes into a style of behaviour that is clearly caused by impatience or bossiness, disengage physically by making no eye contact (apart from occasionally reassuring him in a confident manner if you feel it is necessary) then carrying on. If the behaviour continues, turn your body side on or away from him until he settles down. This is how you say, 'When you scream, back arch, hit, kick, etc., I will wait until you calm down before we carry on.' It helps him understand that as soon as he's calmer, you'll come back and help him and discourages common patterns of behaviour like eating for three minutes then throwing everything off the tray and insisting on getting down immediately. This strategy helps you teach him to stay in his high chair longer, and thus improves his ability to eat a more balanced meal, which ultimately impacts on his mood and sleep.

If you feel stressed about your child's tears or the origin of those tears, always go back to assessing the situation the child is in from an adult's perspective. Waiting for you to tell him when it's time to get out of his high chair, or off the change table, is a perfectly reasonable expectation to encourage right from six months of age.

Understanding your child's cries

Respond appropriately to encourage appropriate communication

What communication are you encouraging?

Babies are amazingly complex and intelligent. They experience the same emotions we do and they can have clear ideas on what they'd like to do and when they'd like to do it. Because they're just grasping the concept that they are separate entities from others, they tend to get a little annoyed when people don't automatically know what they're thinking or, indeed, don't want to do exactly the same things they want to do. This means babies will not hesitate to communicate with parents, and will spend most of their days trying to express how things make them feel.

As your child's brain develops, so does his ability to not only make choices but to act upon them, whether it is to pick up and shake a rattle or to have a piece of cheese out of the fridge. And your baby will use crying as a way of talking as well as expressing his emotions. When you interpret all his cries as fitting neatly into only a few set categories – where the trigger is either emotionally or medically based, like fear or distress, pain or hunger – you show you don't understand how complex and clever your baby is. A good proportion of babies between six and seven months don't display a need for clear parent-governed lines of communication, which is often expressed by being unsettled, grizzly, grumpy, or distressed. However, the need to listen to your seven- to eight-month-old baby becomes an important observational skill to ensure you don't encourage crying or tantrums by misreading your baby's bold and confident attempts to guide those around him.

By the time babies are celebrating their first birthday, they have a very strong understanding of their abilities, of what they would like to do, and have become very efficient at communicating those needs to their primary carers. Be sure to always give your child a clear indication you've been able to understand his cry by giving it a verbal sentence or definition.

This helps your baby start to learn early phrases. An example of this would be when your baby cries and gestures to be picked up. You respond by saying 'Alex wants up. Mummy pick you up', before using your up cue.

When responding to your baby's cries however, be cautious about giving a certain style of inappropriate or undesirable communication from them, like back arching, screaming, head banging, or hitting, a value in their vocabulary. Imagine you are asking your baby to wait in their high chair while you wipe down the tray and complete the meal time. If your child was to start screaming, or back arching, or hitting the tray, then your automatic response might be to remove them from the situation that is upsetting them. But ask yourself:

- Is it appropriate that he learns to wait while you wipe down the tray? (Yes.)
- Is it asking too much of him? (No.)
- Is it a skill that will be useful to him in other situations as a life skill? (Yes.)
- Should he scream, back arch or hit the tray at the end of each meal to get picked up? (No.)

If this behaviour occurs, remain conscious of the outcome you want to achieve. If you want to discourage behaviours such as having a tantrum, screaming, crying, hitting or back arching, then it's crucial not to give these behaviours a definition or predictable positive outcome for your baby. Strive to do the opposite of what he expects the behaviour to achieve, such as wipe down the kitchen table, put your hair up or pat the puppy dog until the behaviour subsides. With under-two year olds you should not leave the room, or move around the room too dramatically or to where he has difficulty seeing you. Just stay in the room and carry on with your chores until he stops the behaviour. This can take a little bit of time so you need to stay calm and patient. But in the longer term your child will learn that you only respond to his calm behaviours, and he is only picked up when you say the words 'up, up' and *not* when he's screaming, smacking, or back arching.

To respond with body language – such as looking at him, moving faster to complete a task, leaning in to cuddle him in a bid to stop his tantrum – or to pick him up in response to inappropriate or undesirable patterns of behaviour is to literally teach him to continue the behaviour for you to co-operate with him. This obviously does not apply to a baby who has got a sudden fright, who's extremely excited when someone he loves comes home unannounced, or he's accidentally hurt himself or been hurt. We're only talking about not teaching him to behave in a manner that will ultimately have people scowl at him, make you exasperated or frustrated with him, or pigeonhole him as a certain type of child, which impacts on his self-esteem. Be honest with your expectations and teach him that you will always follow a routine flow of events to complete a task, and his inappropriate styles of communication are not how you talk to one another in your house.

If your baby is happy and content continue to use your language and always praise positive outcomes. This helps him associate this style of routine language with enjoyable outcomes. Right from the time their child is eight months old I encourage parents to be mindful of what their actions are teaching their baby by:

1. disengaging physically when their child goes into a style of behaviour they do not wish to see continue: making no eye contact apart from occasionally reassuring them in a confident manner, and turning their body in a different direction and simply carrying on with doing something else
2. turning their body side on or away from their baby until they settle down if the behaviour continues
3. distracting their baby once they settle down with a toy or a story until the behaviour stops entirely.

Then they can pick them up or offer them something they were asking for. This is how they say, 'When you scream, back arch, hit or kick me I will carry on with something else, but when you are calm I will come back and engage with you and get you up or give you what you want.'

The importance of boundaries

Children do some of the things they do, and behave in some of the ways they behave, because they don't know the consequences of their actions, or the impact those actions have on others. This is normal and natural. Sometimes they are happy to oblige, sometimes they're less than impressed with your plans, even if you know they are good plans and in their best interests.

Children are naturally impulsive, and will run onto a road to chase a ball, grab a burning candle because it's eye-catching, and turn on a hot tap because they've seen you do it. Equally, they will squirm and tantrum when you change their nappy because they'd rather get down and play even if that may result in nappy rash and pain. This is because they don't have the capacity to think in terms of consequences and only respond to the moment they're in. You, as their guardian, are responsible for deciding when their impulsive actions are in their best long-term interests.

Some people claim children behave in certain ways because they 'need' to do all the things they do. I firmly believe children only do things and behave the way they do around certain events because they haven't been shown an alternative or a better way. They have no way of knowing that the consequences of some of their impulsive actions will be detrimental to them or others.

The same principle applies to setting basic boundaries on any given day, such as those around sleep and other basic needs like nappy changes, getting dressed, sitting in a pram or letting you feed them. We live in a time of tremendous judgement and pressure to perform and be 'perfect' parents. I've seen many parents so focused on trying to keep their children happy at all costs that they abdicate their 'knowledge' of what truly makes a child happy. They look to a tiny child, not even two years old, for guidance on a subject the child doesn't yet know or understand.

Some parents accept certain behaviours, no matter how exhausting, unpleasant or inappropriate they are to the child, the family or those around them, regardless of the long-term effects those patterns of behaviour will have.

This means a child who needs desperately to sleep because he's tired is allowed to stay up half the night, or a child who needs to eat nutritious food because he's clearly hungry is allowed to drink milk whenever he demands it. It means a child who is having a tantrum or screaming on a change table is allowed to crawl all over the floor rather than learn how to lie still and be calm and patient.

Finally, it means that when the child turns four or five and his parents decide they no longer like him doing any of the things he's grown up being taught is right, they tell their child to 'grow up and stop acting like a baby'.

A fairer, more honest and healthy approach would be to decide, as a family, which behaviours you want to avoid, or correct, and what the boundaries are within your house and family. Boundaries are good!

In fact not only are boundaries good, they are the absolute key to balanced and happy babies and toddlers, and essential in preparing a child for life. Boundaries help a child learn patience, persistence, social skills, expectations of others, self-control, empathy, and safety, as well as providing opportunities for you to encourage the great sleep and healthy eating necessary to promote optimum growth and development so your precious child can be all he could ever possibly be.

Anyone who says children shouldn't have boundaries fails to see the vitally important role they have in a child's life. To not provide boundaries, particularly around the areas of health and safety, is neglecting your duty of care by failing to provide the best possible state of health for your child to develop and learn at peak capacity. Boundaries act as emotional safety nets, reassuring children that when they feel out of control or overwhelmed or overburdened in a world full of choices, they can safely turn to you and you will take over, unburden them and keep them safe.

Those safety nets should be set close, like training wheels, while a child is young. As the child matures and starts to develop the capacity to cope with the responsibility of choices and guiding others, the nets can be slowly withdrawn to allow a child to steady himself and try out his new skills. You will still need to keep an eye on him, though, and if you feel he's tired, stressed or in a challenging position, you may decide to tighten up the safety nets until he settles down again.

Setting appropriate boundaries or house rules also sets your child up to have a healthy expectation of others' respect towards him, and helps him learn what he can expect in return. At first our children know nothing of our western culture or its social ways. We mainly function through the day, and sleep at night. We have cultural and social etiquette and boundaries, and generally need to be in a reasonable mood to cope with the day-to-day trials of life. So, unless you plan to move in with the Moiré tribes people, our little children need to 'learn' how to live in our western culture, and it is up to us as adults who understand the consequences of our actions to teach children how to function within those boundaries.

It's unrealistic to expect a child to have an automatic understanding of how a toy works when he first sees it, or how to go to sleep in his cot, or lie still while you change him, or play on the floor while you wash the dishes, so he relies heavily on you, who knows more about this amazing world he's part of, to tell him what to do, and how to best do it. You need to show him what's going to result in the best outcomes for him when he steps out into the world. You're the ones who want to teach him all these things with love and respect and patience. Children need clear guidance with their play and their behaviour.

It's important to give him a day he can predict, so he's freed of the burden of telling you how to make him happy, because you already know he needs to be loved, to feel safe, to sleep, to be nourished, and to feel free to explore and play to enjoy and learn about the world around him. Only an adult can find that balance when things go a little awry.

Be confident: make decisions, and help him through those decisions until he too understand the benefits of some of your ideas and plans.

7

Understanding play

All children love to play. And while play may look like nothing more than good fun, it is absolutely vital to a child's development. That said, play is not a *goal* or something a child has to *achieve*. Instead, it's a journey of discovery, fun, laughter and opportunities to develop skills. Helping children play is about discovering what they enjoy and building upon those experiences. It's about introducing them to the world and helping them build the confidence to explore it.

So what has play got to do with sleep? In a word, *everything*, and, hopefully, by the time you've read this book, you'll understand how and why.

But first let's look in detail at why play is so important. Then I'll set out:

- the link between play and sleep
- stages of play
- styles of play
- role play
- independent play.

Why play is important

Between the ages of six and 12 months, children will begin to hold a block, developing their fine motor skills in the process. Then, with jerky movements, they begin to connect one block to another, developing their eye–hand co-ordination, spatial awareness and physical development.

Through practising this task, children also learn to cope with the sensation of frustration, and develop the skill of patience. When they've mastered these new skills they will eventually build a small tower.

Even the simplest forms of play foster healthy development in children. Play provides opportunities for them to be in control of their surroundings in a way that empowers them right from the tender age of six months. Play provides them with opportunities to make lots of noise, express themselves freely, be entertained and have fun, all the while developing the skills of patience, repetition, persistence, completion and transitioning. All these skills are needed for confident socialising when they go to childcare, playgroup, kindergarten or preschool.

Play also teaches children independence, co-operation and, as they get older, how to share. Children discover they won't always get the outcome they want so they learn how to compromise. Play teaches them to ask for assistance, and helps them develop the communication and social skills essential for integrating confidently into any normal social environment.

Play and sleep

Good challenging play is also a great sleep inducer. The years I've spent encouraging an environment rich in opportunities for children to explore and play has yielded great results in the area of sleep development and maintenance. Having established and refined these strategies I strongly believe in the importance of creating a fun play environment filled with challenging and interesting opportunities to explore and play every day at home.

In particular, I incorporate a critical style of play into every daily routine in the morning that I call independent playtime. An unstructured free play that incorporates all the skills your child needs to master and encourage sleep skills. In order for you to respectfully repair your little one's sleep concerns, this one area must be incorporated into their daily routine. The following chapters will equip you with all the tools and skills you need to empower your baby with the very crucial skill of confident independent play. This skill is your baby's ability to feel comfortable and safe within her own skin, within her own space and have the emotional tools to cope in any environment.

The stages of play

Understanding the types of play babies are capable of helps you understand *them* better, which in turn will give you the confidence to establish a play environment that caters to their needs. It will also help you balance their learning opportunities and make watching them learn a truly eye-opening experience.

The different ways young children play were first classified in 1932 by the sociologist and researcher Mildred Parten, who identified the following stages:

- unoccupied play, where children simply observe, or appear to be performing random movements
- solitary or independent play, where children play by themselves, showing no interest in the activity of others
- onlooker play, where children show moderate interest in others' activities but do not actively participate
- parallel play, where children play happily alongside others doing a similar activity but do not play *with* that other person (this form of play provides parents with an excellent opportunity to learn what interests their child so they can emulate that play and gradually expand it)
- associative play, where children play with others but without organisation
- co-operative play, where children play with others in a co-ordinated fashion, often with rules or other organisational elements.

It appears children work their way through these stages as they develop. However, older children will still engage in solitary play, while even quite young children can be capable of simple forms of associative and co-operative play. What's important to understand is that all six kinds of play are vital for children's development, and they learn skills in one kind of play they can apply in another.

Styles of play

Mildred Parten's stages of play continue to be the scheme by which people understand how children play. But when I'm discussing play relevant to the development of skills in the area of sleep repair, I focus on three particular styles of play. These three important skill setting styles of play are:

- one-on-one play: where a family member sits down with a baby or toddler and plays either with or alongside her. This may be a form of parallel, associative or even co-operative play, depending on the situation and the child;
- role play: where a child watches as another person enacts a scenario using toys or shows a child how to play with a toy. This may be a form of parallel play or associative play, and is very useful for teaching a child all kinds of things; and

- independent play: where a child plays by herself without too much carer intervention. Learning to play independently is key to learning how to sleep through the night.

One-on-one play

One-on-one play is the intimate play you engage in with your baby and generally involves eye contact, physical closeness and time. One-on-one play can involve many different activities, from doing household chores such as cooking, making the bed or watering the garden together. It could be dancing or singing songs and doing the actions together. One-on-one play can even be a special trip to the post office or fruit shop. These trips can become a language-rich one-on-one interaction so long as your focus is on having a fun playtime without distractions.

This kind of play should happen regularly throughout every day. It gives parents the chance to provide language-rich experiences, and promotes parent–child bonding. It also provides teaching opportunities to encourage a positive association with play through fun, laughter and learning what is interesting to your child.

One-on-one play is a favourite with parents, siblings, extended family, friends and babies alike. It is usually well developed in most homes I visit, and a healthy bond and strong sense of trust has always been fostered as a result.

Role play

Role play is the style of play a parent might engage in when introducing a new toy, or coming home from work after missing their child all day. This play usually involves a toy and generally follows a simple path: the adult attempts to show the child how to use the toy by using it themselves with lots of enthusiasm and fun. The play generally follows the child's interest, with the carer offering an activity for enjoyment as much as learning. In role play, you play enthusiastically alongside your child and either actively engage their attention or not.

Role play is an important and valuable style of play as it can be used to teach a child how to use their toys in more enjoyable and challenging ways. This helps ensure they get the most out of their play, and empowers them with strategies for the more challenging but equally important independent play.

Using role play to calm an unsettled child

Role play is ideal when your child is happy and content, but it's also a useful tool for calming her when she's unsettled or stressed. In fact, playing enthusiastically and confidently by yourself next to an unsettled child can be one of the quickest ways to calm her, whatever the cause of her tears.

If the only thing you do to help your child to calm down is to pick her up or breastfeed her, you're teaching her that is the only way to calm down, which is just a learnt pattern of behaviour. So why not empower her by teaching her other ways to calm down, and make at least one of these new strategies a routine she can use that doesn't completely rely on you? Then, if you need to go out and leave her with your mother, husband, wife or sister, she has coping strategies that don't depend on you. Even more importantly, it means that if you say goodnight and leave the room, and she gets cross momentarily at the request (which is pretty common), she knows how to calm down quickly without you picking her up or breastfeeding her.

By using role play in these kinds of situations you show her that by playing happily with her toy she can calm down and feel happy again. This is equipping your baby's emotional tool kit.

For this kind of role play, sit down near her and, staying calm and confident, enthusiastically play with one of her toys. Remember you are *not* asking her to look at you or the toy – you are not saying your child's name or waving the toy under her nose. You're simply playing in a solitary or independent fashion alongside her until she calms down, becomes distracted and then settles.

It's also important to play with the toy in a way your child can copy or master later. This might involve banging two blocks together, spinning the wheels on a car or scratching the textures on a toy. For toddlers it might involve building a little tower of three blocks, knocking them over and looking surprised. Whatever you choose to do, it should involve up-beat tones and vocalisation (which may look like you talking to yourself or the toy), so use a happy voice and vibrant expressions.

A repeated pattern of behaviour and sound will often distract your child and draw her attention. Even when she's making a protest or crying, she will stop briefly and have a chuckle at a repetitive action and sound, before resuming her crying.

The final part of this strategy is to be consistent and, above all, patient. When I use this strategy with children and we've worked through tears or protests for a period of time, parents tell me they would have given up long ago and never seen that it was possible to calm their child in that way.

Each time you use this strategy it will become easier and easier for your child to calm down quickly and start to play. Eventually, you will be able to use this form of play to defuse a situation before the tears start.

Using role play to teach self-settling

This is obviously vital for sleep, so your confidence and consistency here will mean your child will learn the all-important, 'Lie here calmly until you fall asleep' skill. It will be something you've both already worked through at a less stressful event, like daytime play, where they learn to listen when they are not feeling tired.

Independent play

Between six and 12 months, the first style of play you are likely to see is solitary or independent play, where a child plays by herself, showing no interest in the activity of others. Independent play can be clearly identified in young babies and often remains an important and active style of play for the rest of their life.

Independent play should make up around one-third of your child's play opportunities during the day, including a concentrated hour of play each morning when your child is at her absolute best. Remember, it's about balance, so not all play should be independent. But seek to encourage that hour of independent play in the morning, then allow your child to choose between playing with you or pottering off and playing on her own if she likes at other times of the day.

Are we giving our children enough space to play independently?

When I was growing up, running a household was more labour intensive. Few homes had the conveniences we now take for granted – microwave ovens, dishwashers, four-minute-cycle washing machines, etc. Takeaway food was a rare treat, household bills had to be paid in person, and grocery shopping was done at several shops, not a one-stop supermarket.

Consequently, our parents did not have as much time as we do to spend sitting and playing with our children. But they were a well-organised bunch, so a daily routine or schedule (whether intentional or not) was essential to get all the chores done. I remember my mum crawling around the floor with me and my sisters, but I also remember adventuring all over the house while Mum busied herself with the chores. I also remember making the trip with Dad to the bank each week and waiting and waiting and waiting while he paid the bills and organised the family finances.

I'm thrilled we now have so many products and conveniences to make our lives easier and give us more time. But the down side is that our children, especially first-born ones, are no longer learning as a matter of course the simple skill of playing independently without the need to be entertained.

Interestingly, second or later children often have a far greater ability to play independently. This is probably because, as families grow, parents get busier, giving subsequent children the time and space to learn how to play by themselves without adult intervention.

In many of the homes I visit today, babies struggle when put down for just a moment, and become stressed if their mum or dad stands up and walks one or two metres away to grab a glass of water.

There are other factors to be considered, too. In many families both parents work. With time such a precious commodity, they take every opportunity they can to play with their baby and shower them with attention. But this can add to the difficulties babies develop around play from an early age.

Parents are often stunned to learn that their baby can play on her own in daycare, yet doesn't display this skill at home. But in fact a child needs to learn how to cope in all environments.

Even if our time is limited, we need to create a balance of opportunities for children so they can develop the independent skills they need to grow and develop. We need to give children the opportunity to discover the joy of a quiet play with their toys, and empower them to feel comfortable and safe on the floor or in a play environment where they can still see their carers without feeling anxious.

The importance of independent play

Learning to enjoy independent play without constant parental intervention is key to your child developing the skill of sleeping through the night. However, when it comes to independent play both children and parents may need encouragement. Children need encouragement to try to play without constant assistance or attention; parents need encouragement to allow their child to play independently without fearing for her safety or comfort. After all, fearful parents engender fearful babies who can't play independently because they believe they are in an unsafe situation.

To learn to play independently children need enough time and space to practise and get the hang of it. Giving them this time and space is about parenting from a place of love, based on a child's true needs, rather than parenting from a place of fear, based on their short-term demands. A baby's true need is to be given an opportunity to experience the balance of all styles of play, including learning to play independently. Without these opportunities they may become clingy, unable to cope unless they're in someone's arms or immediate vision. This is just as imbalanced a strategy as never playing one-on-one with a child.

By six months of age, children who haven't been exposed to independent play may feel uncomfortable when their parent steps out of their line of sight. This is because they have not developed trust in their parent's communication or had the opportunity to feel the emotions associated with playing in another room from their parents. As a result, babies may 'play it safe' and cling to their parent.

Often, by the time I come into someone's home, these babies are terribly anxious about their parents walking away. This can result in the parents losing confidence in their parenting so they look to their baby for guidance. The baby, in turn, becomes burdened with the exhausting job of running the flow of the house.

If this is you, it's okay: it's repairable no matter what age your baby is, though the strategies are particularly effective with children under two years of age. By helping a child feel safe enough to play independently you develop strong language-based communication as well as provide her with the ability to trust that she can predict your movements, so even when you're not right in front of her she has confidence in her own space.

Independent play is the most basic skill your child needs in order to feel safe and comfortable in her cot for sleep, though the first time your child practises independent play should be during playtime, not sleep time.

Do children need toys?

If play is the route to balanced, healthy physical and mental development, toys and a stimulating environment are the means by which the desire to play is ignited. Toys encourage a longer attention span for playing alone, which promotes an elevated interest in play because of previous successful and fulfilling encounters. By providing an environment that is rich in age-appropriate challenging activities, you will encourage your child to want to explore her environment more.

One-on-one enthusiastic role play will help your child develop strong and confident play strategies and warm and happy associations with each particular toy. Via role play, your child learns how to play with particular toys and will then be keen to practise her skills. This gives her the opportunity to discover what she likes, and what she *is* like. Therefore, variety in play, such as a good selection of toys, will help facilitate healthy independent play.

8

Developing independent play

Setting up your home for independent play

Babies and toddlers are relatively new to the world they find themselves in. So to a baby their home may be extremely interesting but may also seem oversized and sometimes overwhelming. Cluttered spaces, wide open spaces or blocked sight lines can all cause a small child to feel unsafe or anxious. And when a child has those feelings he's unlikely to want to play without you right there beside him.

Find a suitable area

If you'd like your child to play independently, the first thing you need to do is set up one or more areas in your home where he can feel safe and relaxed enough to be put on the floor while you get on with other tasks. The key is to find an area where he can keep an eye on you, a place where he can feel relaxed enough to not feel the need to watch you to make sure you don't suddenly disappear.

The area you choose may be dependent on when you want your child to play independently, and therefore where you're likely to be at that time. I'm a strong believer in independent play in the morning when children are at their best and parents are busying themselves with cooking or other chores. I would therefore recommend choosing an area near the kitchen to set up your child's play area, though the kitchen itself is not necessarily a safe environment while you're cooking.

If you live in an older dwelling, your kitchen may be separate to the main living area, in which case see if there are spaces outside the kitchen where your child could play with a clear view of you. Alternatively, you might utilise the far ends of the kitchen, away from the cooking area, which may mean moving the bin or a breakfast table for a few months until he's become more comfortable with playing while you're busy. If you live in a modern house you're likely to have a kitchen that overlooks a main living area, which is ideal.

Tidy up and create sight lines!

The next step for creating a play area is to make it clean and clutter-free. If the space has accidentally become part-office or part-storage room, for example, put away or sell the old printer and computer on the floor in the corner, and sort through and throw out things that are broken, no longer needed or should be stored elsewhere.

Your baby will benefit from this sort out. Often parents say, 'We know we need to tidy up, but we don't have time because of the baby so we just can't get around to it.' Well, if you're waiting for your child to start playing before you begin your spring clean, you're going to be waiting a long time. Rather, to encourage your child to play independently (and so free you up!) you need to create a simple, clean environment in which he can feel comfortable enough to explore.

In the same way a cluttered and disorganised home will discourage a baby from playing, excessively over-furnished rooms can create visual obstacles between you and your child, giving him the feeling you are too far away or inaccessible. On the other hand, a vast open space may leave him feeling exposed, vulnerable and isolated. Either type of environment can make it difficult for parents to step away and give their children the opportunity to learn a new and enjoyable routine.

When I visit families to help with their babies, I often help redecorate to create a clear pathway between the parents and their baby so there's a visually open environment to foster an emotional sense of closeness. A kitchen bench need be the only large obstacle between parents and their baby.

If your baby is struggling to play independently, move the furniture about to create clear sight lines and walkways. If you have extra dining chairs or large one-seaters overfilling the room, move or remove them entirely while you spend a few weeks teaching your unsettled baby how to play. Tuck dining chairs in under the table and, if you have an extendable dining table, reduce it to its minimum size. Tidy up the position of footstools, magazine racks and coffee tables.

If the room is big, make it feel smaller

If you have a vast space to fill, try to create a more intimate play area. Utilise larger items of play to create the feel of a big playpen but don't block your child's path – leave him space to potter off and explore if he feels comfortable to do so. Large soft pillows, baby play frames and soft floor coverings spaced at a close distance will create a warm, safe and inviting space for him while you're busy nearby.

Safety issues

I encourage parents to do their chores in the morning while their child practises independent playtime, but it's important to ensure they are completely safe. The Safety 1st website (www.safety1st.com.au) lists many tips on how to make your entire house safe for your children and you.

Some families use a playpen for their child's safety. I'm not a fan of playpens, and usually eliminate them from play sessions when I help a family re-establish effective independent play. This is because they tend to get messy, which affects opportunities for effective and challenging play. Also, when a playpen is used for older, more mobile babies it's often used in place of effective communication, such as setting simple boundaries like, 'Wait for Mummy', 'I'll be back' and 'No touch'. However, if your baby is happy to play in a playpen, you're communicating well and all is working well, there's no need to eliminate it.

While I don't like playpens, gates are great for setting safe boundaries. A gate can often make cooking safer, and it is a good idea to use gates to keep play outside the kitchen, so long as your child can still see you. Gates can be useful to stop patterns of crying. Think of when they follow you to the bathroom and cry at the door. By simply establishing a new pattern, such as a short-term absence cue, and by placing a toy at the gateway, your baby may start to follow you crying, but then be distracted by the toy at the gate and sit and play while he waits for you to return.

Gates also offer older children the chance to play with a toy without fear of it being destroyed by their baby brother or sister. This playtime dilemma can cause older children to snatch, push or have tantrums, as well as fuelling a baby's mistrust about play. Some parents regard gates as an unpleasant necessity which is reflected in the way they talk about the gate. It's best to foster warm, positive associations with gates by covering them in sparkly, well-fixed stickers, getting really excited about their installation, and ensuring your child has something to do each time he encounters it. If you make a habit of pointing to the stickers and counting with a big happy smile, your baby will mimic this pattern and enjoy the encounter.

When you place a favourite toy at the gate, walk through and close the gate behind you, then lean over and briefly tinker with the toy. If your baby is relaxed and content about you leaving, just use your short-term absence cue.

Toy storage to promote better playing and easy packing away

If your child is old enough to access his toys independently, set up a toy storage area he can use to make packing away easier for you and your toddler. It also helps keep toy pieces together, which is important if he is to get the most out of play, as incomplete toys may affect his concentration span and ability to complete a task.

Investing a small amount of time in setting up good toy storage will have lasting benefits. The aim is to make the storage easily accessible for your child, while keeping toy pieces sorted and together. This means no stackable crates, and large toy boxes should only be used for cars, dolls or dress-ups. Instead, go to a hardware or storage shop and buy a light plastic frame which contains three or four small, removable drawers. Look for drawers:

- your child can safely remove without the constant need for your intervention
- you can stick a visual prompt on to show what goes where.

A series of drawers means you can circulate the toys you provide, keeping play fresh and exciting.

The items that each drawer can hold could be broken down into the following types of categories, which can be adjusted to suit your toys:

- Construction, such as Duplo.
- Puzzles and problem solving, such as nesting cups, sequence rings, pop-up toys and jigsaw puzzles.
- Role play, such as cooking utensils, toy phones, car keys, etc.
- Transport, such as trains, planes and automobiles.
- Fisher-Price Little People.
- Toy animals and small life accessories such as trees, rocks, coloured paper for water and grass, mats with cars and people.
- Language materials, such as books, felt board, magnetic stories.

- Music.
- Balls.
- Dolls and dolls' accessories.
- Junky toys.

Once you've arranged the toys into appropriate drawers, label them so your child can determine their contents. To do this you could set up the toys from each drawer so they look attractive then take a quick picture and print it up. Stick each picture on the front of your toy storage area with clear contact. Now your child has easy access to his toys, and setting up and packing away will become a joy for all. If you buy several drawer systems, put one or two of the multi-drawer systems away for two weeks, leaving the others to play with. This way you can circulate toys to keep them fresh.

Creating play stations

Once you've tidied up and rearranged an area and made it safe, you're ready to create some 'play stations'. A play station is an area clearly defined with a simple play mat. Each mat is equipped with around four age-appropriate toys, and each mat targets a specific style of play, meaning each of the four toys should come from the same developmental area. The four toys should be evenly spaced in the play station, with one toy on each corner of the mat.

Set up three or four play stations (depending on the size of the space) in well-spaced positions with clear walkways between them. The idea is to create a flowing, inviting, refreshing play environment for your child. You are also creating a routine he learns to expect and, ultimately, feels safe and empowered within.

If the space allows, you may want to arrange the play stations to approximate your child's natural path towards you, with the first play station placed furthest away and the next a little closer. The idea is to create an environment of exciting distractions if your child makes a beeline for you. This also ensures he can gradually move towards you as he becomes more tired as the morning progresses.

Choosing appropriate toys

When it comes to setting up play stations for children, don't buy too many toys or your child may feel overwhelmed and unable to make a choice. Carefully choose good quality toys, keeping the following in mind:

- Don't be tricked by marketing claims that a toy will somehow make your baby super bright. All play is valuable and encourages healthy development. Exploring a cardboard carton can be a very educational experience.

- For babies ten months and older, look for a toy that offers multiple tasks. A toy where a child needs to work out how to make something happen with an action is better than a toy that does things with a simple push of a button or a single insertion of a small ball, which will soon be boring to the child.
- Look for toys with longevity, which can be adapted to the various skill levels of different ages. Two examples are the Safety 1st Bouncin' Baby Play Place, which starts as a fun play walker, then converts to an early stage figure-eight train track; and the Fisher-Price school bus, which starts out as a fun problem-solving toy for babies then turns into a small social-play piece of equipment that matches the Fisher-Price Little People range.
- For babies under ten months, go for less busy-looking toys with softer colours that explore concepts such as colour, shape, texture and sound.
- Think about the things you do often and buy similar toys. For example, if you talk on the phone a lot, get your child a phone. He'll already know what to do with it from watching you, and it will be extremely desirable to him.
- Make toys using everyday household items. Familiar objects are usually the things children enjoy playing with the most.

Making play stations inviting

Some babies are happy to have a few toys on a play mat positioned anywhere their parents put them. Others require more encouragement, stimulation and planning. Most parents who experience difficulties with their babies' daytime play say their babies have shown this tendency from a very early age. Some report that their baby is the only one in their play group who has never played on the floor, or has never just drifted off to sleep mid play or on a pram ride.

If this sounds familiar, you may need to invest a little more time in creating a fun play environment that draws your baby's attention and encourages an active interest in his surroundings. Each play station should look appealing, so fan books out and place one open on a big teddy's lap, clearly role-modelling reading. Semi-construct a block tower. Tower or lay out nesting cups in a sequential line. Doing this will increase the chances your child will start to play without much intervention or the need to work through difficult behaviour.

Positioning

Immobile or slightly mobile babies can be positioned differently at each play station. Ensuring a balance of tummy time, back time and assisted sitting fosters an enjoyable, fun play session and encourages a healthy attitude towards play.

Positions include:

- lying down with toys in reach
- lying down with toys out of reach
- sitting down with toys in reach
- sitting down with toys out of reach.

Start by putting toys within reach, then gradually place some at an adequate distance to promote reaching or tummy shuffling. As your child becomes better at sitting, go from putting a toy in his lap to several toys within reach to provide him with more of a challenge to problem solve and reposition himself to access the toy.

Encourage your child to play for around ten to 15 minutes at each play station, then give him a cuddle, relocate him and spend a few minutes playing with him. If your baby is very engaged with his play, there may be no need to move him. However, be careful not to push your baby to play for more than a reasonable length of time in any one place. If you always leave him too long he may feel the need to cry to have you come and move him, which teaches him to cry during playtime.

If, on the other hand, you provide an environment where he trusts you will come and play or come and give him a cuddle or move him, he can happily focus on play and confidently wait for you. This will quickly increase his attention span, mean he's more likely to play for longer without continually trying to engage your attention through crying, and mean he develops positive associations with play.

Tummy time is important so persevere!

Many babies don't like lying on their tummy. Some are so used to being held upright or being in BabyBjörn-style carriers that lying on their tummy feels new. Others associate lying on their tummy with the pain and discomfort of colic or reflux. For others, siblings may have made the environment unpredictable or stressful.

Whatever the case, tummy time for babies is *essential* to encourage them to learn to push up, roll over, sit, crawl and eventually pull themselves up to a stand. Tummy time also gives babies the chance to practise allowing their carers to put them down. If you put your baby down on his tummy or back for floor play you'll be able to establish realistic expectations for settling him on his back at sleep time. It's better to develop this ability during playtime, when you're there to guide him, than at sleep time when he has a lower threshold for coping.

A child is bound to become confused if, having complained about being put down during playtime, his parent picks him up, only to put him down and leave him to cry at sleep time when he's tired and feeling most vulnerable.

Sitting

Sitting up is a complex task for babies, and it can take quite some time for them to master it. Babies occasionally topple over when they first start to sit, which can be frustrating and, in some cases, painful. Most babies develop the ability to sit at between four and seven months. This usually coincides with achieving skills such as holding their head up or rolling over. Even the most seasoned sitters will occasionally topple when they are distracted or preoccupied, but by around seven to eight months, 90 per cent of babies will be able to sit up unaided for an extended period.

To ensure your baby doesn't associate sitting with toppling over and bumping his head, you will need to do the following three things each time you sit him down:

1. Distribute his weight by ensuring the centre of his weight is balanced on a solid base (to do this, take his nappy from behind and give it a firm pull to help him sit on his lower bottom and upper legs rather than further back on his bottom).
2. Ensure the environment is safe if he falls – surround him with pillows and move any objects that might hurt him if he falls.
3. Be considerate of his personal space and ensure siblings have clear boundaries regarding what is and isn't appropriate.

What do they learn?

Transitioning from one play station to the next helps extend babies' attention spans and builds a healthy association with play and independence. It's a vital skill that should be well established by the time they go to school, where the praise and acknowledgement they receive for their self-direction enhances their confidence.

It also teaches children from an early age how to set up their own play. By the age of three, children who successfully transition in play are setting up their own play stations, which establishes their leadership play skills and draws the attention of other children in a positive and healthy way.

Hence, the benefits of setting aside 15 minutes each day to create a fun play environment for your child are astounding – and well worth the trouble.

How long should they play for?

Aim for a total of one hour of independent play for your child with around ten to 15 minutes at each station. So, after he's played for a period of time, go and join him, play for a few minutes, then transition him to the next area. Spend one to two minutes establishing him at the new station then go back to your chores, using your flow of communication. After ten to 15 minutes, move him to the next play station.

Packing away

Design your play stations so they can be set up once a day and then packed away at the end. Packing up each time marks the transition from that part of the day to the next, such as lunch. For the remainder of the day, play can be less formal and deliberate as your child potters happily among his toys or with his family.

Play stations and siblings

If you'd like to establish play stations for an older child as well, similar principles apply, but there are a few things to remember. First, be aware of the example you and your older child are setting for the baby. Your older child cannot constantly demand your attention while you establish a different set of expectations for your baby, which is independent play. Parent both children with the same philosophy.

Set up three play stations for your older child. The first could be a fair distance from your baby's play stations to give the children space. It could be a parenting corner with a dolly or teddy. Children like to copy what you do and your older child can mimic you looking after the baby. The area might have a baby cot (a cardboard box is fine), a high chair (use a small chair) with bowls and spoons, a change table (a foot stool or step) with nappy, empty pots of cream and a couple of singlets.

Another play station can be put up high on the dining table to prevent an overzealous crawler from destroying it accidentally. This could be a basic problem-solving activity such as a puzzle, or a basic construction set, such as Duplo.

The final play station could either be in your older child's room, on the floor at a distance from the baby, or in an adjoining room. Music and movement is a favourite with two year olds plus, so offer a small CD player with their favourite music playing and some instruments like bells, a tambourine and a xylophone.

You could also incorporate a small language area for both children. Reading is a lovely thing for them to do in the same space without the risk of conflict. All you need are some soft pillows, hardback books and a couple of teddies. Request that they sit and use soft voices. Sit with them both and establish a 'no touch the baby' policy until the boundaries are understood and they're both settled and content. Keep an eye on your toddler and always define the statements above.

Any loud or physically active play, like music and dancing, should occur in an area away from the baby, or in the next room so your older child has the freedom to express himself, and your baby isn't disturbed by the hullabaloo. If your baby has been stressed during independent play and you are trying to re-establish trust in playing again, reiterate the 'no touch the baby' boundary. The older child can play with the baby when you're able to supervise but personal space boundaries must be established when you're not there to protect your baby from well-meaning but very fast and overwhelming big brother or sister.

With that in mind, be cautious about how you set your boundaries. Don't ever raise your voice. Politely make your request and, if he does not listen, remove him from the play zone and only let him return when he is willing to listen. If he returns and does not do as you've politely asked, remove him from the play zone again. Each time you remove him, go back and play with your baby. Repeat this until he ceases the undesirable behaviour.

The reasons for not raising your voice are for setting a good example and establishing appropriate communication skills in your house. Also, if you raise your voice, you've lost control of the situation. This makes it difficult for your baby to confidently allow you to guide him as he may see you as unpredictable.

Twins

In my work with multiple-birth children, I've often found one twin is more reliant on the company of his twin for comfort. While this is fine, parents tend to *always* make sure the more reliant twin is close to his sibling, which can cause the independent twin to feel responsible for keeping his sibling happy at playtime. Twins' close physical relationship is almost always fostered, but providing *both* babies with the practice and skills to play on their own is crucial. Strategies such as head-to-toe or feet-to-feet play ensures both your babies' needs are catered for. A typical sequence of play stations for non-mobile twins might be:

- visual connection but playing separately
- feet-to-feet play
- head-to-toe playing beside one another
- head-to-head play (where they are cheek to cheek without actually touching)
- lying beside one another (parallel facing the same direction allowing for smooching and spooning).

Once twins are able to sit, their positioning might be:

- floor play, where they have a visual connection but play separately
- sitting up with feet-to-feet play
- Bumbo seats, where they can reach each other's hands next to one another but facing different directions with their own toys on suspended mobiles on each side
- doughnut play seat, where they can sit next to one another and have full access to one another.

Examples of play stations

In the following pages I've listed age-appropriate play stations designed to provide balanced play experiences for your child for a week. These toys are just suggestions – base your choice of toys on what you have at home or your child's interests.

Each set-up consists of four play stations. Use the same ones for about a week, because repeatedly playing with a toy helps your child master the skills required; the more familiar he is with his toys, the better he'll be at making play enjoyable.

As weekends tend to be busy family times, you probably won't set up the same play stations, unless you're having a quiet one. But it's a good idea to decide on the coming week's play station set-up on Sunday night. The new set-up should be fresh and new for your baby, so get inventive and imaginative.

Play stations for a baby aged six to seven months

If your baby is not yet mobile, set up your play stations so the more difficult or least favourite style of play (usually tummy play), is furthest away from you, and is the first location for play. This ensures you offer the most challenging task when he's at his best, usually after a sleep and a meal, and when he's ready to be down and playing. Gradually, as the morning or play session progresses, move him and change his position, progressing to less physically demanding styles of play based on his position, taking into account his concentration span of five to 15 minutes.

At this early age, targeting specific areas of development is not as easy as it is with slightly older children, as much of the equipment designed for home play offers blended developmental opportunities.

PLAY STATION 1 (FURTHEST FROM PARENT)

Development target: Blended developmental opportunity
Position: Tummy
Duration: 15 minutes (rotating him once to encourage seven to ten minutes at each end of mat)
Toy examples:

- Lamaze My First Mirror placed to one side to encourage him to support the weight of his head and use his upper-body strength to investigate the sight of his own face.
- Fisher-Price Tappy the Turtle to encourage reaching, pushing for a response and problem solving.
- Textured snake or dog by Lamaze to encourage reaching, discovery through exploration of textures and sounds.
- Small water-filled ball with a duck floating on the water to encourage pushing, pulling, reaching.

PLAY STATION 2 (SECOND-FURTHEST FROM PARENT)

Development target: Blended developmental opportunity
Position: Back
Duration: 15 minutes (rotating position of A frame on mat once, encouraging seven to ten minutes at each area of play)
Toy examples:

- Fisher-Price A frame/Lamaze crossover mobile play gym.
- Fisher-Price A frame placed beside the baby so the spinning, fixed side attachments become the baby's main visual focus.
- Activity board propped up safely on opposite side

PLAY STATION 3 (SECOND-CLOSEST TO PARENT)

Development target: Blended developmental opportunity
Position: Seated on Bumbo seat (never place the seat on an elevated, raised or uneven surface, or on other seats or in cars or baths – use only on the floor surrounded with pillows)

Duration: 15 minutes (rotate the position once at ten minutes if necessary)
Toy example: Play gym with hanging activities of varied lengths, sounds and textures.

PLAY STATION 4 (CLOSEST TO PARENT)
Development target: Blended developmental opportunity
Position: Sitting up with pillows behind
Duration: 15 minutes
Toy example: Safety 1st Bouncin' Baby Play Place – the activities fixed to station are adequate. (The beauty of this activity centre is its longevity; when your baby is old enough it turns into a large figure-eight train set and all the fixed items on the activity centre can be pulled off and complement the train set.)

Play stations for a baby aged eight to ten months

Once your baby becomes more competent at sitting, he's likely to become more frustrated when lying on his tummy or back. This is particularly so for babies in busy homes with an older sibling. Despite his ability to sit, it's still important that he develop the skills required to crawl and sit up.

At this age, targeting specific areas of development is becoming easier, but many types of play and equipment designed for home play still offer blended opportunities developmentally. The general idea at this age is to put a little thought into your set-up and not just put out random toys in a pile on their play mat.

PLAY STATION 1 (FURTHEST FROM PARENT)
Development target: Blended developmental opportunity
Position: Back
Duration: 15 minutes (rotating baby once, encouraging seven to ten minutes at each end of mat)
Toy examples:

- Lamaze Chime Garden to encourage reaching, grabbing, spatial awareness, eye–hand co-ordination and problem solving.
- Lamaze textured snake or dog to encourage reaching, discovery through exploration of textures and sound.
- Small water-filled bottles with glitter to encourage pushing, pulling, reaching.
- Interesting shakers or rattles.

PLAY STATION 2 (SECOND-FURTHEST FROM PARENT)
Development target: Blended developmental opportunity focused on problem solving

Position: Sitting up with pillows behind
Duration: 15 minutes (rotating angle after ten minutes but ensure they are facing towards you)
Toy examples:

- Lamaze Multi-Sensory Clutch Cube.
- Fisher-Price activity board or Fisher-Price Brilliant Basics Walker-to-Wagon within reach.

PLAY STATION 3 (SECOND-CLOSEST TO PARENT)

Development target: Blended developmental opportunity
Position: Sitting up with pillows behind
Duration: 15 minutes (rotate the position of the seat once at ten minutes if necessary)
Toy examples:

- Baby play nests and baby play doughnuts and cubes.
- Fisher-Price discovery beads.
- Soft toys with textures to explore and a material book placed in baby's lap and around the sides of the mat to encourage reaching.

PLAY STATION 4 (CLOSEST TO PARENT)

Development target: Physical development
Position: In Jolly Jumper (please follow manufacturer's safety guidelines carefully)
Duration: Ten to 15 minutes
Toy example: Activity provided by the station.

Play stations for a baby aged ten to 12 months

Once your child becomes mobile you may need to invest more time ensuring he finds his environment challenging and stimulating, and to encourage him to play independently rather than walk to you. If he always seeks you out, adjust your communication style to set clear boundaries and expectations around his behaviour during this hour of play. The aim is to turn a challenging task for your baby into a fun, predictable play routine quickly. At this age, targeting specific areas of development is easier with clearly defined types of play and equipment.

PLAY STATION 1 (FURTHEST FROM PARENT)

Development target: Cognitive, problem solving
Position: Sitting upright and able to happily reposition himself
Duration: Self-directed for any duration or parent-guided for ten to 15 minutes

Toy examples:

- Fisher-Price pop, push and slide toy (other manufacturers make this kind of toy; where you push, slide or turn a lever to have any one of four animals pop up).
- Fisher-Price cookie jar shape sorter.
- Lamaze spin 'n' stack rings.
- A simple transfer task (as in from one container to another).

PLAY STATION 2 (SECOND-FURTHEST FROM PARENT)

Development target: Language
Position: Sitting up, crawling
Duration: Self-directed for any duration or parent-guided for ten to 15 minutes
Toy examples:

- Tent with tunnel attached.
- Books made of material.
- Hardback books.
- Soft toys and pillows.

PLAY STATION 3 (SECOND-CLOSEST TO PARENT)

Development target: Gross motor, music
Position: Beside coffee table or on couch for cruisers or floor mat for non-cruisers
Duration: Self-directed or parent-guided for 5–8 minutes plus
Toy examples:

- Crocodile xylophone.
- Shakers, like maracas.
- Bells.
- Tambourine.

PLAY STATION 4 (CLOSEST TO PARENT)

Development target: Blended developmental opportunity
Position: Sitting upright, crawling, repositioning himself
Duration: Self-directed or parent-guided for ten to 15 minutes
Toy examples:

- LeapFrog LeapStart Learning Table: activities fixed to station are adequate.
- Cooking utensils like big spoon and bowls as he comes towards kitchen.

Play stations for a crawling, cruising or walking baby aged 12 to 18 months

You'll still need to set up four play stations for children in this age group, though position is no longer an issue as they're likely to be mobile and able to position themselves by now. As they will be able to access things from a standing and sitting position you can use different surfaces and areas to create a fun area. Chairs, coffee table, couches and floor activity stations will keep them entertained for a long time.

Each play station should target a specific area of development. This helps your child to transition from one activity to another at that particular play station, because the activities develop the same skills.

Target a different area at each station such as cognitive problem solving, social or role play, construction, discovery, music, fine motor skills, gross motor skills, language, and concepts such as colour, shape, size, weight, movement and texture.

Play stations for 18 month olds to two year olds

This is when your foundational work means your child has established great skills and is enjoying exploration and play. These activities are, and should continue to be, both store-bought toy activities and imaginative home-made ones designed to encourage exploration. You've spent time playing with your child and allowing him to govern play, or role playing skills with each activity while you govern play. Creating balanced independent playtime with one-on-one activities, he's starting to be entertained by exploring the world around him and learning from others.

Now is the time to turn your attention to role play in all its forms. While activities and stimulation to develop all areas of development should be encouraged, once children reach this age there's a natural desire to do as they see, which usually means they like to get domestic. They will have areas of interest you can use as cues for activity ideas, and while it's important to offer lots of different experiences for them around play, their interest in focusing on one activity and mastering their skills should not be interfered with.

Each of the play areas remains the same, but start offering more challenging activities and extending his play experiences by combining activities. This will teach him to blend activities and make the most of his play environment.

COGNITIVE/PROBLEM SOLVING

- Coloured pegs with four plastic pots: attach a coloured piece of paper at the base of each pot and start to show him how to sort and categorise the pegs by colour; he can either place the pegs in the pot or attach them to the side.
- A bucket of autumn leaves and some large plastic insects: show him how to find and collect the bugs in a bucket and offer a safe, large

magnifying glass to extend the play, showing him how to use it by using it yourself.

- A long piece of sticky contact taped upside down on the coffee table, sticky side facing up, and lots of different textures, themes and pictures in a container for him to stick on the tape: try coloured circles one day, pictures of healthy foods another day, felt another day, or cellophane. You can name and date his art and put it up at home for him to admire and show to others.

SOCIAL/ROLE PLAY

- Fisher-Price Little People range (particularly the farm).
- Toys'R'Us Just Like Home activity sets such as broom/mop/dustpan set, toy microwave, 120-piece food set, crockery set, shopping trolley, cash register.
- Old wallet with old discount cards or a handbag and simple dress-ups items like hats and shoes.
- A small pram, bath, high chair, capsule, change table with accessories.
- A little kitchen with pots and a small table and chair set.
- Simple homemade clothes line (set up in a corner so he can't walk into it) with pegs, a bucket of bubbles and some clothes. Supervise any water play.

CONSTRUCTION/DESTRUCTION

- Extend block play with toy animals and coloured paper for water or grass.
- Toys'R'Us wooden block puzzle train.
- Large Duplo with cars.
- Fisher-Price Exersaucer.

LANGUAGE

- Add numbers, colours and shapes at a safe size if popped in mouth.
- More complex books.
- Safe cubby house/tent retreat as their quiet language corner: set it up under the dining table or on the couch with a clear boundary of bottoms on seats to keep them safe from toppling off.

Playing in, out and about

Independent playtime in the cot

A key part of any program to achieve long-term sleep repair is cot play. You should teach your child to play independently in his cot for 15 or 20 minutes after he wakes up. If you can't ask him to play in his cot when the room is light and he's fresh after a sleep, you can't possibly ask him to lie quietly while he drifts off to sleep.

By learning how to happily play in his cot a child also learns to sleep there without stress and tears. It's important for even the best sleepers to develop this skill so they can maintain good sleep during illness or holidays – playing in the cot should be a part of every child's waking ritual until they're four or five. It's *never* too late to establish this simple post-sleep routine and the rewards are many.

In fact, playtime in the cot is a lovely time for your child because he's in the one place in the entire house that is his. Don't assume that because you might not enjoy this kind of activity that your baby won't either. Your attitude about cot playtime will fuel his attitude. If you act like he must hate it, he will. If you treat cot playtime as the lovely time it is, then he'll eventually come to enjoy it.

How and why it works

When children experience sleep disruptions they often expect their carer to come in and pick them up to feed them, pat them, hold them or take them out of the room to start the day again. This is especially so if during the day their carer picks them up when they request it (often by crying). So babies may cry at night because they've accidentally learnt this is the way to request they be picked up.

When your child learns to play in his cot he is learning to listen to you. You make a simple request and you govern the outcome of that request. Importantly, your child is practising these vital listening and co-operation skills when he's at his best – after a sleep. This way he doesn't have to learn how to cope with being alone in his cot when he's tired and it's dark.

By teaching him to play in his cot after sleep you establish a routine that becomes so familiar he soon pre-empts this part of the day, giving him the feeling of being in control. This enables him to feel comfortable with the skills needed to go to sleep in his cot and to cope with a request to go back to sleep if he's woken early and needs you to attend and leave again.

Once a child has mastered independent cot play, you'll be able to come and go from the room without causing distress, and he'll begin to develop self-settling skills.

How to encourage independent cot play

By now you will have determined your child's sleep requirement, so when your child wakes up in the morning you will know whether it's

at the specified time, in which case you won't expect
to sleep.

When your child does wake up, listen for him playing happily
ting after the expected sleep time is complete. If he's not chatting a
playing, he might resettle himself if he hasn't had enough sleep.

Leave him for as long as you can, or as close to the maximum sleep time designated for his routine type before you go in. If it becomes clear this isn't going to be possible because he's crying an emotion-based cry, wait your natural ten-minute pause (see page 354) before going in and establishing cot playtime.

It's important not to *rush in* just because he's crying. Instead, try to enter the room with your waking cues during a lull in the crying. Immediately ask him to sit down if he's standing.

Be careful with your body language. Then say, 'I will get you some toys.' Establish playtime by placing the toys in the cot within his reach and then hand him one. A good trick here is to hold the toy so it interrupts eye contact, helping him to focus on the toy rather than you.

It doesn't matter what toys you introduce during cot playtime. The more fun and enjoyable the better. Just be aware of safety issues, so, for example, don't give him toys in the cot he can climb onto.

If you've established playtime in the cot without much drama, casually and confidently use your short-term absence cue: 'I'll be back', before stepping out of the room for a minute or two.

If your baby makes a noise and starts to cry when you go to leave, don't hesitate or turn back, just keep going. To hesitate or turn back will teach him to cry every time you go to leave the room if he'd like you to stay. He'll soon discover he's perfectly okay, and that cot playtime can be a really enjoyable time of the day.

Remember, his cot is the only place in the entire house that is truly his space. So don't be so frightened of the learning process that you deny him the opportunity to discover the joys of playing quietly in his cot. Wait 30 seconds to a minute after you've left the room if he's very upset, then reassess whether you need to go back in or should give them a little more time to calm down.

If he's still crying and you feel he needs some reassurance, step back into the room casually and confidently, saying 'I'm back', and ask him to sit down and either go back to pottering around the room, or sit by the cot and re-establish cot play again. When re-establishing play, always stay confident, as your response to his crying tells him if he's safe or not.

When they're having trouble

If your child is having a really tricky time because you're not picking him up when he demands, you may need to take a more gradual approach.

Sit down next to the cot if he's unsettled. Stay confident, even if you feel unsettled by his cry. Be patient and don't get frustrated. He's little and is learning something new. He will mirror your response, so if you just get on with parallel playing through the cot bars, using happy tones and expressions, he'll eventually be distracted by his toys.

Keep eye contact to a minimum as he can see it as an open invitation to communicate and may boisterously ask you to pick him up. Even after you've clearly answered him with an honest response it's best to make it clear with your simple 'Sit down, wait for Mummy' cue, then look at the toys while *you* play on your own through the bars to try to distract him. Look like you're having fun, whatever his response.

When babies want to be picked up by someone, they often get irritated if the person doesn't appear to understand their request. If you play with a toy yourself after saying, 'Sit down, it's playtime now', it's more likely he'll calm down and be distracted by the toy you're playing with. Remember, you're not demonstrating the toy to him, you're playing with it by yourself. Play with it in a way he would. This could be banging two blocks together while you make a repetitive 'u-u-u' sound. If you play at his level he'll most likely be instantly interested in what you're doing.

Once you have his attention, don't look at him too quickly or ask him to join in. Take it slowly as you stay happy and busy playing. Once he's calmed down and started watching you, casually place the toy in his lap without looking at him, then quickly pick up a new toy and continue playing happily on your own. This way, he's more likely to pick up the first toy and copy your actions. Having established playtime, you are now playing parallel to him, rather than co-operatively. Play by yourself to role play the type of play he should be doing in his cot.

He may get angry and try to stand up holding the cot bars. If so, ask him to sit down. Remember to define your language. Block his hands from reaching the bars and, even if he gets cross, continue on with your play. Make sure you remain enthusiastic and chatty enough to distract him from his mission and catch his eye.

As he becomes more confident about playing in his cot on request, you can gradually pull back your involvement. Over a three-day process:

- stop verbal chatter while you sit next to the cot playing parallel
- start to play on the floor with your toy rather than through the cot bars

- sit side on to the cot and fold washing or read a magazine while he plays
- crawl over to the change table to tidy the bottom shelves.

If you can stand for a while at the change table, even if he has a little cry, just keep busy and allow him to calm down. If he tries to stand, clearly ask him to sit down and wait for Mummy. Your language should be consistent enough by now that he will sit when you ask him. If he doesn't sit down, tap his hand with one finger while repeating your sit down cue. If he still won't let go, release his hands from the cot bars by sliding your thumb under his palm. Thank him for sitting, even if he's cross at you, offer him some toys by having a little tinker with one momentarily, then go back to the change table, even if he's having a little cry.

Now begin to move around the room without talking to him, even if he's crying. Sing quietly to yourself so you appear confident, to encourage him to feel okay about not being able to control your actions. This is setting appropriate feedback to your baby about his natural emotions and feelings and telling him which ones are fine and which ones need extra reassurance or intervention to resolve.

Be realistic about what you are asking him to do – you're not asking too much of him. If he's in a loving, safe home, this simple request, if done in a respectful and consistent manner, is absolutely within reason and worth working through.

Once you can move around the room, start to come and go from the room for one- to two-minute intervals using your short-term absence cue, 'I'll be back'. Increase your absence time gradually. Remember to not run back in when he cries. If he stands as you leave, pretend you don't see. This way the only response he gets from standing is you leaving the room, which will discourage him.

When you re-enter the room, don't make it seem like you're saving him from playing in his cot, even if he's upset that you aren't picking him up. Instead, walk in with a smile and tell him 'I'm back' in a happy tone. Avoid using a sympathetic or apologetic tone or you deliver the wrong message about cot play and what *you* think of it. Simply and confidently ask him to sit down if he's standing and sit to parallel play through the bars or go back to the change table and keep yourself busy. Don't enter into too much conversation with him unless he's very settled and happy to play. If you try to chat while he's still making demands, he's likely to ask you to pick him up.

Finally, if he's playing happily in his cot, chatter and interact intermittently, remembering this is still meant to be an independent time, but you can go over and join in playing from time to time, and go and get extra toys from another room. A good strategy to get a slightly older baby more enthusiastic about you leaving the room for short periods is to identify a few small toys he really enjoys at non-sleep time. Offer to get the toys, with clear language cues such as a confident 'Mummy go get it! I'll be back' and head out of the room to return with the toys.

When and how often should baby play in the cot?

If you're maintaining good sleep patterns once you have repaired sleep, the main aim is to govern your baby at the completion of sleep time. So if you can offer one cot playtime a day of between ten and 20 minutes and he's content to play, and content to let you leave the room, then it isn't necessary to do it at every sleep. If, on the other hand, he gets upset when you try to govern the outcome of sleep, maintain cot play as often as you can until he's happy to play for you again.

If you're in full recovery mode stick to the recommended times for your new routine. If your baby has woken early and you're not going to attempt to resettle him, it's important he has a longer cot play. If he's woken and is playing happily in his cot for a good period before you have to go in to him, he can easily have a short cot play for a couple of minutes if you're in a rush. Regardless of how well he woke and played independently, have a little cot play after you've entered the room so he has realistic expectations for the middle of the night should the need to resettle arise.

Packing away after cot playtime

When you've decided it's time to pack away, you need to create a predictable routine that your baby can recognise as the transition that always precedes getting out of bed. This is vital for several reasons:

- You govern the end of sleep time, which prevents him from becoming confused during the night.
- He feels in control of the situation because he's able to predict your behaviour.
- He can predict the end of sleep effectively, so at no point during the night does he expect to get up until this process is completed.
- You can practise listening and communication skills.

Who decides when it's time?

The decision to pack away should be yours. To hand the control of this time to your baby tells him that you are waiting for him to cry before you start packing away. This will cause him to become upset when you do not respond to his requests at other cot management times. That said, if you can see that your baby is playing happily, you can decide to end cot play whenever you choose.

The routine

The pack-away routine should follow a predictable pattern. First, perhaps, your baby might hand you the toys so you can pop them away in the same place. Then fold up any wraps or loose sheets and pop them at the end of the bed. Finally, put any extra accessories such as a dummy in their usual place ready for the next sleep.

When you're first establishing a cot playtime routine, be patient if your child cries when you start to pack away. He needs to learn to wait, and you need to stay calm and confident as you follow through on your plan to establish a predictable packing-away routine. Don't move faster than you would if he were cooing happily; you need to teach him not to get cross or cry at you to pick him up sooner.

Getting him up may seem an easy task, but take care not to confuse your baby. This is a time when you should play your wait game, as at all times when completing a parent-governed task. Once the wait game is complete, pick him up using the up cue with a big smile and fun snuggle and carry on with your day.

While you're establishing cot play it's probably best that, if possible, the same parent attend during cot time, including settling, resettling, waking and playtime. If this is not possible, you both need to be on the same page, using the same clear language cues and other strategies.

If your baby is happy for your partner to say hello, have a little play, then use the short-term absence cue before leaving, you can both be part of cot playtime.

Sitting in the high chair, pram and shopping trolley are all opportunities for your child to learn the skill of waiting patiently. The skill of waiting and being patient, of calmly looking to only the environment for entertainment, helps your child learn how to relax and be comfortable in his own skin. It's a skill that's vital if your child is to lie in his cot waiting to drift off to sleep. Therefore, it's important to develop it by confidently using your wait game and gradually improving his attention span through the use of your bag of tricks (see page 118).

Playing in the high chair at home

It's worth taking the time to encourage your child to have an extended quiet sit and play in his high chair at least once a day. For some children this is easy, but for others some encouragement is necessary to help him relax and enjoy this time of the day. High chair play offers your child the opportunity to practise these skills in the non-confrontational environment of your home with you guiding them.

Parents often tell me their child doesn't like solids and will only eat two spoons of food after much fussing and soon after their attention span wanes and they demand to get down. This results in a hungry, grumpy baby who within 30 minutes is snacking on breast milk instead of developing an appetite for his next nutritionally balanced solid-food meal. The problem does not lie with the food or the child's ability to eat but his need to be guided to sit patiently in his high chair.

A balanced eating plan for babies and toddlers is essential for optimum health, a good night's sleep and a happy demeanour. It's also just as important to develop an ability to comfortably look to their carers for guidance around this area. Once again, make decisions based on your child's true needs, not what he demands or *thinks* he needs. If you know your baby needs to sit longer in the high chair so he'll eat more effectively but he's unable to because he's become too demanding at this time, you will need to help him learn to sit patiently in the chair.

By learning to play independently in the high chair your child also learns to sit patiently and trust you to guide him. High chair skills are also important to develop if you wish to maintain the quality of your family life, and go out to restaurants or visit friends or enjoy outings to shops that coincide with a meal time.

The foundation for healthy eating should start at six months. It's harder to start a healthy eating plan when your child is three years old because he'll already have developed poor habits. If you start healthy behavioural patterns around eating from six months of age, your child will learn to eat the right foods and behave in the right way. You will be free to enjoy the social occasions that occur at meals by the time he is three. As a parent, it's your duty to ensure you identify the things that may be impacting on your baby's ability to have a good meal, and the inability to sit at the table for long enough is definitely one of the most common problems around meal time. The second most common problem is snacking. Once poor eating patterns have begun, usually due to the inability to sit for too long or excessive or inappropriate snacking, you may find that meal times for your baby become tied up with poor associations and almost always with rejection of food, which you will need to repair.

To restore the balance around this daily event look closely at developing refined communication with clear boundaries around positioning:

'Sit down, wait for Mummy/Daddy.' Remember to define that statement. Don't teach him that 'sit down, wait for Mummy' means arch your back or hang off the side of the high chair, or pull your legs up and get your arms out of your buckles. 'Sit down and wait' needs to mean 'Sit and focus on play', and *not* 'Try to get up from sitting and have a tantie.'

The most appropriate time for high chair playtime is after dinner. The last solid meal of the day gives children a final little energy boost which they can expend on a little play in the high chair while their food settles.

Once your child has finished eating, check he's still comfortable, his buckles are still done up and he's sitting forward with his feet facing the front. If he can't reach the tray because he's too little, pop a towel under his bottom before you buckle him in at the beginning of the meal, or a soft towel behind his back so he can sit forward comfortably.

If he's older and tries to shuffle around in his seat or arch his back, calmly and patiently reposition him using your clear and friendly cue, 'Sit down and wait for Mummy'. Define the statement by showing him how you'd like him to sit. Stay enthusiastic and confident, even if he's being a little stroppy with you.

Bring out a toy that you know is a favourite and establish playtime. Ensure you offer toys for which you've already helped him develop personal play strategies through role play at one-on-one play during the day and lovely associations so he's really interested in what you're offering him. If he's still resisting, start playing with a toy beside him. Stay confident and make the play look exciting without it looking like you want him to play. Follow your parallel play strategies until he is playing.

Now you have two choices depending on your baby's reaction to being kept in the high chair. If he starts playing happily in the high chair, stand up and take his high chair over to the sink, where you will be tidying away after his meal or beginning to prepare your food for the evening meal with your partner. Chat away happily to him, talk about his toys and play, about the day you've had together and about what you're doing. As he gets more involved in his play, you can talk less.

If he's cross because you haven't picked him up, stay where you are and help him move past this feeling. It is common for a baby to resist high chair play initially. If, however, you identify this as too hard for your baby it's worth investing some time to help him feel okay with your loving guidance. It's a basic requirement for a balanced, respectful style of family communication. If he refuses the toy by pushing it away, or by taking it off you and throwing it, acknowledge what he's said: 'Okay, Charlie doesn't want that toy.' If he's still refusing to play after five minutes of trying to establish playtime in the high chair, you can decide it's time to carry on with your chores and bring his high chair into the kitchen anyway and carry on and he can sit and wait for a little while watching you. If he's still cross at you when you do this, follow the 'Still having trouble?' instructions below, only put more emphasis on happy singing to yourself and looking busy. The more enthusiastic you sound and preoccupied you appear, the more likely he will become distracted.

About ten to 15 minutes of high chair play after a meal is reasonable for six to nine month olds and can gradually be increased to about 20 minutes by the time they are 12 months old. Once high chair play is finished, the wait game can be used before getting them up for a bit of a rough-and-tumble, extra-fun, energy-burning playtime before evening bath.

Still having trouble?

When helping families suffering with sleep and daytime blues I find that if the babies haven't mastered playing in a high chair within a few minutes and persist with crying, the mums and dads always say 'Now what? Should we get him up?'

It's really important to be conscious of the time it takes a baby to learn something new. The first time this is done it may be unfamiliar to him, and he will need to get used to not getting out of his chair the moment he's finished eating like he's used to. That takes time. You're changing his old self-instigated routine into a parent-guided positive routine and, like anything new, it may involve a few tears, but they are temporary. Babies usually learn a new routine in a day and settle in like it's been around forever when you're consistent and remain confident. This means, don't teach him to cry to get out of his high chair. Play with him and establish play until he's calm, then get him up using your wait game.

The most important thing to do now is be patient, persist, and practise. Continue to encourage play. It doesn't happen immediately for all babies so if he is showing signs of getting cross because you haven't picked him up, be patient, and remain confident and reassuring until he finds the predictability in this expectation and starts to settle down. It may take a couple of days. Remember not to teach him to cry to be picked up.

Don't feel bad for asking him to have a play in his high chair. It's not mean or unfair, it's just a normal life skill and request. It's also the same thing you'll need to be able to say when he wakes at 2 a.m., having no concept of time, and he asks to get up for the day. You will need to have established times of the day where you say, 'Not now bubby, Mummy/Daddy will tell you when it's time to get up', and he needs to understand that, know how to cope with it and know what to do. If the first time you ask your child to accept that request is when he's in the cot at night, then sleep-time stress is guaranteed, which is what we are working to avoid through this playtime in the high chair strategy.

Stick to the recommended timeframe of your daily routine and, if necessary, spend more time sitting with him playing than trying to move away to do your chores. By the time the play session is finished, always complete the task by packing away and using your wait game to create predictability. This ensures he doesn't learn that he needs to cry to get up, and helps him trust that he can relax and you will always let him know when playtime is over. It also gives you the opportunity to govern the end of the event in a non-confrontational way. This makes you predictable and makes the routine of high chair play consistent and comforting for him.

If your baby is under ten months, and starts a high-pitched scream between pauses and it doesn't sound like the usual happy squeals you hear, you can be sure he's yelling at you. Make sure there is nothing wrong, that he is comfortable and hasn't done a poo in his nappy, then carry on with your initial request for playtime. If the screeching persists, ignore it. Don't give him attention at this time or you will teach him to scream to get your attention, and that would be awful for him and unpleasant for you.

Chat and sing to encourage busy playing, but stop singing and chatting briefly to indicate you won't continue if he screams. Once the behaviour subsides, chat and sing again. Persist patiently with this until the pattern stops. This may take one to two play sessions, and the patience (and perhaps ear muffs) that were required to establish a more pleasant style of communication will be well worth it.

If your baby is ten months or over, it might be that you have a serious bossy boots on your hands (and they do get very bossy sometimes), so you'll need to implement a new cue, 'Too loud for Mummy's ears'. Once you've said this, either turn his high chair around so it's facing away from you, making sure he can no longer see you even when he looks around or turns away. Cease verbal interaction for about a minute as well. If you show him that the opposite of what he expected happens when he screams, he will quickly discover that your attention comes when he's interacting with you through chatter and happy sounds, not the other way around. After a minute has passed, turn him back towards you and greet him happily again and offer him an 'illegal toy' (something that is not one of his toys), perhaps something great off the bench like the whisk, measuring cups, or a broken TV remote control or mobile phone, then carry on.

The Daddy factor

It can be disruptive to a new routine when Daddy, or any member of the family, arrives home mid play. It's important to encourage a baby to play in his high chair for his daddy. If every time Daddy walks in the room, even on a day when he stays home, your baby insists on being picked up by him, a routine pattern is being set up where your baby thinks it is normal to always be picked up immediately by his daddy. That one expectation can be very confusing during any attempts to resettle him back to sleep at night if he's woken, so aim to create a balanced and honest set of conditions for him through the day.

Start to change the way Daddy (and other members of the family) responds to your baby when he enters the room during the day, for example, when the child is playing on the floor. Sometimes Daddy might use the up cue and get him up, sometimes he might sit down to play only, and sometimes he may just chat to the baby and then carry on with chores. It's important that he chooses his response before entering the room and then follows through so he doesn't fall into the trap of changing his mind every time baby cries when Daddy tries to pursue any method other than picking him up on demand, which just teaches him to cry to be picked up. Once a blended style of requests is established during floor play and your baby has learnt to wait for the cues as to what Daddy will be doing that play session, you can use the same style of blended requests at high chair playtime.

Once your baby is better at playing, you can use your pre-emptive language to tell him Daddy will be home soon, and he needs to 'Sit down and wait for Daddy'. That means when Daddy comes in, he can come and sit and play before following the pack away, wait game and up cue routine. Eventually Daddy will be able to enter the room after your baby has been given some simple pre-emptive language and your child will smile and babble away happily but continue to play until everyone is ready for the next part of the day. This takes the burden off the baby, and helps the house flow more peacefully.

Playing in the high chair at a restaurant

Obviously, establishing a good pattern of expectation in the high chair needs to be worked on at home first. Once you've achieved this you will be ready to go to a restaurant. If your baby is too little to sit in a high chair, which is rarely the case by six months, it may be more difficult to encourage a long play in his pram. This is simply because he cannot see you as well when he's down in his pram and may become frustrated quickly with that arrangement. By six months of age however, a high chair (slightly reclined until seven months and upright thereafter) is generally a perfect location to encourage a fairly decent playtime in a restaurant.

There is generally a flow to the way your time in a restaurant unfolds. Here it is along with some hints to make the most of your time so everyone is happy:

- Don't forget your playtime bag of tricks (see page 118).
- Try to choose a restaurant that isn't overcrowded.
- Try to pick a time that lines up with one of your baby's meal times.
- Make sure he gets a high chair to sit in or you won't be able to get a long enough playtime out of him to get through a whole meal.
- Once you arrive at the restaurant make sure you start using your clear language cues like, 'Sit down, wait for Mummy'.
- When you first sit your baby in the high chair, just let him sit there with nothing so he has a chance to take in the sights and sounds of the restaurant.
- Get the menu immediately and order fairly efficiently. Longer, more relaxed meals come as a privilege over time, once your little one has developed good associations with fun, fast restaurant experiences.
- Ask the staff to heat up your baby's food, if it's not already warm, and while you wait for your meal to be served give your baby his dinner.
- After your baby has eaten, your food will probably be served, so give him the spoon to play with and sit back and relax and enjoy your meal.
- If your baby is eight months plus he'll be interested in what you're eating and you can safely pull out a Cruskit or, if he's older, choose something appropriate for his age off your plate and allow him to have a munch. By now he will have food, a spoon, and possibly a small lid from your baby-food container to keep him entertained as you all chat together and to him.
- Don't leave him out of the conversation; babies enjoy the social interaction of a chat at a restaurant as much as you do.
- Once you see him starting to tire of the eating concept pull out your bag of tricks (see page 118) to extend his concentration span for a little longer. Gradually work through your bag of tricks while you wait for your dessert.
- When all the tricks in your bag have been used up, offer him some of the interesting and unique things from the table: a menu, napkin, etc. This is when you know his time in the high chair is fast drawing to a close. Once he grows tired of these objects, it will be the final

stretch of your time in the restaurant. This is generally the time your dessert or a final drink has arrived and when most babies come out of the high chair (after a quick pack away, wait game and up cue). He can now sit on your lap until it's time to leave.

- If you choose, you can set a boundary so that your baby *never* gets out of the high chair for the first five visits to a restaurant, which often sets a tone for happy extended playing from then on, but it depends on how long you like to be there. Just be certain never to get him up because he's having a tantrum or he *will* have a tantrum every time he goes to a restaurant.

Pram play

For a baby, going for a walk in his pram, with the sun shining and birds floating above his head, is one of the most delightful parts of going on an adventure with his mum and dad. But the opportunity for a baby to relax and just lie back is slowly becoming a lost joy. A by-product of some modern parenting strategies is that children are burdened with guiding their parents and as a result lots of babies struggle with feeling comfortable when someone is pushing them around for a relaxing stroll. It's a lovely time of their day, though, and you need to establish it or re-establish it to ensure your baby's delight in interesting adventures.

It's important to establish playtime in the pram for two main reasons. Firstly, it's nice for them to be able to have a relaxing outing to the shops without stress or the need to be carried everywhere. Secondly, it's another opportunity for you to practise your sleep-time communication skills with him at a non-confrontational time of the day.

I generally suggest mornings be reserved for physically demanding home independent playtimes, with afternoons the best opportunity to provide a lovely wander in the pram. The reason for this is fairly simple. Your baby will be asleep at 7 p.m., and won't wake until 6 or 7 a.m., then he'll want a snuggle and breastfeed or to have breakfast in his high chair, then another sleep. Can you imagine how frustrating it would be after being physically inactive for 14 to 16 hours to be asked to sit patiently in a pram while you do the shopping in the morning? After a long day of playing and growing and learning, the afternoon can become quite difficult for him from around 4 p.m. onwards, so this is an ideal opportunity for him to put up his feet and happily watch the world go by as his energy levels drop off and his tolerance for playing and co-operating starts to diminish.

This doesn't mean you won't have to work through some old patterns of behaviour that occur at pram times. Many babies settle into pram time immediately when the routine and communication skills are adjusted and they no longer have to guide their parents; however, while we are targeting the best possible time for pram play, there is always a possibility that some negative routine may already have been established. Because babies are creatures of habit, they will continue to exhibit their usual pattern of behaviour because it's all they know to do.

Use your pre-emptive language, so your baby knows he's about to have a wander in his pram with you. Ensure you've implemented and practised your 'Wait for Mummy/Daddy' cue at home so he'll be able to look to you for guidance with ease from the moment you pop him into the pram. Be cautious about a few basic things:

- Make sure he's comfortable: don't overdress him with bulky items that make it difficult to sit or move freely and equally don't leave him feeling so exposed and loose that he arches his back and slides around hoping someone will pick him up so he can feel more secure.
- Sit him upright, and make sure his buckles are done up firmly so shoulder straps don't rub his cheeks or slide off his arms. If he still needs a little help sitting, have the pram slightly reclined, but by nine to ten months of age all babies respond positively to a clear message when you sit them upright.
- Turn him so he can see the world. While it's lovely for us to watch our babies, it can be a whole lot more interesting for him if he has more to look at and is not travelling backwards.
- Do not start your pram journey with all his toys already in his lap because by the time his attention span has reached its limit, you'll have already used up all your distractions. You are looking at providing a graded exposure to stimulation and distraction as you progress through your trip to the shops, so take your bag of tricks (see below) and only use it once he's had a lovely long wander admiring the view first.

It's lovely to just allow your baby to sit without toys as he settles into his pram and takes in the world around him. If he makes the odd complaint, carry on with your journey without intervening. If an older baby of ten to 12 months is turning in his chair and this results in him crying while he reaches up to you for attention, help him turn around and sit facing the front and ensure his buckles are firm enough to prevent this pattern. As you travel, take the time to stop and point out balloons, signs, and other babies in prams. By taking his focus off demanding you pick him up, to looking at the many things of great interest around him, babies will often suddenly discover how interesting the shops or a walk in the park can be.

Once you can see he's finding the chore of sitting for a prolonged period a little difficult, dip into your bag of tricks. Always ensure you have a selection of toys that ranges from some interesting ones, some favourite ones, and some 'illegal toys', like an out-of-use (but safe to play with) mobile phone, or a broken remote control. Slowly introduce the toys, ensuring you save the best toys for last.

This expectation that a child can play happily in his pram is totally fair, even for babies as young as six months. Children can develop this skill in a matter of days, going from squirming, grumpy, crying little babies with their arms outstretched trying to be picked up, to relaxed, content, happy little people busily pointing to all the interesting things around them and, as the pram session continues, they focus on playing happily with one of their bag-of-tricks toys.

Still having trouble?

For parents on full recovery, an unsettled baby in the pram is a common problem. The following strategy will help establish a more positive association in a baby towards his pram and extend his patience when on an outing. If your baby is still finding this time a *real* challenge, it's time to go into slow motion. Graded exposure will ensure he can learn that these journeys can be short and achievable and will start to help him change his expectations of this time from negative to positive.

Start off with brief periods in the pram in your local neighbourhood. About 30 minutes before you head off get excited about going for a walk in the pram. Use pre-emptive language to set the tone of your journey. If you're nervous, your baby will be nervous. When heading out it's important to follow through and define your original request to 'Sit down and wait for Mummy'. Be sure to keep your baby focused on what's ahead, like looking for a cat or a bird. Your baby will have encountered cats or birds by six months of age, and you will have taught him the sound they make, so when you say 'Where's the bird gone, tweet tweet?' you will catch his attention and have the opportunity to keep him calm. Continue to talk about everything you see around you, sounding happy and enthusiastic. This will distract your baby and he will start to calm immediately.

As you are rounding the corner to go home, say, 'Nearly home, nearly time for up up.' This cue will become familiar and serve as an instant settler for an impatient bubba. Complete pram time by using your wait game.

Crying when you stop the pram

Good communication is vital to ensure you're able to have a lovely trip in the pram and the occasional stops don't open the floodgates of baby fury. Introduce some of the new language streams you've practised. Always keep your baby informed. So before you go on a shopping trip where you may be stuck in a typical queue for up to five minutes, you'll have already started to play the wait game.

When you walk around your neighbourhood introduce a new cue: 'Stopping. Wait for Mummy'. When you say this pause the pram briefly, and when he stops demanding you move on, say, 'Off we go'. If he starts to cry and protest when you stop briefly, use your wait game and see if he will settle, then resume your walk. If he gets very cross at you, go around to the front of the pram, get down on his level and ask him to wait. Try to distract him by pointing to some of the interesting things in the environment. When he stops fussing or crying say, 'Good waiting, bubba. Off we go' and head on your way quickly before he starts to cry again.

Repeat the strategies above, extending the length of your pause as your baby gets better at this game. Remember it's a game, so create a fun feeling about stopping and waiting so your baby is more likely to smile and wait in anticipation of a fun take-off rather than complain about the fact you've stopped.

Prams in a large shopping centre

Occasionally, a baby or toddler may find busy environments like a big shopping centre much more stressful than a pram trip to shops up the road. The reasons for this may be varied, but bear a couple of things in mind. Don't generalise all unsettled pram behaviour into the category of stress. If he always battles with you about the pram, which he should be able to happily ride in until the age of two and a half, then his behaviour should be managed as mentioned in the above section of pram play. If, however, you find he is behaving in an unusual way in a large shopping centre environment, take some steps to try and reduce stress.

I often find that providing a visual or physical security helps babies feel less exposed and vulnerable in a large crowd and calms them down almost immediately. Something as simple as a blanket or muslin over their knees and tummy or around their shoulders can be comforting for babies. Attaching your baby to a comfort item like a teddy bear can be a great way to help him cope with the sensation of being vulnerable in a shopping centre. Alternatively, if you have a pram that reverses direction, it may be helpful to turn him around to face you. Usually, facing the wrong way in the pram can cause tears and boredom but for a child showing signs of stress in a crowded environment, this may be helpful for a short period until this passes.

These episodes are generally rare and short lived, but it's important to remember that you're working to move your child past these kinds of concerns. Don't stamp your child with a tag like 'He doesn't like crowds', or no longer expose him to that environment. Just reduce the stress of the situation until he becomes a little more comfortable within that environment.

Shopping trolley play

Just like enjoyable pram play, getting a child to sit patiently in a shopping trolley can be challenging. For all the same reasons that pram play is important, it's good to encourage your child to experience and adjust to sitting in the shopping trolley when you ask him to. While a well-timed routine with consistent communication is generally enough to settle a baby down during a shopping trip, occasionally you may need to go that extra mile to ensure a successful and happy outing.

As discussed in the pram play strategy, you need to select your times for going supermarket shopping carefully. Afternoons are always best for outings as quiet sitting in the morning is a challenge for a baby who has been asleep all night. Even if your baby is sleeping poorly at night, allowing him to be inactive all morning by being in a pram or shopping trolley to compensate for that poor night's sleep will either create or perpetuate cycles of poor sleep and early waking. Why would he ever need to change the poor pattern of sleep at night or early waking cycles at 4 to 5 a.m. when he gets to sit all morning in a pram? So make the mornings physically active and the afternoons the time for pram and shopping trolley play.

This time can be fun, and is a wonderfully rich communication opportunity. Even though you are busy and trying to get your shopping done quickly, it's a great time to involve your child. Talk about the things you're buying, point out pictures and colours on labels, give him special things to hold, and stay happy.

Before you set out make sure the trolley is comfortable and predictable for your baby. A Clean Shopper (www.cleanshopper.com.au) is a good idea to soften the hard edges of the trolley, keep germs at bay and help stop small toys or drinking cups from slipping down through the bars, creating frustration for your baby. Watch for positioning problems that may create frustration for your baby and keep him sitting forward with buckles firmly fastened.

I often see babies tell their mother they want to be picked up by raising their arms. Instead of answering the baby, the mother launches into a frantic race to finish her shopping before the baby loses the plot. The better way to handle this effectively is to make sure you're not dawdling, so be organised before you leave home. Have a list, and watch the time. Then it's important to show your baby you've heard his request to be picked up and intend to answer him. Your answer should be either a clear 'yes' or 'no'. When you embark on a supermarket trip, it's not a good idea to establish a boundary of being picked up unless you're happy to do it every time you go to the shops. It's not okay to say one week, 'Sure I'll pick you up', and then get frustrated when he demands it every time. This is being unpredictable and inconsistent and creates a clingy baby and tears. It's best to establish a predictable rule that while you're in the supermarket, he doesn't get picked up.

When he asks you to pick him up, take his hands and lower them to his lap and say in a loving way, 'Not time for up up now, hands down, wait for Mummy.' You will have been practising this wait game and routine at home, so it's time to implement the positioning request at playtime. Define your statement. 'Sit down, wait for Mummy' doesn't mean 'Ask to be picked up'. Place your baby's arms down on his lap and say, 'Hands down, wait for Mummy', reach for your bag of tricks and ask in an excited tone, 'Oh, where's your lion gone? Rroooaaar.' This will give you ample opportunity to distract him, say you've heard him but you can't oblige his request right now, and show him an alternative for when he feels like this in the future.

If it keeps happening, remain calm and consistent and repeat yourself until he understands that 'Sit down, wait for Mummy' doesn't mean 'If you cry long enough, I'll get you up'. Be careful not to teach your baby to cry for a long time before he gets up. Once you've made your request to wait, follow through and complete your shopping trip with the same expectation in play. If you feel on the brink of giving in, it's better to finish up your shop early, pay and leave, then pick him up outside. This ensures you don't teach him to cry loud and strong for you to pick him up. Within one to two shopping trips, your baby will happily accept the predictable conditions of the trolley and your shopping blues will be a thing of the past.

Nudie playtime

Nudie playtime is an important part of a baby's day for a number of reasons. As the day draws to a close, a child's body is depleted of fuel and energy as sleep and food sources dwindle after the demands of a long day on a growing body. Because of this the final meal of the day, dinner, provides a sudden glucose high that promotes a naturally elevated mood. For years parents have been told to keep children calm for the last portion of the day. Though this is partly true, fighting their bodies' natural urge to use up the fuel just consumed creates one of two problems:

1. The baby will be difficult to manage, often appearing grumpy, and it's difficult to calm him down and keep him quiet, so it's easy to blame a spouse coming home from work for overexciting him.
2. It may promote night wakings because when food is consumed it converts to glucose, which is energy.

The fuel from dinner is only needed to sustain babies until it's time for a full night's sleep, so it's good to burn off the excess with a quick play before a bath. If your child's natural energy levels remain low after a meal, it's important to try and pull on any fuel reserves he has in his body to give him a final burst of energy to make the last hour of the day enjoyable for him.

Change the tone at the end of the day

Often full-time working mums or dads miss out on having fun with their babies if they're encouraged to be very quiet when they come home – the 'hush hush' zone. However, if a parent makes it home in time, nudie playtime can be a very enjoyable one-on-one time of the day, and a great way to end a day positively. It gives working parents a chance to enjoy interacting with an excited, giggly baby who's just eaten.

In addition, by promoting rough-and-tumble play, your child becomes more confident with his gross motor skills, develops spatial awareness, boldness, strength, and a love of high-output exercise.

Protection from predators

By promoting an open nudie playtime, where children have fun and feel confident in their own space, you set healthy body boundaries that enable a child to learn from an early age what is and isn't normal physical contact. Because children are creatures of habit, a change to any kind of interaction at nudie time will evoke a strong response and an initial resistance. This acts as a deterrent, making up one part of your child protection plan.

Sadly, we live in a world where innocent children can be the victims of predators. During nudie playtime it's worth instilling two simple language cues as soon as children can use the words 'stop' and 'no' by playing games that allow them to use these words. Empower children with ultimate control over their body with 'no' then 'go', or 'stop' then 'go' games. Predators are notoriously cowards, preying on children they deem as helpless. If a child says 'No' or 'Stop', an adult predator would perceive him as having a concept of right and wrong, which is likely to make them stop out of fear the child may tell. Also, by making it a normal response that you stop when they request it, it is more likely that children will accidentally say, 'Uncle didn't stop', even if they've been told not to tell anyone. This two-step plan, hand in hand with parental vigilance, offers great protection for children.

Instil an expectation around your baby's body even before he can talk. As you blow on his tummy, or tickle him, end with a clear 'Stop Mummy' and raise your hands next to your head. Once you roll him over to Daddy he can have a tickle and roll him around and then say 'No' before raising his hands, then passing baby back to Mummy again. As he reaches the age where he can use single words, you can say, 'Mummy is going to tickle your tummy. Say "stop" when you want me to stop.' Be careful to allow them the opportunity to say 'no' or 'stop' if they are laughing by not relentlessly tickling them. So always pause in any tickle game to allow him time to catch his breath and move away if he wants, or if you can see he's trying to stop you. Encourage the words with the cue 'Say stop/no'. The moment he says it, raise your hand off him and say 'Mummy/Daddy stop'. If he wants to continue, encourage him to say 'go'. A child who cannot say 'go' will come and lie in front of you ready for more tickles, and this is your cue to use the word 'go'.

Always respect the words 'stop' and 'no' the first time your child says them. Do not make them repeat it. Even if he says 'no' as soon as you go to start again, it must be respected. You can play this game in reverse with older toddlers too. Daddy and toddler can tickle Mummy until she says 'stop' or 'no', then everyone stops. It's a simple game that leaves your children empowered with control of their body.

Confidence building around gross motor skills

By providing an active nudie playtime you promote jumping, rolling and climbing, increasing your child's confidence in his body and movements. Every day should have a silly time, when the only intention is to have fun and he has your undivided attention. Having this at the end of the day means everyone looks forward to it because it involves laughter, togetherness and a final closeness before bed for the night. It ensures the day ends on a great note, and your baby is ready for a relaxing bath, feed and kiss before getting tucked into bed pooped after such a fun day.

Teaching them when to stop

During nudie playtime toddlers, in particular, can get very excited. This is when they don't know how to express themselves and may become rough in a way that we would deem as aggressive, like hitting, biting or pinching. It's the same sense of joy and excitement that comes when they are playing with their little friends or you pick them up to have a fun play and they whack you, or bite their friend lovingly on the cheek. Nudie playtime gives *you* a chance to say 'stop' when things go too far so your baby learns what are and are not good expressions of excitement.

Practise the 'lie down' game and cues

The secret to teaching toddlers to sleep often comes down to their ability to lie down. While some other sleep strategies involve lying children down a hundred times or more while they cry for hours in their cot, it's better to teach them what the term 'lie down' means. Playing the 'lie down' game creates a positive association around lying down, and enables children to accept this request at sleep time without stress. Simply play on the bed, then say 'lie down' and everyone must lie down. They must stay lying with you until you say 'up time!'

Playing in the car seat

Promoting playtime in the car can be difficult. Unfortunately, when children aren't big enough for their chair to be safely turned to face the front of the car, some find the process of going backwards in a car extremely uncomfortable, so a long drive can have lingering effects. Once an appropriate routine is established, where children are sleeping well and a balance of communication is part of their lives, it becomes much easier to tackle this area.

While your child is very young and has to travel backwards, ensure any long trips are around his usual sleep times. Make sure some toys are attached to his seat, and he's well hydrated before you leave. Keep your bag of tricks next to you on the car seat so you can access it at traffic lights.

Once your child is able to face forwards, you will see an immediate turn around in his ability to cope with a longer car trip. Regardless of the direction his car seat is facing, graded exposure to toys is your best option to extend his attention span and ability to cope for longer periods in his car seat.

When you set out on your journey, start with no toys at all. This will give your baby the chance to take in his surroundings. Only allow him to fall asleep if it is within your routine. Allowing him to sleep whenever he likes during the car trip will make him more tired because it will disrupt his ability to sleep at the next designated sleep time, which will cause unhappiness. A misplaced nap, even as brief as five minutes, in a baby with a low sleep requirement can take up to two hours off his sleep in a 24-hour period. This means your poor tired baby cannot, no matter how much his body wants him to, fall asleep or, worse, stay asleep longer than 20 to 30 minutes because his power nap has taken away his ability to do so.

If he's not at a designated sleep time when you need to travel in your car, don't dress him too warmly or it will make him sleepy. Also ensure he's not wearing bulky, irritating items of clothing that restrict him. This is a common cause of tears on a car trip because every time he turns his head he gets a fluffy collar in his mouth.

The general flow of a car trip should involve gradually exposure to his toys. But remember: safety first. Too many mothers reach or look back and take their attention off the road while driving. As most new mums are always tired, this is a recipe for disaster. It's better to let your baby cry and stay focused on the road than risk an accident. Mirrors are available so you can see your baby, even if he's facing backwards, without turning around while you're driving, so consider buying one.

Unfortunately for some babies, long car trips just don't agree with them and parents have to plan their travel carefully. Many children suffer terribly from travel sickness. If your child throws up a lot during or after a long car trip, talk to your doctor about using something to help settle his tummy so he doesn't have to feel so uncomfortable. If he's not throwing up, and only showing signs of frustration, impatience and crying, there is no magic wand. If he's still upset despite your bag of tricks you may have to find opportunities during the day when he sits with you and learns how to play in a stationary position. A good settling routine with books will help him start to enjoy quiet play and this should help him with car travel.

If your child generally has a problem sitting in one place, such as a pram or high chair, you may have to wait until he grows out of it. In this case, lots of happy repetitive singing, and perhaps something unusual to hold like your water bottle, may help keep him occupied while you're driving. For a longer trip, when you might have the luxury of two adults in the car at once, it's sensible for someone to sit in the back seat if your baby predictably finds travel difficult. Obviously, with a long car trip, regular breaks and time out of the car are essential to keep babies fresh and happy. Stop for all their normal feed times, and if you are in the car all the way up to and including one of his main sleeps of the day, stop, feed him, change his nappy, follow through on his settling routine before taking him to the car, buckling him in, covering him over with a cotton blanket and saying your sleep cues.

If the sensation of falling asleep has been uncomfortable or associated only with you holding him to help him cope, repairing sleep issues will almost guarantee car travel issues will stop because you've equipped him to cope independently with feeling tired, so even a drowsy car trip will no longer represent stress to him.

9

Nutrition and meal times

Sleep and nutrition are intricately linked. When you don't sleep very much, you can become quite hungry, and when you sleep a lot, you are generally less hungry. This happens with babies and young children as well. When you provide children with additional food to compensate for poor sleep, their bodies start to depend on excess volumes of food, giving them excess energy, restricting their need for sleep. This perpetuates a pattern of poor sleep. On the other hand, if you have a child who is sleeping large amounts you will find her dietary intake is lower. Equally, the timings of meals and snacks play a critical role in sleep. Excessive snacking on carb-based snacks mid morning can steal sleep away from your following morning between 2 and 6 a.m. Nutritional intake also impacts on sleep, and there is no culprit greater than low iron intake and absorption. Poor iron intake creates prolonged wakings at night. Therefore, a balanced eating plan with a balanced diet is critical in any daily routine so is a vital factor to work on. Let's now explore in detail the intricacies of diet and nutrition so you can start to correct your sleep issues the respectful way.

Meal times should be a positive experience for you and your baby. If meal times are happy, stress-free events, you will both reap the benefits, which include:

- a well-nourished, happy baby
- a baby who understands what you expect during meal times and enjoys the experience
- a harmonious home and family life
- a baby who sleeps through the night.

However, when it comes to feeding babies, everyone has an opinion. Three common ones are: 'Babies must be eating lumpy food by seven months of age'; 'Toddlers must learn to sit without distractions'; and 'Babies must be feeding themselves by 12 months.'

As a parent, it's *your* job to decide what's best for your child! Using your common sense and knowledge of good nutrition, teach your child which are healthy food options, and make decisions about the things that will damage her appetite for a nutritious meal later in the day. Just because many children will ask for crackers doesn't mean they should eat them. Babies and toddlers need strong, clear guidance from their parents or carers regarding when and what they should and shouldn't eat.

In this chapter I'll look at what and how much your child needs to eat for a balanced diet that helps her sleep through the night and how to start her on solids.

Getting the balance right

Many people think the final solid meal or milk feed of the day is the one that helps babies sleep better at night. In my experience, achieving a nutritious, balanced diet that includes eating of solids, good milk intake and great water hydration *throughout* the day is what helps a baby sleep well at night.

Children need iron to sleep well

I believe that a major cause of sleep disruption in babies and toddlers is low iron levels. It's important, therefore, to ensure children receive a good source of iron every day, so they can sleep peacefully.

The best source of iron for a baby or toddler is meat (you can start them on chicken) combined with vegetables and blended well. You can begin to serve this once a day at lunch time when your child is six and a half to seven months of age.

At the same time, eliminate or significantly reduce milk feeds at night (unless otherwise instructed by your doctor). This will help build up a baby's appetite for solids during the day.

Encouraging an appetite

When you need to repair meal-time difficulties, it's vital for you to have first established a balance in your baby's food and milk intake during the day and at night. This ensures an appetite that will help a child feed well. So often I have people say to me, 'I was going to wait for her to start eating better during the day before I tried to drop the night feeds', but excessive night feeds prevent children from eating solids through the day and it becomes a vicious cycle. If children have an increased calorie intake through the night as a result of excessive milk feeds they will be unable to eat effectively through the day. In order for them to eat more effectively through the day, it's necessary to actively eliminate some of the night feeds so as to build their need for solids through the day.

It's normal for newborn infants to need feeds every two to three hours, but as they grow and their capacity to consume higher volumes of milk increases, their need for feeding that regularly 'should' naturally decrease (unless milk feeding has become an association to go to sleep or they're on a snack cycle of demand feeding). By around six to seven months, with the introduction of solids, babies' need for night feeds should diminish naturally. Babies should only develop a need for two milk feeds a night 'again' if solids haven't been introduced by six to seven months, or one milk feed a night if solids have been introduced but no meat has been introduced. They should need no milk feeds through the nights if solids and meat have been introduced.

This need for night feeds is based on nutritional input only, and is not designed to be a guide for settling or resettling. Low daytime nutrition can be corrected by eliminating two key triggers of poor appetite:

- Excessive calorie intake through the night disrupting daytime appetite – if your baby (six to 24 months) is having excessive milk feeds through the night, defined by the need for more than one or two night feeds between 7 p.m. and 7 a.m.
- Excessive snacking (on snack foods or excessive milk feeds) through the day disrupting the more nutritious meals.

The above are repaired by stopping all night feeds from 2 a.m. until 6.30 or 7 a.m. on the day you plan to start a positive eating plan. Then you need to commence one of the balanced meal-time plans highlighted below.

How many solid meals?

Make sure you offer good healthy-eating opportunities throughout the day. The number of solid feeds I would recommend are:

- six to seven months: two to three solid meals (including a lunch of meat and vegetables, a vegetarian meal and/or a fruit meal)
- seven to eight and a half months: three solid meals (as above)
- nine to ten months: three solid meals and two snacks.

Lunch should be the biggest meal

The biggest meal of the day for children should be lunch and it should include a source of iron in the form of meat, and a balance of vitamins and minerals. To avoid or correct sleep problems, don't give children sandwiches for lunch until children are over two and, even then, only if they can eat a healthy salad and meat sandwich.

How much milk do they need?

Whether milk is from the breast or bottle is up to you, but a good number of milk feeds per day for different ages is:

- six to seven months of age (if they are not yet eating meat or haven't started solids): four to five milk feeds
- seven to ten months: four milk feeds
- ten to 12 months: three milk feeds
- 12 to 18 months: two milk feeds
- 18 to 24 months: one to two smaller milk serves as snacks.

As a child gets older, milk feeds can remain in breast or bottle form, or can be offered in a cup.

Children don't need to drink all the suggested quantities of milk. Instead, at least two-thirds of the recommended quantity is probably the minimum they should drink, with 240 millilitres being the maximum per serve. Once babies have decided they don't want any more, try to get them to lie still and offer them one last amount. If they refuse, that signifies the end of the feed.

Milk, solids and snacks

Solid meals and milk feeds should be separated, apart from breakfast. Low-sleep-requirement babies will need a morning- and afternoon-tea snack at a younger age than higher-sleep-requirement babies. By eight to nine months lower-sleep-requirement babies may need a Cruskit with avocado or something similar in the afternoon as well as their milk feed, and by around nine to ten months a light fruit snack is needed as well as their milk feed in the morning. Higher-sleep-requirement babies burn less fuel during the day as they spend more time sleeping and therefore may not need morning or afternoon tea until they are weaned off their mid-morning and mid-afternoon milk feeds at around ten to 12 months.

The need to add a solid snack in the weaning process is easy to identify: the child is not lasting well to lunch or dinner. If she is hungry, grumpy or showing tired signs without the need to sleep well before a meal is due, it's a clear sign that the milk is no longer sufficient as a between-meal feed, and she will need something more to sustain her in the long gaps between breakfast and lunch, and lunch and dinner. The need for solid afternoon tea to be introduced as well as her milk often occurs before the need for morning tea. This is only a guide and babies may need slightly more or slightly less than is suggested.

Snacking

Children often crave carbohydrates as a means of sustaining themselves when they are tired due to poor sleep. The best way to correct this is to ensure children's meal times are well-spaced and their diet is balanced. It's important not to try to correct poor sleep cycles by providing additional feeds or snacks because by doing this you risk perpetuating the cycle.

Low-sleep-requirement babies over eight and a half months may need some fruit for morning tea if they appear hungry more than two hours before lunch. They can also have a snack for afternoon tea (such as toast or a breadstick plus yoghurt or cheese, or fruit). High-sleep-requirement babies from the age of ten months can also have fruit for morning tea if they appear hungry long before lunch, and a snack for afternoon tea.

Excessive snacking disrupts children's appetites and need for sleep, so it's best not to give them a snack during the two hours before lunch or dinner because:

- healthy balanced meals provide energy that lasts longer and therefore often helps children stay calm and content
- snacks are often higher in kilojoules and less nutritious than a healthy balanced meal, so are only effective for short bursts of energy
- continued snacking and poorly balanced meal intake may result in behavioural difficulties
- snacking too often during the day is a way of replacing or compensating for poor sleep and therefore perpetuates poor sleeping patterns.

But surely something is better than nothing?

We all know that when we've snacked during the afternoon and then sit down to a healthy dinner we don't need to eat much to feel satisfied. When we've been busy all afternoon and haven't snacked we feel hungry and want to eat a nutritious dinner.

The same applies to children. Avoid overfeeding them with snacks, and they will start to eat effectively at meal times. Children will not starve themselves, and if their appetite is built for a healthy meal, they will begin to eat better. For these reasons 'something is better than nothing' is not true because eating something at the wrong time leads to them eating nothing at the right time.

Don't give snacks to help them cope

Parents sometimes give children snacks to help them cope with unpleasant feelings such as boredom. This is an effective tool occasionally, such as on a plane, or to keep children calm and content in restricted locations they can't move around freely in. But snacking is an unhealthy and unbalanced approach to coping with emotions.

It's crucial that children learn how to be patient in a pram, or while a parent washes the dishes, or while they're sitting and looking around for interesting things. Being bored or having to 'wait' are normal experiences: we wait in the pram, bath, at traffic lights, for food to cook, for people to arrive, or to fall asleep. Telling children to eat when they have to wait results in poor skills for coping with unpleasant feelings.

Instead, assess what children are feeling and work on developing healthy solutions. This way you will equip children with multiple tools for coping in a variety of situations in a more balanced and healthy way.

Water is important, but when?

Providing proper hydration is one of the most important ways to help children sleep well at night and remain happy for the entire day. Some tantrum-style behaviours in toddlers can be attributed to them not drinking enough water. It's therefore important to keep suggesting they drink water by sitting them down and holding the cup for them and guiding them in a confident parent-guided line of communication.

Water should not take the place of healthy meals, however, so it's important to avoid providing drinks 30 minutes before a solid meal, especially when trying to restore or repair meal times. Children often confuse hunger with thirst, and ask for a drink. If a meal time is only half an hour away, hold out until after they've eaten.

If your child would like a drink during the first ten minutes of a meal, try to only provide a sip so she doesn't fill her tummy and ruin her appetite.

Don't compensate for poor sleep with excessive food

When balancing children's meals to help repair sleep time, the simple principle is: the food children consume needs to be in normal healthy amounts required by their body as fuel to grow, heal and develop as well as to be active and energised throughout the day. As that fuel source starts to deplete, children who resist sleep may appear to want food to correct the way they are feeling. When that food is not offered you'll see a natural desire from the body to sleep more effectively. This is how to repair sleep in children fighting sleep and demanding food in its place, but children may need to go through a day or two of hunger until their sleep is fully repaired.

Do not be tempted to compensate for poor sleep by offering your child additional food, or additional sleep at other times. It is better to work with babies' bodies and their need for sleep rather than working with children's temperaments and their desire to stay awake. When children start to feel true tiredness from their poor sleep because food is not a compensation tool, they may appear more tired than usual. At this point, keep them awake until their normal sleep time is due, and let them know what they are feeling: 'It's okay, bubba, you're just tired, you can have a sleep in your bed soon to make you feel better.'

Equally, when children become hungry because they are having 'normal' and healthy gaps between meals instead of constantly grazing and keeping their appetite subdued, they may not know the feeling of true hunger and may become very agitated. Again, it's important to tell them what they are feeling: 'It's okay, bubba, you are just hungry, Mummy will get your dinner soon.' On those first few days, help them cope in the lead-up to meals by keeping them still and distracted. Toddlers may enjoy their favourite DVD, for instance, while sitting in their high chair for ten minutes before their meal. Be careful they don't fall asleep as their blood sugar starts to naturally drop before their meal.

Be flexible

All children are different, and parents need to remain flexible and find out what works for them and their children. For example, some babies find it difficult to eat lumpy food because it appears to trigger or overstimulate their gag reflex and makes them retch. If this occurs with your child, she may prefer to go straight from pureed food to finger foods. There may be a transitional period in which she's spoon-fed pureed food for longer, and then has the opportunity to choose from steamed vegetables or small shredded pieces of chicken or meat off her tray. Once she becomes efficient at finger-feeding herself a portion of food adequate for her age and stage of development, you can reduce or cut out the spoon-fed pureed food. The key is to do what makes meal times happy and healthy.

Some children prefer eating items individually, with foods such as pumpkin and carrot in separate sections of their plate. Others are happy to have food blended together. You'll soon work out what your child prefers, so go with that, especially in the beginning.

If you discover your child has a sweet tooth and you're having trouble feeding her vegetables, add some pureed fruit to the vegetables. Once the child becomes accustomed to the textures and flavours of the foods, gradually reduce the volume of pureed fruit to vegetables until it is eliminated.

Babies also vary in the volume they need to eat. The best way to judge the right quantity of food is to go by pre-packaged jar sizes for their age group. That doesn't mean you need to feed your child jar food (although sometimes it can be more convenient or hygienic), but jar foods vary in size based on age, and provide a useful guide to quantity. Work on the premise that anything less than your child's age-group suggestion size is not adequate. For example, a 12 month old eating the equivalent of a nine month old's portion is not eating an adequate amount.

Some babies are hungrier than others, and jar quantities are not adequate for their body's needs. Avoid giving up on solids and reverting back to milk too quickly as babies can become lazy and may always opt for what they know best and what takes the least amount of effort, which is to breastfeed or drink from a bottle.

Children can vary greatly in their ability to feed themselves. Some need to be spoon-fed meat and vegetables until they're two or over to eat an adequate quantity of vegetables and have enough iron each day. Others happily progress to lumpy foods but prefer to eat only meat with their fingers and may need feeding for a little longer so they eat a healthy portion of vegetables. Others will eat large quantities with a good balance of finger foods from an early age and don't need to be fed via a spoon for long. In these cases parents should still pop some food into their baby's mouth from time to time to maintain the pace of the meal in those first ten minutes.

However it works for your baby, be flexible. There is enough to worry about as a parent without thinking your child has to meet other people's deadlines.

Promote a healthy attitude towards food

Good food should be fun all day! Involve your child in grocery shopping. Let her hold fruit and vegies for you and don't worry if she licks, smells or tries to bite the food. Incorporate pictures of food into her play by cutting out pictures and making a collage or having drawings of food you've sketched near them at meal time.

Provide positive role-play opportunities by eating good food in front of your child. So, for example, when you make her some steamed vegetables, make enough for you too, and let her see you 'bite', 'chew' and really enjoy the food.

Positioning and strategy for bottle feeding

If you're introducing a bottle, it's best to do so in the early months of life, even if it contains expressed breast milk. This ensures a baby can be fed from a bottle as she gets older, which will help you keep her well hydrated with water as she grows.

If your baby is showing initial resistance to bottle feeding at six months, make sure you always let her know that the taste will be different to breast milk by saying 'new taste, bottle'.

Another trick is to offer the bottle when you know she'll be quite hungry – perhaps the first feed of the day – and get Daddy to give it. Be persistent and don't compensate by offering milk from another source, unless she's had no milk at all.

If after several days of trying you're not getting anywhere, raise the white flag and move on. Your child will need to graduate straight to a sippy cup for her milk feeds and water. While this may take a little bit longer, it's perfectly fine. Whatever you do is your choice, and whether you transition to a bottle or a cup while still breastfeeding will not impact upon her feeding routine nor result in early weaning.

It's also important to make sure your baby doesn't find sucking a bottle too difficult so make sure you use the appropriate teat and that the top is not fastened too tightly. When your baby starts to drink you should see a steady flow of bubbles trickling into the bottle as she sucks. If the bubbles don't start within 30 to 60 seconds, the lid is too tight. Without breaking the feed, slightly loosen the top until you see the bottle is drawing in air. (A lack of air flowing into the bottle is the main cause of projectile vomiting in bottle-fed babies, because it forces them to break the feed regularly.)

Positioning is also important when feeding a baby with a bottle. Once a baby has learnt to sit or lie still to have her nappy changed you can use the same language to ask her to lie down for her feed. Make yourself comfortable in the corner of a couch and put a pillow under the arm your baby is going to lie on for support. Say, 'Lie down. Wait for Mummy' then lie her down so one of her arms is tucked securely down your side or behind you. Angle her body into yours and hold her firmly. If she's waving an arm in the air, use your non-feeding hand to hold on to her hand. Initially you may need to hold her hand quite firmly so it doesn't flap about, but once the feeding has started, she will be more settled.

Establishing bottle feeding is similar to introducing solids. Make sure you define your positioning request. Some children will sit up, get down and crawl around the floor before having a suck again. This doesn't result in a good healthy feeding opportunity, and will make the time it takes to feed a child too drawn out. Instead, make sure your baby stays on your lap for the entire feed and, unless you sit her up to wind her, which is not so vital by six months, she needs to remain there until either the feed is finished or you're satisfied she's had enough and is full.

Introducing solids

Whether children are six months or 16 months old, they will need to go through the same process to learn how to eat solids. Remember, children have no concept of consequences, so they don't realise that to refuse food now will disrupt their sleep or have an impact upon their happiness later. Children will only try to retain the governing line and, therefore, the outcome of meal times if they are not given clear communication and a predictable pattern to follow. A successful outcome requires a parent who takes charge in a confident, enthusiastic and persistent way.

Here is a step-by-step guide to starting babies on solids.

1. Always install and fasten the high-chair harness correctly. It's both unsafe and disruptive to meals to have your child in her chair without adequate safety devices in place or without them being fitted well.
2. If you are introducing solids for the first time, or are correcting a disrupted meal-time behavioural pattern, remove the high chair meal-tray altogether.
3. Recline your child so she can relax back into her seat. Make sure you tell her before you do this, and always recline her slowly. If she becomes unsettled, hold her hands and make it a fun thing to do, a little like the way you would vocalise and smile as you slide her down a slippery dip. You can recline your child up to the age of 12 months.
4. If the high chair does not recline, and you have a baby under nine months of age, put her into a bouncer/rocker chair for meal times. Don't forget to remove the toy bar first so it doesn't get covered in food.

5. If she tries to sit upright by getting up on her elbows or pulling on the sides of the high chair, help her relax by putting her hands back into a comfortable position in front of her. This involves physically releasing her hands from the side of the chair and gently saying, 'Lie down, bubby. It's time for lunch.' You'll have been managing this kind of behaviour during nappy change so she should be accustomed to and trust the request.
6. If there's going to be a battle about who is governing the outcome of meal times, it's better to have it when you're putting her bib on or asking her to relax in the chair rather than when you are feeding her.
7. Once your child is safely in her chair or recliner, get yourself comfortable. Be prepared for a little bit or a lot of mess. This doesn't last for long, and it is well worth the clean-up required to achieve relaxed, settled meal times where your child happily sits and eats while having a chat and playing with her toys. To not address an existing poor meal-time routine because you don't want a little mess will result in ongoing meal-time battles.

Recipe suggestions for first spoon-fed meals

Many people think they need to offer a new taste sensation to their child at every meal, but children usually respond better to the predictable, especially when they're unsettled. Instead, stick to a few simple recipes until you've established trust at meal times before broadening their food repertoire a little each week.

Always begin with a small range of puree meal suggestions in infant and toddler cookbooks and gradually progress from pureed foods to lumpy foods *if* your child can tolerate them. If not, it's okay for your child to go from purees straight to finger foods if that works best for them.

The most common mistake parents make when blending meat and vegetables for their child is to overcook the meat so it doesn't bind properly with the vegetables. This results in the meat sticking to a baby's tongue and making her gag, cry or vomit. In order to avoid this, start with three simple recipes and remain predictable and consistent until she settles down and starts to trust the food you feed her again.

Here are three recipes to get you started. These simple, smooth, creamy mixtures will ensure children get a good mix of vegetables and protein to help them get into eating.

Mixed vegetables and pasta or rice

500 g pumpkin
2 large potatoes

3 large carrots
2 zucchinis
1 cup mini pasta stars or rice
formula, breast or cows' milk (optional)

Peel and chop the vegetables into similar-sized pieces and steam until tender. Place in a food processor and puree until creamy smooth and no lumps remain.

Boil pasta or rice until tender. Remove, drain and rinse thoroughly in cold water. Add to pureed vegetables and blend in the food processor until smooth and fluffy.

If you feel the blend is too sticky and needs to be fluffier, add a little bit of milk, about 10 to 20 ml, to help you achieve the right consistency.

Mixed vegetables and chicken
500 g pumpkin
4 to 5 Red Delicious apples (optional)
2 large potatoes or half a sweet potato
3 large carrots
2 zucchinis
½ to 1 small chicken breast (do not use mince)
formula, breast or cows' milk (optional)

Peel and chop the vegetables into similar-sized pieces and steam until tender. Place in a food processor and puree until creamy smooth and no lumps remain.

Cut the chicken breast into cubes of similar size. Add chicken to a saucepan with 3 cm of boiling water and poach it until it *just* turns white all the way through. Do not overcook or it won't blend well. Once the chicken is white through (cut and check one of the larger pieces) remove from the water with a slotted spoon and place in a small cereal bowl. Place a bread-and-butter plate over the top of the bowl containing the chicken and allow the chicken to steam in its own heat for a further five minutes.

Add the chicken to the pureed vegetables and blend until the chicken is completely mixed in with the puree. It should look like tiny white flecks in the vegetable mix. The entire mix should be fluffy and completely smooth.

If you feel the blend is too sticky and needs to be fluffier, add a little bit of milk, about 10 to 20 ml, which will help you achieve the right consistency and ensure the chicken and vegetables remain blended together. Do not add water as it can cause the chicken and vegetables to separate and you will end up with the chicken clinging to your baby's tongue.

Mixed vegetables and sirloin steak
500 g pumpkin
2 large potatoes or half a sweet potato

4 to 5 Red Delicious apples (optional)
3 large carrots
2 zucchinis
sirloin steak, about the size of the palm of your hand (do not use mince)
formula, breast or cows' milk (optional)

Peel and chop the vegetables into similar-sized pieces and steam until tender. Place in a food processor and puree until creamy smooth and no lumps remain.

In a skillet, cook the steak on a low heat until it's cooked through but not overcooked. Watch the meat to ensure it is cooked and no longer pink, but remains moist and soft. Remove from the heat and place on a plate to settle for five minutes.

Cut the meat into cubes and add to the pureed vegetables, and blend until the two are well combined. It should look like a darker blend of vegetables mixed with tiny brown flecks. The entire mix should be fluffy and completely smooth.

If you feel the blend is too sticky and needs to be fluffier, add a little bit of milk, about 10 to 20 ml, which will help you achieve the right consistency and ensure the steak and vegetables remain blended together. Do not add water as it can cause the steak and vegetables to separate and you will end up with the meat clinging to your baby's tongue.

Encouraging balanced eating

The first spoonful is often the most difficult for babies. This doesn't mean they don't want the food, it's just a warm-up process they go through, and probably occurs because of a lack of forewarning about taste, texture and temperature. Make sure you always inform them respectfully, and this first-spoon battle won't last long.

If a child has never been able to accept spoon-feeding, and is not eating adequate quantities, or has a severe aversion to food or your guidance at meal time, go back to a very smooth puree for their meals and spoon-feed it to them. Not every baby is able to cope with lumps. There's a school of thought that recommends babies start eating lumpy food by a certain age, and this is achievable in *most* cases. However, when you come across a child who finds lumps in puree or mash vile, it's okay to bypass lumpy foods and keep spoon-feeding them purees for a little longer while they establish good self-help skills around finger-feeding themselves, and just skip straight to solid finger foods when they are ready.

It's not really surprising that some babies can't tolerate the texture of lumpy mash. Just as not all adults enjoy the same textures of food, not every single child will like the same texture of food. It's far more important to determine what suits an individual child best. Some babies do the 'text book' recommended thing and progress happily from pureed food to fork-mashed food to finger foods without batting an eyelid. Some babies take a little more time to get used to puree and find the concept of fork mash challenging to get used to. These babies may eat a more vigorously mashed version and eventually eat finger foods. Some babies will take time to settle into puree but gag, retch or vomit at even the slightest lumps in their food. These babies rarely get used to lumps in their food and will move directly from puree only to puree and finger foods.

None of these feeders is better or worse than others, or should be defined as 'good' or 'bad' eaters based on it; they just have individual likes and dislikes. There should never be a 'blanket' strategy for children under two when it comes to feeding because it isn't balanced and doesn't take individual needs into consideration.

When are they ready to learn to feed themselves?

When your child is allowing you to feed her, you can introduce a spoon for you and a spoon for her. Until then you should be the only one to have a spoon at meal time.

If your child is eating efficiently, you can start to allow her to feed herself, but always retain the capacity to offer a spoonful now and then by following through with your management strategies.

If your child's eating becomes poor again and she starts to get bossy about you feeding her, take the spoon off her and re-establish parent-feeding to stop the behaviour, and try again later. She will be far less happy, day and night, from hunger than she would from not being able to have a spoon for a few more weeks.

What you want to achieve is confident parenting, where your child understands that you expect her to eat for you as well as on her own, and that if she's fussing or having a tantrum you will assume the feeding role. The reason I'm so clear about this is that small children can become unhappy and unsettled when they don't eat properly. When you take the fussing part out of meal time and they are busy playing and eating without fighting and crying, they will become more happy and content through other parts of the day, and will sleep better at night.

Achieving happy, healthy meal times

The first thing you need to know about feeding solids to babies and toddlers is that until the age of two, their concentration span while eating lasts for a *maximum* of eight minutes. This doesn't give you much time to get nourishing food into them.

Therefore, for meal times to be effective, where your baby happily eats a nutritious meal chosen by you, you'll need to guide her via a parent-governed line of communication. You'll need a good high chair, some meal-time boundaries and a 'bag of tricks' (toys) to get her through those last few minutes.

Feeding solids: the process

The first spoonfuls

Dip the spoon into the food so there is just a little bit on the spoon.

Tell her it's dinner time and she's eating chicken and pumpkin (for example).

For the first mouthful, wipe the spoon on her bottom lip and tell her what the food is again, for example: 'New taste, chicken and pumpkin.'

Your child will lick her lips, giving her a chance to taste the food she's about to have. For the first few mouthfuls have just enough food on the spoon so she can gradually build up the size of the mouthfuls over the first minute.

Once she has the flavour in her mouth you can increase the quantity of each mouthful. This is the same for feeding a six month old as for preparing to help an 18 month old re-establish their meal time and eating.

Keep it coming

Because a baby's attention span with eating is between three and eight minutes long from when they first taste their food, you need to keep it coming consistently and repetitively, without pausing. While she's swallowing one mouthful you should be preparing the next spoonful, encouraging her about the yummy meal, and remaining emotionally available and engaged with her. As soon as the spoon is full, tap her bottom lip once, and pull the spoon back a little, preparing her for the next mouthful.

If your child is storing food in her cheeks, put the spoon side on to her lips and tap on her bottom lip to encourage swallowing. If she still won't swallow, a little massage under her chin should move the food and trigger the swallow reflex. Smile like you are tickling her, or as if you are squeezing her beautiful cheeks.

Between mouthfuls, if she doesn't realise she needs to open her mouth, use the side of the spoon to push down on her bottom gums to break the natural suction of her mouth, then quickly tip the spoon so it is angled slightly downwards (side on) but into her mouth and slide it in, turn the spoon so it is in the correct forward-facing position quickly, then wipe the food onto her palate as you remove it.

Just wipe her mouth with the spoon every few mouthfuls; otherwise, it can be irritating for her. Remember, it doesn't matter what she does with the food at that point, so long as you keep up the pace of the meal.

In the early days some food will come out of her mouth and some will be swallowed. This is normal and is to do with the muscles in the tongue being more used to suckling milk. These spills do not indicate dislike of food.

Some babies will enjoy sucking the food off the spoon after they are first introduced to solids. This can be an effective feeding strategy, but if your child has been having difficulties, follow a more confident parent-directed style of feeding.

Maintain a brisk pace

When people watch me feed their baby for the first time, they are surprised at my pace. I do slow the pace of meal times eventually, though not until feeding has been repaired and the child is enjoying meals.

When repairing stressful meal times it's important, after that first spoonful, to increase the pace quickly so the bulk of the meal is finished within three to five minutes. This involves filling the spoon, putting it in her mouth, then immediately filling the spoon and bringing it back to her mouth, tapping her lip and into her mouth, repeated until the meal is over.

By increasing the pace you ensure meals are achievable and over quickly for a child. A quick pace is also in line with her milk feeding patterns of suck–swallow, suck–swallow. Finally, by getting food into your child quickly you ensure that if she feels uncomfortable with the sensation of hunger, her appetite is quickly satisfied so she doesn't associate the sensation of extreme hunger with being fed, and learns that food solves the feeling of hunger and stress rather than causes it.

What to offer first

If a meal contains sausages or chicken or something that requires a fair bit of chewing to get through, and you know your toddler is likely to opt for that before vegetables, only provide a small amount of the chewy item and ensure she has some vegetables in that first ten minutes before you offer any more meat or sausages. You have a very brief window of opportunity to feed your under-two year old and it is not in her best interests to only eat a sausage at a meal. Look for balance to ensure she is having vegetables as well as meat at each meal time.

Meal-time mess and flow

During the first meal of your new meal-time management, you may become spray-painted from head to toe with pureed vegetables, and your baby's face and hair may well be caked in her lunch. Remain positive and when she's finished the meal show her the bowl and say, 'All gone, bubby, good eating. Mummy get you some dessert/face washer to wipe your face.' Some parents give up feeding their child because of the mess it creates, but if you remain positive and encouraging and follow the basic meal-time rules of 'hands down', 'out of mouth' and 'sitting forward', etc., you will quickly find your baby starts to accept the food, and the face painting and pumpkin hair will become a distant memory.

Re-establishing feeding after a drink of water

If your child absolutely needs to have a sip of water during a meal, it can be difficult to re-establish the meal. Some babies and toddlers, particularly fussy ones, may stop eating and choose to end a meal with any indication of a transition. Each time this occurs, to re-establish the meal understand that 'the first spoon' is always the hardest, and you need to re-establish the taste, texture and temperature again while watching your pattern of response to her behaviour around being offered the spoon.

The role you play in their attitudes towards meal time

You have a crucial role in helping your child feel positive about meal times. I can turn a baby who gags at the sight of a spoon and is therefore failing to thrive into a baby who loves their meal within a day for under-12 month olds, and in a couple of days for 12 to 24 month olds almost solely by using a patient, confident, encouraging, persistent approach to meal time.

This entire strategy of learning how to eat from scratch again is designed to be a confident parent-directed and -governed style of communication so all your language should be statements, not questions. Once you have a confident, happy, enthusiastic tone around meal time, your child will adopt your same mannerisms.

Being enthusiastic is an important way to communicate with babies, as are clapping, cheering, specific praise, and one-on-one attention, all of which are very encouraging for babies.

When parents ask me, 'Do we still praise her even though she hasn't eaten much?' I always say 'Yes!' Children respond better to encouragement, to your belief in their ability and to positive input about meal times than they will to anything else. If she's eaten so poorly you can't even draw on a single mouthful of food to be positive about, acknowledge what she did do: 'Thank you for sitting in your high chair bubba, that was a little bit tricky but thank you for trying.'

Keep your cool

If you dread meal times, your child may become anxious about this time too. If you get frustrated, angry or impatient she won't understand and will become stressed at the thought of eating. Even something as simple as a huff, heavy sigh, eye roll or talking under your breath in an exasperated tone will affect her.

The key is to keep your cool, have clear expectations of her and follow through. If you approach every meal with a happy tone, positive language and an enthusiastic air, your child will quickly develop the same attitude towards meal time.

Tips for happy, healthy meal times

A good high chair is important

One of the best things you can do to help make meal times stress free is to invest in a good-quality high chair. Many high chairs look cool with sleek edges and designs to suit a modern home, but some may offer little or no security for babies starting to eat solid food. A safe, secure, adjustable high chair can make all the difference.

When you're buying a high chair, look for one with the following features:

- Adjustable height positions.
- Adjustable reclining seat.
- Padded seat liner that can be removed for cleaning.
- Removable, dishwasher-safe tray.
- Adjustable lap and shoulder harness to make transition to dinner table easy.
- Castor wheels for easy mobility.
- Ability to fold up easily and compactly.

Any good high chair with all these features will do the job.

Make meal time enjoyable

Make meal times fun by singing songs, chatting about the day's events, talking about your child's favourite people or things, and sharing your enthusiasm for food.

Let them become familiar with the spoon

If your child has an issue with the spoon, offer it as a chewing object whenever possible – while in the bath or car, or during floor play.

This helps her become accustomed to the texture, smell and feel of the spoon in her mouth so she can develop a new relaxed association with it.

Adopt a parent-governed line of communication

As discussed elsewhere, children love predictability in their day, because it makes them feel in control and relaxed. To guarantee predictability at meal times, use a parent-governed line of communication.

When asking your child to co-operate with you to eat her food via a parent-governed line of communication you shouldn't sound demanding, frustrated or harsh. Don't get angry if you feel like it's not working or she's having a tantrum when you ask her to eat. A stern or exasperated expression, tone or statement will only unsettle or frighten her. The more unsettled she is, the more calm and soothing you need to be. Drop your voice an octave, slow your speech and sound loving and reassuring. Be consistent with your feeding plan, sound confident, and be persistent with the feeding process: spoon in the bowl, scoop up the food, spoon in the mouth.

Remember the learning ladder of success if you feel uncertain.

Use consistent, repetitive language

Use your flow of consistent language cues to prepare your child in a happy and enthusiastic tone that the meal time is coming up, and to tell her what she can expect to be eating. This is particularly important from eight months of age, and is most definitely a pivotal part of re-establishing feeding with the 12 months-plus age group.

Language routine for meal times

Here's an example of the kind of consistent language you might use before, during and after meal times:

1. **Pre-empting**: 'Jake, it's nearly time for lunch, *nearly time* to sit down in your high chair and wait for Mummy.'
2. **Forewarning**: 'Last one Jake, then *it's time* to sit down in your high chair and wait for Mummy.'
3. **Stating event and expectation**: 'Okay, Jake, it's time for lunch. Sit down and wait for Mummy.'
4. **Defining your statement**: 'Jake sit down while Mummy makes lunch.'
5. **Praising**: 'Good sitting, Jake! Now where's that spoon?'

6. **Following through**: 'Jake, time to eat yummy chicken and vegies.' (Also remember to forewarn them regarding the food's taste and consistency.)
7. **Completion**: 'All finished! Good eating, bubba!' (Wipe face and hands, wipe down tray and use wait game and cue.)

Use language cues to teach self-feeding

Language cues are vital when you're helping your child learn how to feed herself. Consistently use repetitive positive language like 'Scoop it up' and 'In your mouth.'

Once she has a spoon of her own, offer the bowl briefly and say, 'Scoop it up' and wait for her to scoop the food up, then encourage her by saying, 'In your mouth.' Clap and cheer and before you know it she will feed herself beautifully!

Language: Dos and don'ts

- Take care not to influence your child's attitudes with comments such as 'Oh, you don't like that!' or 'You're not going to eat this for Mummy, are you!' or 'Mummy's sorry, she's not very good at feeding you.'
- Always use statements, rather than questions. For example: 'Nearly time for dinner' *not* 'Would you like some dinner soon?' or 'Time to eat the yummy chicken and vegies' *not* 'Bubba try the yummy chicken and vegies?'
- Avoid saying 'Just one more' over and over again or you will confuse your child and encourage her to negotiate, which may cause the meal to end prematurely. Use positive language delivered with an air of confidence. State your expectations clearly at each stage and follow through.

Give them your full attention

While you're spoon-feeding your child, give her your full attention. For those ten minutes, do not be distracted by an older child, the television, the telephone or having a conversation with someone else. Stay focused, confident and happy about the meal. Make sure she keeps her hands down and away from the spoon by using the cue, 'Hands down! Mummy do it' and defining that statement by lowering her hands with your own. This should be a normal expectation at each meal time.

Use lots of smiles and chatter and praise while she gets used to having things like a spoon or solids put in her mouth, even if she's not sure about the process. This may well be the case for a baby when she's first reintroduced to solids, or for an older child who's never learnt to take solids from a spoon before. Be prepared for the normal pattern of swallowing when very new eaters are introduced to solids.

Stick to your guns!

Always target an achievable portion size you would like her to eat, and work through the meal enthusiastically. I've noticed parents give up well before I would, and I've never had a poor result from my meal-time repair strategies. Don't give up! Set a good pace and keep going until the meal ten minutes is up.

Your attitude towards her food and meal times is important. Stay calm and enthusiastic, and have a repertoire of songs and conversation to distract her and maybe even be prepared to have her protest louder than you can talk. This doesn't mean you increase your volume of singing or talking, however. The rule is that the more unsettled she becomes, the calmer and more soothing your tone should be.

Distraction during meal times

Children adore singing and respond well to active communication when they have a little task to do, like finding the dog, 'Where's that puppy dog of ours gone? Blicky, come and say hello to Brooke while she has dinner.' For toddlers, sharing a meal with their favourite teddy, or showing their pet cat or dog how good they are at eating is often a positive way of encouraging good eating. Say something like, 'Look, Blicky, look at Brooke eat her vegetables. Isn't she a great eater', before clapping and cheering, and this will usually be accompanied by your child joining in and looking around to see if teddy or puppy is as proud as you both are. Usually she'll finish her meal and be focused on wanting to eat, rather than trying to avoid it.

Use toys to keep them eating longer

With such a short attention span during meal times, children will quickly lose interest. Therefore, as well as setting a brisk pace, they may need to be given a toy or two from a 'bag of tricks' to string them out a little longer while they finish being fed. Toys can make the process more enjoyable for children and help them to stay calm and relaxed. Importantly, unlike television, toys *don't* appear to transfix children to the point they are no longer aware that they're eating. Just remember to only start to dip into your bag of tricks once their attention span is reached. We never start with toys unless it is absolutely necessary.

Set meal-time boundaries

If your child has established poor associations with feeding she may do things such as blow raspberries, purse her lips, turn her head from side to side, shout and so on. What matters is your response to such behaviours. Never pull your hand away when she blows a raspberry or turns her head or makes a crying sound or screams at you or the spoon. This teaches her that screaming or a raspberry equals no feeding.

Instead, be confident, encouraging and persistent. Keep the spoon near her mouth. If she turns her head, put your hand gently on her right cheek (to discourage her turning her face into your hand) and then follow her mouth with the spoon on a 90-degree angle. If she protests, pop a mouthful in, and continue to feed her, even if she's protesting. Use distractions, offer toys, songs and remain happy. You're teaching her meal time follows the same pattern: scoop it up and in your mouth!

When the meal is finished say, 'All finished! Good eating, bubba!'

While we can't make children eat, we can manage their behaviour at meal time. Use the following language cues and actions consistently and repeatedly to guide your child during meal times.

Behaviour/ boundary	Language cue	Physical intervention
Allowing Mum and Dad to wash hands and face.	'Hands down, Mummy do it.'	Don't allow your child to grab the face washer or try to pull it from her face. Block her hands with your forearm. Wipe a cheek at a time, then her chin and nose.
No throwing food, cutlery, plates, etc.	'No throwing – plate on table.'	Take her hands and help her place the plate back on the tray then make her let go. Hold the plate in place if she refuses to have it on the tray and repeat cue gently.
Always put cup down in a no-spill position.	'Cup on table.'	Use a sticker or drink coaster to show her where to put it. Though this is more important for 12 to 24 month olds it should be encouraged with younger babies, too.

Behaviour/ boundary	Language cue	Physical intervention
No fingers in mouth.	'Fingers out of mouth.'	Take her hands away from her mouth.
No covering mouth with hand.	'Hands down.'	Take her hands away from her mouth.
No leaning sideways off chair.	'Sitting up, please.'	Stand behind her when she gets heavy, or from the front for younger babies and sit them upright. Tighten buckles if necessary.
No snatching spoon from Mummy.	'No, ta. Mummy do it.'	Avoid allowing her to get the spoon, but if she does, release her grip from it without giving her the spoon.
No mouthing high chair while being fed.	'Sitting up, please.'	Stand behind her and sit her upright. Tighten buckles if necessary.
No flapping hands when being spoon-fed.	'Hands down, Mummy do it.'	Block her hands with your forearm as you feed her.

Repairing significant meal-time blues

I live by a simple principle: you can't keep doing the same thing and expect a different result. If your child thinks meal times are a disaster, and food involves stress and anxiety, you need to correct that belief. When I go to a home where the baby or toddler and their parents find meal times distressing, I love showing them it's a time of the day they can look forward to. I'm excited to teach parents how to work through and past even the most extreme anxieties around food and eating. And I am thrilled for parents who, within two to three days, can sit down and spoon-feed their hungry baby without tears or concern from the baby. One of the strongest desires in parents is the desire to nourish their baby, so when they feed their child peacefully for the first time some parents become teary with happiness.

The process you need to go through for a day, or sometimes two or three days, to achieve peace at meal times, however, is usually messy and often involves a lot of bluffed confidence, persistence, singing, chatting, game playing and distraction from you. You may encounter crying, resistance, spitting, food in hair and protests. When I'm working through a poor meal-time routine to re-establish a new eating pattern, parents often look surprised when I persist despite a failure to get much food into their baby on the first attempt, and have a quiet sense of relief that, 'Even Sheyne is finding it a messy challenge.' I assure them that the only reason I am ultimately successful is because I have a plan, I have a goal and I am patient.

When it comes to working past your child's meal-time stresses, assess the environment and meal-time conditions from an adult's perspective. Is there any reason for her to be frightened of meal times, and should food be stressful or unpleasant? If the answer is 'no', she has a misunderstanding and it's your role to correct it. If you never attempt to do so, she will continue to feel the same way about food. So as her guides in life, work past that association and help her move through the stress so she discovers food is enjoyable and she can look forward to meal times.

The only time a process like this can be destructive to a child's association with food is to start, reach a peak of resistance, then quit and not see it through to a positive outcome. When a child has had difficulties with something like severe and painful reflux, it's likely she'll associate meal times with pain. While the pain of meal time is likely to have subsided by six months of age, the association with pain can remain long after the symptoms have gone. You'll need to help her eat solidly and consistently while remaining positive and reassuring. That way, she can see that while she feels uncomfortable with the new meal-time plan, her mummy and daddy are okay, which translates into a message that she's okay too. Ultimately, she starts to see that meal times do not hurt her, and she can start to eat free of anxiety.

When your child does not have a history of pain with eating, however, she may still have developed distrust in her meal time because of something as simple as many flavour, texture and temperature changes without warning. There are lots of reasons meal-time plans can go astray. Often the standard approaches, like 'Let them eat what they want' and 'Let them do it themselves', will do nothing other than keep you and your child in the same place of poor eating and poor associations with eating. This is because you're not teaching her to move beyond that old pattern of association. When you need to restore a very disrupted style of feeding you will need to revert to the full spoon-feeding plan (see page 141). This means that meal times go back to being an entirely parent-governed part of the day for three full weeks until everything settles down, and she becomes familiar, comfortable and ultimately relaxed with and looking forward to meal times again.

Regardless of a child's age, it's important to go back to the eating stage for her *ability* rather than trying to get her to eat like a child her age. This is particularly crucial for a child who's never really learnt how to eat correctly. So if your 16 month old has never learnt how to eat vegetables, go back to very pureed vegetables with no lumps. If she's never learnt how to eat meat or vegetables go back to basics. It is unfair and unrealistic to expect six month olds to eat lumpy foods because they are only just being exposed to food for the first time, and if your child is still in that situation at 16 months, you need to go back to how you'd feed a six month old if the meal disruption is significant enough. Equally, if she can eat solids but not nearly enough, go back to feeding her pureed food to ensure she's eating adequate quantities and then follow it with some finger foods that she can feed herself. Often children then progress very rapidly on to lumpy and then solids foods so do not feel anxious if you need to climb the ladder of learning.

There is no avoiding things with a child; you are just putting them off. So don't put it off any longer. Teach her how to eat.

10

Setting up a suitable sleep environment

When you start teaching your child to sleep you're sure to receive plenty of advice from well-meaning friends and family. One piece of advice you're bound to hear is that babies have to learn to sleep in light and/or noisy environments so they can be put to sleep anywhere.

That may be true when your baby or toddler has learnt to sleep independently and well. However, when he's starting out on the sleep journey you can help him by creating an environment that makes the process as stress-free as possible for him.

This usually means going back to basics, regardless of your child's age. Whether he is six months or two years old, if he's never been able to self-settle or resettle without assistance you need to take into account that the skills he has for the task are equivalent to those of a newborn.

The environmental conditions or aids you introduce to help your child learn to sleep don't have to be permanent. Once he has learnt how to settle and resettle without help you can begin weaning him off these conditions or aids in a time frame that is comfortable for both you and him. But while you're teaching him to sleep, set up the right conditions in a supportive environment so the process of learning in the first few days is as easy as possible.

How the environment affects your child's sleep

The poorer your child's sleep skills, the more overtired he is likely to be. And when babies are overtired they become overstimulated, so they respond to environmental factors more than your average well-slept baby. This makes them more alert or, in some cases, frenetic, which makes the task of going to sleep difficult. In some cases, overstimulation makes the task of resettling, when a baby naturally transitions from one sleep cycle to the next, almost impossible.

The first step in breaking this vicious circle is to reduce or eliminate any environmental factors stimulating your baby.

Environmental factors that can affect sleep

Environmental factors that can affect your child's ability to sleep well include:

- light
- noise
- temperature
- movement
- toys or comfort items such as dummies.

Addressing your child's sleep environment is key to reducing or eliminating tears when you're helping him work through poor and habitualised behavioural patterns at sleep time.

The good news is, ensuring your child's environment is conducive to sleep can be done fairly quickly and easily, and most unsettled babies will respond very quickly to the most basic environmental help, such as restricted or eliminated light and noise, a suitable air temperature, wrapping, and appropriate aids. In the right environment, your child will most likely settle quickly from the first attempt, and the number of times he wakes can be reduced by up to 90 per cent immediately.

Light

Our bodies are designed to respond to sunlight. When darkness falls, enzymes in the brain stimulate the release of melatonin, which induces sleep. When light hits the back of the eye's retina, the release of melatonin is halted and it becomes harder to sleep. Artificial lights, particularly bright downlights, influence the brain in much the same way.

While you might expect bright light to cause such a reaction, once a child becomes overstimulated even the slightest amount of light can affect him. This, in addition to any association he has with being able to make out shapes in his room during a partial-waking phase of his sleep, will be enough to cause him to wake up.

Therefore, when helping a baby to learn how to sleep past 5 a.m., or to sleep instead of catnapping during the day, eliminate or reduce light in his room.

Tips for reducing light

Below are tips for reducing or eliminating light in your baby's room. Some are temporary and can be replaced later by more permanent solutions like heavy curtains.

Block all light entering the room from windows

First, measure the windows in your child's room, including the window frame. Then purchase the required amount of curtain backing (adding 20 per cent to your measurements to ensure you have enough) to completely cover the window and window frames. The curtain backing you need is called P3, which provides 100 per cent light block-out. (NB: Cardboard does not do the same job.)

Using thumb-tacks, secure the P3 backing to the outer edges of the window frame so no light rays can come in. Once done, the room will be almost pitch black.

If you want to install curtains, ensure they have a 100 per cent block-out backing and, if possible, have ceiling-to-floor curtains, and allow extra width so light doesn't enter from the sides. Make them as flush to the wall as possible, and install a pelmet over the top. Alternatively, install a 100 per cent block-out blind behind the curtains so you can reintroduce some light into the room after your baby has learnt to settle and resettle independently.

I don't generally suggest outside awnings and roller blinds to reduce light during sleep training, but both can be useful in a particularly hot room. While costly, they are an alternative to air conditioning and can help children who are prone to irritated airways or suffer from repeated ear, nose and throat infections, which can arise from or be exacerbated by sleeping in air conditioning.

Eliminate all electrical lights

Disconnect, turn off or cover with electrical tape any night lights, clock displays, stereo systems or LED lights on monitors.

Block out all other light sources

Place a rolled-up towel on the floor outside your baby's door to prevent light filtering into the room. Turn off all lights in the hallway and nearby rooms or close doors to these rooms.

Noise

Noise is another environmental element that can affect your child's ability to sleep, so try to eliminate or reduce noise in or near his room when he is learning to sleep.

To immediately reduce noise in your baby's room:

- shut the door
- shut other doors in the house
- shut windows to reduce noise from outside
- don't play loud music or have the television on during your baby's sleep.

Dramatically reducing noise in your baby's room isn't as straightforward as eliminating light because it's not reasonable to expect your family to be silent while he sleeps. Nor can you eliminate the usual sounds from outside the house, such as traffic, birds, planes, etc. Therefore, another solution may be necessary.

White noise

A constant pattern of white noise can really help babies who are super-sensitive to noise. White noise is a sound that consists of all audible frequencies with equal intensity and provides a constant background noise that blocks out other noise. But unlike most other noises, the brain becomes so used to white noise it doesn't register it so your baby can sleep without noticing it.

I tested white noise on myself for eight weeks before I first tried it with babies and toddlers. I played it at the highest volume and initially it sounded like a jet engine and I didn't believe I'd ever be able to tune it out. However, I fell asleep without any more difficulty than usual and found the white noise didn't wake me during the night. Within a week, I had to check whether the white noise device I'd bought was actually turned on.

I was aware of one thing, however. As I drifted off to sleep, I suspect my brain tried to make sense of or decode the noise. As a result, I regularly heard rhythmic sound patterns which were possibly my brain's attempts to interpret the noise. However, these patterns were soothing and therapeutic as I drifted off to sleep so if you also hear patterns of sounds, it isn't the device or CD creating them.

Buying a white noise machine or CD

If you'd like to try white noise to help your child sleep, there are several machines and CDs available. Do some research before buying one to ensure it fulfils the manufacturer's promises.

If you buy a CD play it on repeat all night. Also, as you're running a CD player in your child's room throughout the night, install a smoke detector in the room. Don't forget to block out any light from the CD player.

If you buy a white noise machine, ensure it generates true white noise and not ocean sounds or a heartbeat. Do not buy a white noise machine that includes a ceiling projector or has a bright digital display, as they can create another problem.

How to introduce white noise into your baby's environment

Start by introducing the white noise into your child's play environment. Don't let him participate in the process, just tuck the machine or CD player out of sight.

To begin with, play the white noise at a low volume. You'll be able to hear it when you turn it on. It's not silent but the consistency of the sound encourages the brain to tune out and you'll soon stop noticing it.

Your child may initially react to the sound and look around. Try not to respond in any way and carry on as if it isn't there. When he sees you don't notice the sound, he will quickly tune it out.

If your toddler looks outside thinking it's raining when he first hears the white noise, or he's a little unsure of the sound, acknowledge his curiosity or concern. You might imitate the sound and comment that it sounds like rain, then ask him, 'Shall we look outside and see if it's raining?' Once you get to the window, say, 'No rain', then distract him and direct him back into play and carry on.

As the morning progresses, gradually turn the volume up. Leave it on for a couple of hours and get him used to the sound before introducing it to his sleep environment. When you start using it in his room, put it under the cot and leave it running all day so it's on when you change his nappy, after his bath, or if you walk past his room. In this way it becomes a normal sound in the room he won't think about at bedtime. Eventually, you'll be able to switch it on and off for sleep times.

White noise can help babies learning how to sleep and the devices for it are portable so you can take them on holidays, to restaurants and so on. Once your baby is sleeping better you can gradually reduce the volume and eventually turn it off completely. However, it will still be worth turning on every few days during your child's sleep so it's an option for when you really need it, such as on holidays or during a dinner party.

Temperature

The ideal room temperature for sleep varies. It is around 19 or 20 degrees when babies are swaddled and 21–23 degrees when they aren't. Most babies can't sleep well in a room temperature below 16 or above 24 degrees. Getting the room temperature right can be tricky because air temperature fluctuates a lot, even over a period of a few hours, depending on the time of day, the weather and the season. Nevertheless, try to ensure the room temperature is appropriate, and dress your baby in the appropriate clothing to sleep in to improve his ability to sleep well.

Is your baby too hot or cold?

You'll probably be fairly familiar with how air temperature varies in your house during different seasons and weather patterns, so you'll need to decide whether to have heating or cooling in your baby's room at these different times. This will also vary depending on your need to swaddle your baby or not. A swaddled baby using my technique will always sleep best when the room is 19–20 degrees.

Start by following your instincts. If you're kicking off your covers during the night because you're too hot, your baby is probably feeling the same way, so you may need to dress him in lighter clothing or install a cooling device in his room. Similarly, if you're too cold and looking for extra layers at night or putting on the heater, you may need to dress your child more warmly or put a heater on low, monitoring it, in his room to prevent him from getting too cold – which can lead to him rolling on to his tummy and curling up in a ball to stay warm, which is a high-risk factor for SIDS.

Before introducing heating or cooling, gauge the air temperature in his room using a simple thermometer or buy an all-weather-system house thermometer, with a portable main-base station and one or two separate thermometers that you can read remotely. Keep the main-base station in the living area or your bedroom and place one of the thermometers near your baby's cot so you can check it at any time without entering his room.

A note about humidifiers

If you do decide to use heating or cooling in the room, such as air-conditioning or a heater, be sure to use it in conjunction with a humidifier to keep the air moist to prevent your baby's mouth, lips, nose or airways drying out. This can, in turn, help prevent many of winter's snuffles, sneezes and wheezes.

If you have reverse-cycle air-conditioning

If your baby's room has reverse-cycle air-conditioning controlled by a thermostat, achieving an ideal air temperature should be easy. Simply set the thermostat to around 20 degrees and switch the air-conditioner on 30 minutes prior to bedtime to ensure an ideal air temperature before your baby goes to sleep. If your air-conditioner isn't fitted with a timer, you may have to turn it on and off manually.

Again, don't forget to use a humidifier in the room to maintain air moisture and prevent your baby's mouth, lips and nose from drying out.

Using a heater in cooler months

If your baby's room gets cold during the cooler months use a heater to warm it. The most convenient and safe kind of heater is an oil-filled column heater with a thermostat and timer, so you can control air temperature and the heater itself.

If your heater doesn't have a temperature gauge, consider purchasing a thermometer, as mentioned earlier. However, maintaining a constant air temperature is more difficult when your heater has no thermostat, so if you can afford it, splash out on a heater that monitors air temperature and adjusts itself accordingly. There are many affordable ones available.

If your heater has a thermostat, set it to 19 or 20 degrees and turn it on around half an hour before your child's bedtime. If not, still turn the heater on half an hour before and ensure it's around 19 or 20 degrees.

A timer allows you to set the heater to switch on and off, saving electricity and giving you more control of the temperature in your baby's room. If your heater doesn't have a timer you can buy one cheaply and fit it at the powerpoint.

Again, don't forget to use a humidifier to help prevent your baby's airways drying out if you are using a heater to warm your child's room.

Heater safety-first

- Never allow anything to lean on or touch the heater when it is on, and never leave it within reach of your baby.
- Do not use a radiant bar heater.
- Ensure the heater is designed to turn off automatically if it falls over.
- Dust all heaters, fans and air-conditioners regularly. Clean air-conditioner filters in hot water regularly and dry them in the sun for a few hours.
- Install smoke detectors throughout your house, including in your baby's room, and ensure they are working correctly.

Using a fan in warmer months

If your child's room isn't air-conditioned, you may want to use a fan to help keep him cool while he sleeps. Use a free-standing fan with either a built-in timer or a timer fitted at the power point. Set the fan to medium and don't direct it towards your baby. Instead, point it at a wall so the air flow bounces off and runs down over the top of his head lightly to keep air flow around him without drying out his nose or lips. If your baby's room regularly goes above 22–24 degrees a fan is not adequate if you need to swaddle him.

Appliance safety-first

Never allow your child to touch the fan or heater. Once you've established clear communication you can teach him not to touch the appliance. Until then, keep the appliance turned off and unplugged, except when he is safely in his cot. When you turn it on prior to bedtime, remember to keep the door shut and ensure your child cannot enter the room without you.

Appropriate sleepwear

Many parents worry they are dressing their baby too warmly or lightly for bed. This is easily solved if the air temperature in the room is between 19 and 20 degrees for a swaddled baby and between 21 and 23 degrees for a child dressed in clothing. If so, you can pop your baby into a cotton long-sleeved and full-legged outfit. This can be in the form of a safe, baby sleeping bag and long-sleeved top; or a full-body swaddle with a singlet; or a singlet under a long-sleeved cotton pyjama top and pants plus socks.

If your baby is over 12–16 months and doesn't need to be wrapped, use a light or heavy weight sleeping bag, depending on the season. Sleeping bags discourage standing up, keep your baby at just the right warmth, help prevent climbing out of the cot and act as a lovely pre-sleep cue. Avoid sleeping bags with a removable lower button-on foot portion. As wells as the dangers associated with buttons, a baby can get his feet caught outside the sleeping bag, defeating the purpose.

A baby tends to have more difficulty sleeping if his arms or torso are cold, so when it's cold I suggest warm, long sleeves under a sleeveless sleeping bag. In summer, a light, long-sleeved cotton t-shirt under a light-weight, cotton, sleeveless sleeping bag will help a baby to sleep soundly.

A child under two should only sleep in anything less than a light-weight long- or short-sleeved cotton shirt in extremely hot environments. A baby should only sleep in just a singlet when he's out and about in hot weather, such as in a pram.

When room or body temperature fluctuates

It would be a lot simpler if air and body temperature remained constant, but your baby's body temperature can fluctuate as a result of hormones or tiredness.

When your baby gets cold during the daytime sleep

Being too cold is a more common cause of children's daytime sleep problems than being too warm. So while it's important not to overheat children, we should also make sure they are not cold.

If the room temperature is ideal, your first step in helping your baby sleep is to add an extra layer of clothing to his torso and arms. A child will always need long sleeves at night, but may actually need an additional layer for days compared with the early portion of their night sleep.

When your baby is warm at the end of the day

The other most common body-temperature fluctuation occurs when a baby first goes to bed at the end of the day, when he is often warmer than usual. Therefore, keep him a little cooler towards the end of the day, reserving any warm layers of clothing such as long-sleeved tops, sleeping bags or swaddles until just before your bedtime at 10 p.m. to ensure he goes to bed at a cooler temperature, allowing the environment to gradually warm him.

If your baby is naturally a warm baby, give him a cooler bath at the end of the day. Ensure his room stays at around 20 degrees until around

10 p.m. In the warmer months, cool it for 30 minutes before you put him down at night. In the cooler months, don't turn on the heating until 10 p.m. to ensure he doesn't overheat in the first few hours of his evening sleep. If the room is 18 degrees or below, heat the room half an hour before bed, but be careful not to make the room too hot initially. Just take the chill out of the air.

Alternatively, use a free-standing fan in your baby's room for the early part of the night with a timer at the power point or an extension lead long enough to plug in outside the room so you can turn the fan on and off easily without risking waking your baby. Unless you have a particularly warm baby, turn off the fan after 10–11 p.m. if his room is a healthy 19–22 degrees.

Cool a room half an hour before you put a baby to bed rather than once he goes to bed or he may become too hot and wake up quickly as a result.

When air temperature fluctuates

Air temperature in a house can fluctuate, particularly at around 4 or 5 a.m. when it can drop dramatically. This happens to coincide with when a baby is approaching the final stage of his night sleep. As a baby cannot regulate his temperature by pulling coverings on or off, he has to rely on the air to keep his body at a comfortable temperature. If he becomes too cold, he will wake and instinctively cry to warm up.

However when you first put him to bed at night he's warmer than he's likely to be later. Therefore, it's not really practical to dress him in preparation for a 4 a.m. temperature drop without risking him being too warm when he goes to sleep.

You can put a blanket on him at 10 p.m. though you can't be sure it will stay on him until early morning. To manage the 4 a.m. temperature drop in the cooler months of the year, dress him to cope with the first part of the night, then work with the early morning room temperature to prevent him getting too cool. If you have a heater with a thermostat and timer, set the heater's timer so it comes on and regulates the room by around 3.30 a.m. This ensures the room is at the right temperature when he comes to the next light stage of sleep.

Movement

My key advice to parents about how to help their children sleep with as little stress as possible, and avoid him waking, is to wrap or swaddle their babies tight.

After your baby is born you hold him in your arms. You might hold his face up close to your neck to provide comfort. And you might even whisper 'Sssshhhhhhhhhhhh,' to calm him. What you've *taught* him by using these instinctive calming tools is that being held firmly is comforting.

Swaddling your baby has a similar soothing effect as holding him and is one of the most important comforting tools we have. I call the swaddle the 'surrogate cuddle in the cot'.

Even for children as old as 12–16 months who 'hated' being wrapped as a tiny baby or prefer to sleep on their tummy or move around in the cot, the swaddle can make the difference between crying and not crying much or at all. The swaddle is great for these children and for babies who can self-settle but have short sleep cycles or regular wakings that require intervention from a parent or carer.

Nevertheless, often when I swaddle a baby his parents will tell me he 'hates being wrapped' or 'can get out of every wrap'. Most of those parents change their mind when they see how much their baby loves being wrapped because, if done properly, it keeps him snug as a bug for his entire sleep.

If your baby is under 12 months of age and has been struggling to go to sleep or go back to sleep, or experiencing multiple or premature wakings, he will benefit enormously from a firm swaddling wrap similar to that used for a newborn baby. Firm swaddling allows babies aged six to 12 months plus to feel secure and comfortable. A wrap will also stop him from startling himself awake with sudden limb movements and discourage babies who are unable to lie down by themselves from automatically sitting or standing up before they've woken up fully.

It takes just one or two sleep sessions for most babies to adjust to the swaddle. They can then go to sleep without crying and stay asleep for periods of 11 or more hours. I see this even with children who have been unable to sleep for longer than 30 minutes to an hour at a time prior to wrapping. Most parents are staggered by the level of comfort it provides for their child.

Another comment parents make is that as soon as they lie their baby down to wrap him he starts to cry and fight. However, rather than the wrap being what these babies are fighting, it's the message the wrap delivers that it's time to go to bed, something many children prefer not to do. A genuine sign of not liking a wrap is when a baby wriggles out of it and stops crying and sleeps better when free of it, which I rarely see during sleep repair.

Try not to impose your adult views on the swaddle. When your child becomes upset and you hold him to calm him down you don't do it to restrain him but to comfort him. You did not teach him that cuddles represent restraint. Swaddling has long been a normal part of a baby's life in most cultures and countries because it is the most effective comfort and sleep-inducing device available.

If your baby needs to be held, won't sleep in his cot, or stands and screams in his cot to be picked up, is in your bed, or wakes over and over again and is unable to sustain sleep, then firmly swaddling him *will* be the quickest way to help him get to sleep and stay asleep.

The trick is to wrap your baby firmly enough so he remains swaddled for the entire sleep so his environment remains the same from settling till he wakes up.

Think of swaddling as a *temporary* surrogate firm cuddle in your baby's cot to make him feel safe while he's *learning* to go to sleep in an environment that is new to him. Later, when he's learnt how to sleep he won't need to be wrapped.

If you're still doubtful, check progress after the third day and night of swaddling, remembering that if your baby complains it's likely to be about going to bed rather than about being swaddled. In most cases, after three days and nights of being swaddled, babies are settling and sleeping beautifully.

So if your baby is under 12 months of age, DO *NOT* DISMISS THE WRAP. Even an extremely unsettled 14 to 16 month old can be comforted by a leg wrap, Safe T Sleep (see page 166–7) or the tuck-in techniques I'll describe.

Who should be fully swaddled?

I recommend swaddling any babies between six and 16 months who are:

- transitioning from being dependent on others to help them fall asleep to self-settling and self-resettling for the first time in their life.
- under 12 months and waking repeatedly during the night or sleep for no more than 30 to 40 minutes at a time during the day
- constantly calling out to be held while they go to sleep or resettle
- wanting regular feeds and snuggles to go back to sleep – these babies are often a little cool and the warmth of the swaddle is the same as a cuddle
- between six and 12 months and constantly stand up at sleep time and are unable to lie down again, or are standing up automatically before they've opened their eyes when they reach the semi-conscious state of surface sleep.

Who doesn't need to be swaddled?

If your baby is older than 12 months and is settling and resettling independently but sleeping at odd times of the day and night, he doesn't need to be swaddled. Instead, adopt a sleep routine that suits his daily sleep requirement. You also don't need to swaddle your child if he is 12 months or over and just needs a dummy to put himself to sleep. Just teach him how to get the dummy himself (see page 180).

What kind of wrap to use?

The best kind of wrap for swaddling should be as large or larger than a cot sheet and made of very light, thin muslin. Simply buy a few metres of very fine cotton muslin. I have the local dry cleaners make up two wraps to the dimensions of 1400 mm × 1800 mm. Have at least two wraps so you can wash one and use one, or in case you need a double wrap.

If you are concerned your baby will get his arms free no matter what you do, you could try to use a double swaddle. I have developed a wrap DVD that will clearly teach you escape-proof wrap technique, which is also available on my website.

Before you swaddle

Before you swaddle your baby:

- If his mattress has a plastic side, ensure the fabric side is on top.
- Make sure his bath isn't too hot, as he won't sleep if he's overheated at the end of the day, and swaddling will warm him.
- A wrapped baby must be safely positioned on his back for the night with a Safe T Sleep and tuck-in in place, a singlet, nappy and light muslin swaddle for summer or winter if he is in a full wrap or a nappy and a light long-sleeved top in a one-arm wrap or leg wrap. You can also heat or cool the room to an appropriate temperature. My wrap DVD will demonstrate all of the above (www.australianbabywhisperer.com.au).
- Even on cooler nights, avoid putting any covers on your baby when he is wrapped for the night, a firm sheet tuck-in over the Safe T Sleep with the wrap will be adequate.

The Safe T Sleep

For older babies who are getting too big to be wrapped (13–16 months), but still clearly need the comfort and security that the swaddle provides, use a Safe T Sleep to firmly and securely tuck them in. These would be used for all babies and toddlers that require immediate repair. A Safe T Sleep is like a firm tuck-in that is attached to the mattress, that will not come loose like normal sheets would. This allows you to tuck your baby into place and for him to learn to sleep peacefully without tossing and turning and getting up endlessly, and ensures he never loses his covers. This is possibly one of the most brilliant sleep support devices I've ever encountered in my career which I credit with enabling me to to get stunning results in sleep repair at amazing rates.

'As snug as a bug in a rug': how to swaddle

When you introduce anything new to your child it can cause some upset, and swaddling is no different. It is therefore vital to take the time to help your child become familiar with the swaddle before you introduce it into his sleep-time routine. You can do this by using role playing to ensure he understands what's going to be asked of him and the sequence of events in his new sleep routine. A good time to do this is during cot playtime.

When you are confident your baby understands what is expected and the sequence of events, you will be able to introduce your new daily routine, using your new settling routine, incorporating your new environmental aids like wraps and Safe T Sleeps. You must do it all at once to ensure the correct association is linked to the wrap and the settling routine.

Practise first

Swaddling a baby aged six to 12 months is done differently to swaddling a newborn. You need to ensure the wrap stays in place all night and is a no-movement wrap. It's important when swaddling this age group to wrap it nice and firmly to discourage them from struggling to see if they can squirm free.

It's worth practising your swaddle many times on a large teddy bear or doll before you try swaddling your baby because you need to be able to swaddle a baby quickly and smoothly while you concentrate on sounding confident and reassuring.

You also need to practise to ensure you can swaddle your baby firmly enough that they can't wriggle free for eleven or more hours. If your baby learns he can squirm free on the first or second time you swaddle him, he will try every time so you should aim to get it right the first time so he can stay focused on the task of going to sleep. If you do get it right, he will settle very quickly.

If you are concerned he will get his arms free no matter what you do, I've made a 'wiggly worm arm pockets' wrap insert you can purchase via my website. Otherwise a double wrap may help you get your swaddle just right to help bubby get to sleep as quickly as possible.

Styles of swaddles

I recommend various styles of swaddles and tuck-ins for babies under 16 months, depending on the baby, the sleep issue and their age. I call these four styles:

- the full surrogate hug
- the one-arm wrap
- the leg wrap
- the firm tuck-in.

The full surrogate hug

The full surrogate hug is designed to provide the same security as a car seat, pram, sling, pouch or cuddle, by holding a baby still so he can fall asleep. It is a temporary strategy to help him learn how to sleep in as short a period as possible.

This type of swaddle will prevent a baby from startling himself fully awake during a sudden partial waking (usually between 10 and 11 p.m., at around 2 a.m., and between 4 and 5 a.m. if your baby goes to bed at 7 p.m.) or getting distracted from the task of falling asleep by rolling, kicking, flapping hands, standing and then being unable to lie down, or just generally fussing too much.

Once your baby has gained confidence in falling asleep independently, he won't need the security of a full surrogate hug and you can start to wrap him more loosely, or purchase a Safe T Sleep from any leading children's store.

PREPARING THE WRAP

Spread out the wrap with the long edge running horizontal in front of you (that is, opposite to the way you'd spread out a beach towel to lie on).

Fold down the top long edge by 10 centimetres for added strength.

Position your baby slightly right of centre, so there is a long section of sheet on either side of his body. Ensure the top of the wrap is at the level of the bottom of his ears.

There are four steps to swaddling, each involving the four corners: the top-right portion, the bottom-right portion, the entire left side of the muslin wrapped around his body once, then the final leg wrap from the remaining muslin on the bottom left side of the wrap.

1. THE TOP-RIGHT PORTION

Hold your child's left arm firm and straight by the side of his body and against the mattress, with his thumb facing up, while you gather the muslin from his left shoulder to his nappy. (If you have problems keeping his arm in place while you do the first tuck-in, tuck the arm into a 'wiggly worm arm pockets' wrap insert first.)

Pull the gathered material in your right hand towards the ceiling then firmly across his body keeping all material above his feet, while ensuring his left arm is still securely in place. Your baby's right arm is not included in this tuck-in, but remains lying free beside him.

After you've pulled the muslin across his body using your right hand, firmly hold it against the mattress with your left hand, in readiness to tuck it under his back and bottom. Only when you are holding the sheet firmly against the mattress with your left hand are you safe to release the material from the grip of your right hand. This ensures you don't lose any firmness as the wrap is holding his left arm in place.

To tuck in the material now in your left hand, reach over your baby with your now-free right hand and place it on the left side of the sheet that is still lying flat on the bed. Holding that flat with your right hand, firmly tuck the gathered sheet from his left side under his bottom and back using your left hand.

In addition to tucking the sheet under him, try to push his body further into the wrap now securing his left side. This will ensure he is even more firmly locked in and prevent him from wiggling his left arm free while you are wrapping him.

2. THE BOTTOM-RIGHT PORTION

Find the furthest point on the folded lower right side of the sheet and pull it up and over his legs firmly and tuck under the same point of his lower back (if it can reach) as the first tuck-in you just completed. Again push him into the tuck-in firmly so the sheet becomes tight all the way down his body and his legs are now moving within a loose pocket. Don't worry if his knee bends up; this is generally what happens with a wrap until the final wrap around is complete. Just try to make sure his legs are straight and together when you start the next part.

3. THE ENTIRE LEFT SIDE OF THE WRAP

Repeat the first step, but with the left side of the sheet. Then, with his right side now held firmly in place by the gather of material in your left hand, pull the sheet across the top of his body above his feet, not below them. Use your right hand and arm to firmly sweep the rest of the sheet under his body from the right side back to the left side, and pull on the sheet very firmly to tighten it from the top, all the way down the length of the body, so he becomes well secured and unable to move his arms and legs. This needs to be done quickly and firmly to prevent him wriggling free, especially if you aren't using the 'wiggly worm arm pockets' wrap insert.

4. THE FINAL LEG WRAP FROM THE BOTTOM (YOUR LEFT SIDE)

After firmly wrapping the sheet around him, the long portion of sheet remaining on the lower left side goes around his legs. In a broad sash, lift the sheet up and over his legs then back under his legs, pulling firmly to ensure his knees come together. When you've wrapped the final piece of material around his legs pull it tight and tuck the end into the wrap in a place where it is tight so it can be held firmly in place.

Just before you pick your baby up, tighten up the loose piece of material on your top left and ensure it doesn't come loose when you carry him to his room.

One-arm wrap – variation for ten to 12 month olds

The full swaddle is best but some older babies need a free hand for their self-settling comfort items such as a thumb, dummy, cuddly toy, rag or some other tool to help them go to sleep. Note, however, that this swaddle is designed only for those babies who are already good at using an effective tool to settle and resettle themselves. The 'wiggly worm arm pockets' wrap insert can still be used for their one enclosed arm to help keep the wrap in place.

This wrap is for his legs and one arm and will help prevent your child from startling himself to a full waking during his partial wakings (at 11 p.m. and 2 a.m. and between 4 and 5 a.m.) or getting distracted from the task of falling asleep by rolling, playing, kicking his legs into the air or fussing.

Once your baby gains confidence in falling asleep independently, you can start to do the wrap up loosely and let him just enjoy the comfort of the Safe T Sleep.

This wrap is done almost exactly the same as the full surrogate hug with a single exception: part 3, the left-side section.

Follow steps one and two of the surrogate hug wrap. But in Step 3, rather than keep his right arm by his side, raise it before proceeding to gather the muslin and pull it towards the ceiling, then across his body towards his left side under his right arm. With his right hand free, pull the sheet across the top of his body ensuring it goes above his feet, not below them. Using your right hand and arm, firmly sweep the rest of the sheet under his body from right back to the left side and pull on the sheet very firmly to tighten it from his armpit, all the way down the length of the body, so he becomes well secured and unable to move his left arm and legs. This needs to be done quickly and firmly to prevent him from wriggling free if you are not using the 'wiggly worm arm pockets' wrap insert.

Proceed with final leg wrap of the surrogate hug wrap.

Leg wrap – variation for ten to 16 month olds

This firm leg wrap, used in conjunction with a Safe T Sleep and tuck-in, is a comfort for babies who can self-settle using a comfort item but are prone to multiple wakings. This particular wrap is for baby's legs only and designed to prevent him startling himself fully awake during a sudden partial waking (at 11 p.m. and 2 a.m., and between 4 and 5 a.m.) or getting distracted from the task of falling asleep by rolling, playing, kicking his legs into the air. It is also designed to emulate the feeling and limited movement a pram or car seat provides, which is effective in helping babies settle down and drift off to sleep quickly. Once your baby has gained confidence in being able to fall asleep, you can do the wrap up loosely, and let him enjoy the security and comfort of the Safe T Sleep.

Place your baby on the wrap so the top of the muslin comes up to his armpits. Raise up his left arm so it is out of the way. Then proceed with the first and second steps of the surrogate hug wrap.

Raise his right arm out of the way. Then proceed with the third and fourth steps of the surrogate hug wrap.

The firm tuck-in

The firm tuck-in is designed for babies who can sometimes self-settle and self-resettle, but may also stand and protest for a very long time if the mood strikes them and they are displeased with a request to go to sleep. These babies tend to have a fairly comfortable positioning method already and only need the security of a Safe T Sleep and a firm tuck-in to assist them in lying down and feeling secure. This often corrects wakings through the night immediately by allowing them to feel as though they are being held when they wake briefly in the middle of the night.

It's *very* important this strategy is always used in conjunction with consistent settling, resettling and waking routines. These routines should be role played before using them in your baby's sleep time. Place your baby down on his back in the Safe T Sleep device, allow him to assume his favourite position and do it up firmly. Follow the instruction provided with the Safe T Sleep. Then tuck him in as follows.

I learnt the art of tucking in from my mum, who developed a routine that involved a song called 'Go to Sleep and Goodnight', before tucking us in. I clearly remember lying in my cot, loving the feeling as she bounced my mattress tucking all the sheets in firmly. After she left, I would lie there as still as I could so the bedding would stay all firm, just as my mum had made it. So when I tuck in babies now, I am inspired by this lovely bed routine my parents used on all three of their children, born 13 years apart. And we were all excellent sleepers.

The trick is to get the bedding nice and firm so your baby can feel safe and snuggled each night. Make the bed without your baby in it first. Then tuck them in as suggested below. First, to make the bed, use the length of the flat cot sheet across the width of the cot, rather than long-ways. Then tuck the sheet in on the far side of the cot so there is a lot of length under the mattress. Spread any extra coverings you need over the sheet and tuck them in place on the far side before pushing cloth nappies or a towel firmly down the gap between the tucked-in covers and the cot side to prevent the covers coming loose during the night. Then pull everything from the far side firmly and tuck the covers under the near side of the mattress, just as you did on the far side, ready to be locked into place with towel rolls as well once your baby's in bed. Pull back the near top corner of the bedding and open up the Safe T Sleep, if you are using one, ready for baby to be tucked snugly into bed when you settle him. Now your cot is ready.

When you are ready to tuck in your baby, with the cot side down lie your little one at the top of the cot on the fitted sheet, then gently slide his legs under the neatly made sheets. Slide them down into the firm sheets. When he is in the right position, do up the Safe T Sleep or smooth out his sleeping bag if you are using one before you start the process of tucking in the near top corner of the bedding you loosened earlier. Lift the cot side before you lock his sheet firmly into place by slightly lifting the mattress on your side and pulling and tucking the sheets firmly and deeply under the mattress. The final step is to push cloth nappies or a towel down the gap between the tucked-in sheets and the cot bars along the length of your baby's body. Sliding the nappy rolls down the side of the mattress may be a little challenging, as it should be. It should be pretty hard for you to get them out again also, meaning they are safely secured.

Your baby is now officially 'as snug as a bug in a rug'.

Weaning your baby off the wrap

Weaning your baby off something implies *you* have decided he should no longer have a particular thing as it is now detrimental to his development. If your baby is content in the wrap and sleeping well for the first time in his life however, and you are using a Safe T Sleep and a good tuck-in, then it is clearly not detrimental to them. When you use a temporary wrap, and you suddenly find your baby sleeping all night every night peacefully, don't be in a rush to get rid of the thing your baby has found so comforting. Remember, throw away any preconceived adult concepts about a swaddle. Keep it in place firmly for as long as you like and do not attempt to loosen it until your baby starts to show signs he is ready to transition from the swaddle.

Alternatively, if you're keen to do away with it, wait three to six weeks before you start to look for signs. To find out whether your baby is ready to come out of his wrap, gradually make it a little looser on one hand at a time. If he has one arm or both in the 'wiggly worm arm pockets' wrap insert, then stop using the pockets one at a time, but continue to wrap him as firmly as always. Don't loosen his legs just yet. This is when your baby will tell you if he is ready to sleep without this added security or not. A great indication is that you go in to him the next morning and he has one or both arms out of the wrap and has continued sleeping anyway.

If he is in the process of being weaned from the wrap, make sure he is wearing longer sleeves of an appropriate thickness. Once out of his swaddle, I always transition him into a child-safe sleeping bag.

In this initial self-weaning process, you should still, as always, maintain a surface-sleep window pause of around ten minutes (see page 354) and the appropriate responses to crying before attending to him. Apart from ensuring you do not trigger episodes of wild thrashing by fully waking him accidentally, you are also making sure you don't interfere on those first few occasions as he moves about and has a grizzle and a grumble under the new conditions before drifting back off to sleep.

Once this process begins and your child is starting to sleep with his arms out each night, either do the wrap loosely around his arms, or don't wrap his arms at all.

If in that time his sleep deteriorates again, then he should be wrapped firmly again and not be given the opportunity to self-wean for a further three to six weeks. You will see him sleeping solidly again once you re-do the wrap.

I find that boys want and need to keep the wrap a little longer than girls, but will show clear signs when they are ready to be out of their wraps by wiggling hands out and sleeping on happily.

Once your baby is wearing the Safe T Sleep and is sleeping well with only his leg wrapped, maintain a firm leg wrap until you can come in the next morning and see he has been able to kick it loose, and move his legs about inside the swaddle freely but still sleep. This means he is ready to sleep completely without the wrap and you can just provide a pretend leg swaddle, to maintain the predictability of the settling process. Once he is happy with this, just bypass the wrapping process altogether and pop him into a sleeping bag instead, then the Safe T Sleep.

Comfort items

When I work with babies aged between six and 12 months, unless they already have an attachment to a safe comfort item like a muslin toy or muslin cloth, I don't encourage one because it often takes longer to introduce a comfort item, leaving room for crying and stress, so it's easier to swaddle babies to repair sleep quickly. If babies are over 12 months and have a regular comfort item in their cot or through the day, I encourage that attachment because it helps the settling process. If children over 12 months are transitioning from co-sleeping to an independent sleeping environment, I develop a comfort item association around a safe teddy bear.

If your baby is still under 12 months and has developed a strong attachment to a comfort item, and still falls into the group of unsettled babies who need to be wrapped to help them feel secure and comforted while they learn how to sleep, I'd suggest the one-arm wrap. In extremely unsettled babies, you may need to eliminate the comfort item and replace it with the temporary comfort of the surrogate hug provided by the full swaddle. As this is only a temporary measure, within a few weeks to months when your baby has been sleeping well and is enjoying going to bed and sleeping through the night, you can move to a one-arm wrap and reintroduce the comfort item. Gradually, over the next couple of weeks, your baby should begin to sleep without the wrap as he will be comfortable with the conditions of sleeping in his cot.

When choosing a comfort item, teddy bears need to be a well sewn and high-quality, free of buttons or long ribbons, and have stitched cotton eyes, nose and mouth. Read all tags carefully and always remove any non-essential tag, like the sachet pouch containing extra cotton or the bear birth certificate, and examine the bear for any potential choking hazards.

Remove any ribbons that are not firmly stitched to the bear. Avoid bears which contain stuffing like beads or straw. If the bear starts to come apart at the seams, always have it professionally restored to ensure your baby cannot choke on any filling that may come loose. Don't allow a bear with fur that's showing signs of easily coming away from the product. It's normal for bears to wear down and become bald from excessive loving, but it should be a gradual process. Always try to buy a duplicate teddy if he is desperately in love with his bear so you can wash it regularly to keep it dust-mite free and hygienic.

Toys made of muslin are the safest form of comfort item for children over six months of age to have in their cot because the baby can still breathe if a muslin toy happens to go near his mouth. Muslin-based comfort-snuggle rabbits and bears are widely available but again, looking for a good-quality version is essential.

Dummies

Dummies are a hot subject in debates about parenting. However, judging parents for the choices they make is more destructive than any dummy could ever be. While I try to eliminate dummies from a child's day once he's about six months old, they can be useful if the baby is having a difficult time with reflux in the very early stages of his life or you would like to stretch out the time between feeds a little without your baby becoming stressed. With reflux, the suckling and subsequent swallowing helps keep stomach acids from tracking up and irritating. Because of this, it is understandable that a parent might find a dummy extremely soothing for their baby and decide to use one.

By six months of age, however, if you haven't resolved your infant's reflux with your doctor, then do so. I find that dummies are only ever associations and are never a relief for physical symptoms by this age, which means your baby has a habit of sucking the dummy, not a need for it. The dummy is a solution to certain conditions or feelings he has. Ask yourself what your child uses his dummy for. It can be his solution for coping with being tired, bored, dealing with emotions like feeling grumpy, frustrated or angry, or when impatient on a car or pram trip.

Dummies can affect sleep in two ways. Firstly, if your baby doesn't know how to put the dummy in his own mouth he won't be able to put himself to sleep or back to sleep without your intervention, which is a problem that can lead to a learnt pattern of dependent associations in order to sleep. These children will need help for a minimum of two to three times a night, and if the constant need to call out makes them overtired they can wake even more often. In a worst-case scenario, they can wake as often as every 20 to 40 minutes, 24 hours a day.

Secondly, by allowing your baby to always deal with his emotions using a dummy you teach him to never express himself, to always resolve emotions by putting something in his mouth, and to not learn to feel the range of emotions he would naturally experience at sleep time, like being a little grumpy, or having to be patient and quiet. If you can see your child is over-dependent on a dummy during the day, and it's preventing him from learning to cope with a range of normal emotions, it's time to get rid of it.

If I am addressing significant sleep-time problems in a child aged six to 12 months I remove their access to a dummy using a two-step process. The first step occurs in the lead-up to starting a new daily routine, when I make the dummy a sleep-time-only comforter. In the few days before I start any new routine I don't allow the baby to have the dummy when he's out of his cot. During the homework phase of your PRM (see Dream Baby Profile pages 11–12) you need to make your child's dummy a sleep-time-only comforter. A lot of parents worry their child will cry if they do this. This may occur because the child hasn't yet learnt he can cope with waiting in a pram or feeling a little frustrated or grumpy on occasions and recover without this aid. Be patient because though some babies adjust quickly others may take a day or two. Just don't go back to the dummy once you remove it from his daytime. If your baby hasn't had the opportunity to practise feeling emotions and resolving them without the dummy during the day, it isn't fair to ask him to cope without it at night yet.

Avoid replacing one oral emotional solution to normal emotions with another, such as offering snacks to your baby. Instead, be reassuring and use the strategies in the communication sections of this book. Remember to be consistent during this process. Don't confuse your baby or teach him to cry by sometimes giving him the dummy at a non-sleep time if he *really* cries, because it teaches your baby that 'if you really want the dummy, you need to really cry!'

Once you eliminate the dummy from daytime use, stick to your plan and help your baby work through new ways to cope with emotions. Show him how books can be soothing or find a safe comfort bear, muslin or snuggly toy to cuddle, or play with him until he feels better. He will soon learn that the emotions are okay and he can cope without the dummy. After two days it shouldn't be an issue and you'll be ready for step two, which is to embark on your new daily routine, sleep repair program with the full PRM approach with new environmental comforts like the wrap or tuck-in and without the dummy. Your baby will have had the chance to be exposed to his emotions during the day and, more importantly, to have learnt to cope with them better without the dummy at sleep time.

Please note, if your ten to 12 month old is not suffering significant sleep-time problems and you only need to pop the dummy in his mouth once in a blue moon when he wakes, then it's best to work with the dummy game (see page 180) designed for 12 to 24 month olds than to remove it.

The dummy and sleep time for 12 to 24 month olds

When your baby is between 12 and 24 months you can decide whether or not to get rid of the dummy at sleep time. When you look at true needs versus short-term demands you can see your baby's sleep won't be disrupted if you teach him how to get the dummy himself. If a child has significant sleep-time problems, I tend to not take the dummy away from him as it can act as a real comforter during a major change. I reason that if he's had it this long you may as well use it to your advantage. Then, when he is more comfortable with his new self-settling routines, you can consider removing it from sleep time altogether *if* and *when* it is necessary.

While I would not introduce a dummy to a child of my own unless it was for temporary reflux or feed-stretching purposes, and nor would I sustain the use of a dummy after six months of age, I wouldn't suddenly decide when the baby is 12 months old that because it suited me, the baby could no longer have it. If a child has had their dummy that long, making it a cot-only sleeping aid and teaching him how to get it himself is not damaging to him in any way.

If a baby was absolutely struggling with independence and the dummy pot game (page 180), or the dummy was never that big a deal to the child at sleep time when I arrived to resolve their sleep-time issues, this would be my motivation to take it away at all sleep and non-sleep times. If, however, you decide to keep the dummy as a sleep aid, and want to help him become more independent, establish independence through the dummy pot game. I would still work on the principle of eliminating the dummy at all non-sleep-time portions of the day using the same strategy as for eliminating the dummy for six to 12 month olds.

Be honest with him. Answer his request for a dummy with 'Dummy is all gone. Dummy is for nigh' nigh' time only.' Make sure you've removed it from sight and from where he can get it, and work through his reaction without giving in.

Support your child through the emotions of the situation with a confident voice, body language and positive feedback. Show him another way to make him feel better, like cuddling a teddy or muslin snuggly toy for instance, which might be useful for him in the cot environment. Be consistent and remember to define what 'dummy all gone' means, so don't say it's gone then bring it out because that will confuse him and you won't be able to eliminate it quickly or without tears.

As mentioned earlier, however, if he relies on the dummy for sleep time, there is no need to take it away at sleep time. The main aim is to ensure he knows he is the one who can put it into his mouth, he knows where he can find it, even in the dark, and he understands you'd like him to do it for himself. Empowering your baby with the ability to get his own dummy at sleep time eliminates the need to take it away from him altogether or constantly do the dummy run through the night.

You can do this using language cues and dummy pots. The language cue is simply 'Get your dummy'. The concept for the dummy pot is also simple: you put several or all of his dummies in two soft material pots safely secured to the top corners of his cot where he can always find them, even in the dark. You then teach your baby how to get their dummy by playing the dummy pot game (see box on page 180) and show him where those pots are when it's time to go to sleep. You then establish a settling and resettling routine that incorporates him always getting his own dummy to go to sleep and to go back to sleep. This teaches your child to automatically reach out and find his own dummy when he wakes during the night, and eliminates his need to cry because he no longer needs you to come in and find it for him.

You'll need to play the dummy pot game first at non-sleep times so you can practise the new language and create a positive association around the use of it. Before you start, use your flow of communication to let him know that soon you're going to play the dummy pot game while showing him the pot. When it's time to play, be enthusiastic. You'll need to ask him to wait by using your wait cue so he doesn't just grab the dummies and put them straight into his mouth. While this is the ultimate aim of the game, establish the language cue 'get your dummy' so you can incorporate it into his sleep-time ritual so he must wait.

Once your baby has been introduced to the new language cue of the dummy pot game, you can firmly fix the two dummy pots to his cot, with their bases resting on the mattress so he can reach in and get one without standing up. If your baby moves all over the cot during his sleep put one pot at each end, or put two pots at the top end in each corner and put all your baby's dummies in the two pots. If he is going to have a dummy, he needs to be able to find one at all times during the night, so there is no point in having only one or two dummies.

Show your child the two filled dummy pots before starting his settling routine. There should be no dummies during story time, even if he asks, because it's too confusing for children to not be allowed dummies outside the cot, but then have a different set of rules when it suits you. It also discourages active communication during story reading. By not allowing him dummies during stories, you encourage him to feel comfortable with the tired sensation without the need for a dummy, making the transitioning into self-settling in his cot without the dummy as he gets older, easier. Finally, by leaving the dummies in the cot, you make it so he's excited to go to bed because he has something to look forward to.

If he asks for a dummy, say, 'Soon, but let's have stories first' and head to the couch. Incorporate the cue 'Nearly time to get your dummy' into your settling routine pre-emptive language. Follow your settling-routine position and management if your child protests about not being given his dummy for stories. Once you've finished your settling routine head into his room and continue your routine with his settling song and a cuddle in your arms without giving him the dummy. When it's time to put him into his cot, say, 'Time for sleep, Mummy and Daddy love you' and 'Nigh' nigh', lie down, get your dummy'. At this point, he must lie down before he gets his dummy and, if at any point during the sleep-time process he stands up, take it out of his mouth and put it back in a dummy pot until he's lying down again.

He must lie down (with or without your help) before he can have his dummy back. You can assist him to reach into his pot once he is lying down if he can't find it, but do not give it to him. Don't be alarmed if he takes a large number of dummies initially; he will soon discover it's challenging to work out how to use so many of his favourite things at one time. It's okay for him to hold some and swap them around and try a couple at once during those first days. It will all settle down before too long, and he will go back to just enjoying one at a time.

If you don't want to give him more than one dummy because you'd rather he not have any at all, then it's time to take the dummy away altogether at sleep time. There's no point in doing the game half-heartedly because you're reluctant to give him the dummy. He'll need multiple dummies if you want to ensure he doesn't lose them in the middle of the night and doesn't need to call out to get you to help him.

During those first few days he doesn't have to take a dummy if he doesn't want to, but the request to lie down remains. During resettling times, your routine will be the same, with a minor variation consistent with your original settling process. Once you enter his room to resettle him, ask him to lie down if he is standing, and remove the dummies from his mouth or hands or both and put them back in the pot before assisting him or asking him to lie down again. Have a quick feel around the cot and pop all the dummies back in the pots during those first few days. Continue on with your settling routine and when he is lying down as requested point to the pot, or rattle the dummies in the pot, or guide his hand to the pot again and say 'Get your dummy'. Don't put the dummy in his hand or mouth and don't remove the dummy pots from their original positions as it's important to teach him how and where to reach out to find his dummies so he can become self-sufficient.

The dummy pot game

Sit your baby down on the floor, in his high chair, on the couch or wherever you're comfortable and show him the new dummy pot. If he is prone to crawling off, then you're better to play this game in the high chair, or on the couch where he is between your legs, etc. First you say 'Wait for Mummy' and then show him the dummies and put them in the pot, still encouraging him to wait. When you ask him to wait, block his hands if you need to and have an enthusiastic look on your face that indicates waiting is fun, not a punishment or demand, and follow through.

Once he is waiting say 'Get your dummy' and remove your hands to allow him to get his dummy and pop it in his mouth. If he grabs it, get excited. Clap and cheer, and repeat the cue 'Good getting your dummy' before saying 'Ta for Mummy/Pop' and quickly slipping the dummy out of his mouth and back in his pot. If you do all this with a sense of humour, he will laugh at your antics and you will be able to start the game again. Each time you pop the dummy out of his mouth, always say 'Pop . . . ohhh' and do a little surprise look and jump. If you're repetitious with this, he will think you're pretty funny.

If he is not sure if he is meant to grab the dummy, you're teaching him what 'get your dummy' actually means. The entire purpose of asking him to wait is to get him to respond specifically to the language cue 'get your dummy'. If he is not sure if he should reach in and get his dummy, you can repeat your cue, 'Get your dummy, Jack' and point to the pot and touch the dummies. If he is still not sure whether he should get the dummies, repeat 'Get your dummy, ta for Jack'. You can guide his hand into the dummy pot, or pick up the dummy pot and offer the whole pot to him. Only let your baby take the dummies, and not the pot. He can take as many as he likes when you say your cue, but when it's time to put the dummies back in the pot, you need to help your baby put them all back.

Repeat this game until he is familiar with the cue 'Get your dummy' and knows what to do when you say that. This usually takes five or ten minutes maximum for a 12 to 24 month old. If he is enjoying the game, though, you can keep playing it for a little while longer before completing your packing-away routine. The more challenging he finds this game, the more you should repeat the cues per game, and the more often you should play the actual dummy pot game through the day. It should only take one day for your baby to learn this new game.

A note about monitors

In my opinion, monitors are overused. It's useful to have a monitor to alert you that your baby is awake, crying or coughing. They can also be helpful if you're outside hanging out washing, taking a quick swim in the backyard pool, or when your child's cries are out of normal hearing range.

If you can hear your baby when you're in the main living area of the house, however, you don't need to have a monitor on. If you have a large house, or need to use a monitor to hear your child when he wakes, that's fine. But once you've heard your child, turn the monitor off, or turn it down to a low level. Mothers experience a natural chemical reaction when they hear their baby cry, and if you're already feeling anxious about him waking, the monitor will exacerbate that anxiety, or make you misread your child's partial waking (if the monitor is set at an unnaturally loud level). This can make your day more difficult than it needs to be.

Similarly, if you can hear your baby clearly from your bedroom when he cries out at night, there's no need to use a monitor unless you're a very deep sleeper. Most parents with children who have trouble sleeping are rarely deep sleepers themselves. They tend to be listening to their child's every move, and any natural stirring through the night encourages them to over-interfere with their baby's healthy sleeping cycles. This is a key cause of some of the resettling problems.

If you can hear your child from your room and the living area, but still *need* to have a monitor for a sense of comfort, put it in the hallway outside his room. This means you will only hear genuine crying and not rush in when he's just moving a little bit and having a little grumble as he gets comfortable between sleep cycles.

PART 3

SLEEPING WELL FOR PEACEFUL NIGHTS

11

Understanding sleep

Learning how to help your baby/toddler sleep correctly during the first years of life can be one of the most revealing journeys you embark on. To truly understand your child's needs at sleep time, however, you need to get to know her at a deep level at non-sleep time. Trying to fix sleep-time problems only at bedtime generally fails because they are a symptom of an imbalance elsewhere. Knowing who your child is and what makes her tick will help address problems at sleep time.

To address the cause of any sleep-time problems you need to understand your child's physical needs. You also need to work with her at a psychological level by providing a balanced learning opportunity that isn't confusing or aimed at short-term results. While doing so, you need to cater for your child's strengths and weaknesses. This involves respectfully teaching her how to sleep.

Everyone knows putting a baby to sleep can be stressful, so rather than demanding she co-operate be sure the way you guide her empowers her. This will mean a short-term investment of time and energy to discover how to communicate with her respectfully and honestly so she can learn to sleep independently for the long term. You should establish this healthy form of communication from the beginning of your child's life rather than waiting until she's three or four years old.

A respectful sleep-time strategy is dependent on understanding the following three key factors:

- The physiology of sleep.
- The biology of sleep.
- The psychology of sleep.

These three factors make up a child's world of sleep, and comprise the many things that can affect, both positively and negatively, your child's ability to fall asleep and stay asleep. This chapter will provide you with a complete understanding of what causes sleep-time difficulties in babies, and show you how to repair them. But before that, let's look at the world of sleep from your baby's perspective.

A child's-eye view of the field of dreams

As we know, your child knows nothing about the concept of sleep. She only has associations linked to the sensations leading up to sleep. She develops these associations by seeking guidance from you about coping strategies for when she starts to feel tired. The coping strategies you teach her can either be *dependent* patterns of association, such as sucking a dummy or having you patting, breastfeeding or rocking her, or independent patterns of association like sucking her thumb, playing with a blanket or a tag on her teddy, twirling or rubbing her hair or playing with an ear.

Your child also has no concept of time lapsing. She will naturally stir or come to a partial waking multiple times during any sleep cycle prior to its completion and be unaware she's been asleep or that time has passed. All she knows is that if she experiences the sensation of feeling tired when she goes to sleep and wakes up and opens her eyes some time later still feeling the sensation of being tired, everything should be the same as it was. Even after hours have passed, she expects to have her usual sleep associations available in the same place as before she went to sleep. If those associations have changed while she was asleep, for example her dummy has fallen out or she's no longer being breastfed, sleep-time complications can arise.

If the change is dramatic, such as a parent having left the room or put her down in her cot after she's fallen asleep elsewhere, she will be startled when she wakes up because for her it's as if someone has just vanished. Because of this she may start to lose trust in the sensation of feeling tired at sleep time and resist going to sleep in general. So many parents say to me, 'Sheyne, my baby is so tired but she still fights sleep so much. Why?' Well, a change of sleep conditions between a child falling asleep and waking up is your number one culprit.

All children wake up naturally multiple times during their sleep cycle. When a child wakes up partially or fully and still feels tired, she seeks to recreate her coping strategies for feeling tired. If these associations involve your intervention, she will start crying, which is her way of calling you for assistance in recreating her learnt dependent associations (patting, breastfeeding, etc.). If she cries out every time she wakes you will have to go to her again and again to recreate the conditions she's learnt to rely upon to cope with feeling tired and to go back to sleep. If she has independent associations for falling asleep, like sucking her thumb, she will use those to get back to sleep. So, the only difference between children who can and can't sleep through the night is that one has learnt independent associations for going back to sleep while the other has developed dependent associations.

All babies are perfectly capable of developing their own coping strategies if you give them the time and space to do so, but they won't if you're always there fussing over them. If crying and stress occur while your baby is in her cot, she can start to develop negative feelings about her cot environment. Some babies will become reluctant to go into, or anywhere near, their cot, thus increasing the likelihood of developing a strong, learnt, dependent set of associations for going to sleep, perpetuating the cycle of crying out at night as well as through day sleeps.

Knowing this, think about what tools your child has to cope with the sensation of being tired and going to sleep. Does her only strategy for this feeling require you, or can she be in her cot alone as she drifts off to sleep? If her only method for going to sleep involves you it creates an enormous unnecessary burden on both her and you. Whereas she *can* and *should* feel comfortable going to sleep without you, she's learnt the opposite.

The message you send your child when dealing with these situations is crucial. You need to establish a consistent, parent-governed sleep environment to make sleep time calm and peaceful. To do this you should use confident, loving, reassuring tones, as well as verbal expressions and body language to let her know her cot is safe and that it's okay when she feels tired and is going to sleep.

I'm about to teach you new settling routines and cues to reassure your child if she cries when you put her to bed. These routines will let her know she is okay, you are there and have heard her, but she must listen to your guidance and go to sleep independently. Defining your new settling cues clearly will allow you to give your child the time and space she needs to develop independent settling associations to go to sleep in a supportive and language-rich way.

Under this new routine the conditions your baby goes to sleep in (in her room, with no one else in the room, going to sleep after you've requested it) will be identical to the conditions at all partial wakings during the night, i.e. she will be in her room, without you there, going to sleep by herself as requested. As a result she will sleep through the night without the need to call out because nothing will have changed from when she fell asleep to when she has partial wakings.

The first few times you guide your child to sleep independently through the night, the parent-governed line of your request to go to sleep sets you up for helping her go back to sleep during the night. Should she wake and cry, use the same style of communication as when you put her to bed, saying things like, 'There's no need to fuss and cry. Mummy will tell you if it's time to get up.' She will then be able to understand your request because you defined it at the settling routine.

As well as using confident, consistent parent-governed communication with your child for going to sleep or going back to sleep, it's crucial you ask her to look to you for guidance when sleep time is over and it's time to wake up. Because your baby has no concept of time lapsing, she doesn't know 2 a.m. from 4 a.m. from 7 a.m. Hence if you respond to her crying to get up, which is her way of saying, 'I'm awake, can you come and get me?' by going in and picking her up you will undo all your work teaching her to look to you for guidance and not cry through the settling and resettling process.

Don't get me wrong, I would expect a child to let you know when she's awake by crying. It's your response to her crying that will teach her that crying isn't necessary to start her waking-up time. Instead, you should develop a set of language cues and a waking ritual to indicate the time to get up has arrived. Then your baby will learn to play in her cot when she wakes up and wait for you to come and pick her up. This healthy sleep process is peaceful for your child and for your entire family.

To be truly consistent then, ask your child to look to you for guidance around all three areas of sleep: going to sleep, going back to sleep *and* getting up, by providing her with a settling routine, a resettling routine *and* a waking routine.

The physiology of sleep

Going to sleep is the function of settling yourself to sleep from a stage of consciousness. The settling conditions you provide for your baby when she initially goes to sleep, and how you manage her during her partial wakings, will impact on your child's ability to resettle during a sleep session.

Going back to sleep is the function of resettling yourself back to sleep from a semi-conscious state which is what I call 'surface sleep'. Surface-sleep windows last around three to eight minutes, during which a baby's brainwave activity indicates a transitional sleep-wave pattern. During surface sleep she is partially conscious of her surroundings. A child can develop a habit of expecting your intervention in her surface sleep if you rush in to try and get her back to sleep quickly. If you can give her enough space she will become more conscious of her environment, see everything is as it was when she was first willingly drifted off to sleep after you requested it, and then relax and willingly go back to sleep again.

Waking up is the function of coming to a full state of consciousness from a sleep state. The waking conditions you provide your child can impact on her ability to resettle through a sleep session elsewhere in the day.

Your child's ability to sleep relies on all three stages being predictable and consistent. Based on an inconsistency in your approach to the physiology of sleep you will see two different kinds of settling problems occur: settling and resettling difficulties; or just resettling difficulties.

A child who can't self-settle when she is going to sleep will generally not be able to self-resettle back to sleep either. However some children who aren't able to self-settle are able to resettle when they wake during the night. This is rare, however, and there's a high risk it won't last. Other children are able to self-settle during the day but can't do so at night. This is called a 'routine association problem'. These children are still considered unable to self-settle because the governing line of communication falls on them, making sleep unpredictable.

The most common scenario I encounter involving sleep problems is a child self-settling when *going* to sleep but finding it difficult to self-resettle and go *back* to sleep. Due to this, the child can learn patterns of dependency around resettling on a subconscious level. A parent might be able to put their baby to bed and request she go to sleep on a conscious level, but will need to assist their baby to go back to sleep during the night and day on a subconscious level.

Typically, parents who experience this problem try to enter the room quickly enough so they can prevent their baby from waking up fully and get them back to sleep within minutes. This 'if I'm quick' approach appears to be a good idea in the short term, but in the long term it is the cause of night time wakings that will need to be addressed to avoid disrupted sleep sessions.

The biology of sleep

Every baby needs a certain amount of sleep in a 24-hour period but it's important to understand every baby's sleep requirement is different and you cannot expect a child to sleep more than her body actually needs. An average baby between six and 12 months of age will have a daily sleep requirement of between 13 and 17 hours. A baby/toddler between 12 and 24 months of age will have a daily sleep requirement of between 13 and 16 hours.

Our body's circadian rhythm should work in a harmonious way with nature for us to have good sleep. We rise and warm up with the sun. Our energy and activity levels are highest when the sun is brightest. We wind down and cool down with the sun. We have low to no energy levels when the sun is not present because as darkness falls enzymes in the brain stimulate the release of melatonin from the pineal gland. The release of melatonin is halted when daylight arrives, and we experience wakefulness as a direct result. So we're meant to sleep through the night, and be awake during the day.

As a fresh new life your baby is not meant to go to sleep five hours after the sun goes down and wake up five hours after it rises or, worse still, go to sleep hours after it sets and wake up when it first rises in the morning. As a result, I break a baby's sleep requirement into two distinct portions of the 24-hour cycle. They are:

- Day: 7 a.m. to 7 p.m.
- Night: 7 p.m. to 7 a.m.

I choose these times because the mean time the sun comes up in the morning is 7 a.m. and the largest portion of solid sleep needs to be achieved during the night when it's dark. Nature's and your home environment's alarm clocks – sunlight, increased room temperature, birds chirping, traffic rumbling and people getting up – will, on average, occur around 7 a.m., so you need to put your baby to bed by 7 p.m. the night before to ensure she achieves her night-time sleep quota. As a baby's night sleep should be between 11 and 11½ hours long – and there's no need for her to have night feeds after six months if you've introduced solids into her diet – her day sleeps should then be arranged around the remainder of her sleep requirement.

Establishing a healthy night-time body clock is achieved in the first five years of life. That is, the night sleep pattern established when a child is young remains with her for the rest of her life. To try and have your child wake at the same time when she reaches preschool or school age significantly impacts on her entire day. Making 7 a.m. the normal and natural rising time for your child means her energy will peak between 9 a.m. and 5 p.m. Either side of these hours are wind up and wind down times, both of which are essential to a balanced, healthy day.

The early and late shift

If your baby goes down too late at night (between 9 and 10 p.m.), and wakes up late the next morning (between 8 and 9 a.m.) her day sleeps are shifted to later in the morning and later in the afternoon, which perpetuates a cycle of late settling at night. Equally, if your baby goes down too early at night (between 5 and 6 p.m.) and wakes up early the next day (4 to 5 a.m.), her day sleeps are shifted to earlier in the morning and earlier in the afternoon, perpetuating a cycle of early settling at night. Over a long period of time both these patterns affect a child's body clock.

Stolen partial-night cycles

When a portion of your baby's 11- to 11½-hour night sleep is stolen and used as a day sleep, three typical scenarios are played out:

- Morning sleep-cycle thief: your baby wakes at 5 a.m. and stays awake for two hours, then sleeps between 7 and 9 a.m., which means two hours have been stolen from the night sleep. The sleep between 7 and 9 a.m. is actually stolen from 5 to 7 a.m., and needs to be restored.
- Afternoon sleep-cycle thief: if your child goes to bed at 5 p.m. and sleeps until 7 p.m., then wakes and plays until she goes to sleep at 9 p.m. the sleep between 5 and 7 p.m. is stolen from 7 to 9 p.m., and needs to be restored.
- Evening sleep-cycle thief: if your baby is awake for two hours somewhere between 11.30 p.m. and 3.30 a.m. then goes back to sleep for the remainder of the night, the following day she needs longer day sleeps to compensate for her broken night's sleep. This then steals sleep again from the coming night, resulting in another prolonged waking between 11.30 p.m. and 3.30 a.m.

Catnapping

When a baby sleeps for 30 to 40 minutes and then can't be resettled it's a sign of a routine miscalculation. If a baby's sleep times become imbalanced, looking for tired signs becomes an ineffective tool which can perpetuate the cycle of catnapping because a child who has short sleeps often becomes tired again within a short period of time. Generally, this leads to her being put down again after a short period of time and subsequently she is unable to sleep for a substantial period of time again. This promotes multiple short sleeps, short intervals apart, and you are destined to have failed attempts at resettling.

Upside-down days

Many people are told, 'Your child needs to know day from night!' and are instructed to ensure the child's sleep environment during the day is different from the night by allowing sun into the room.

I don't agree that all babies should sleep in sun-drenched rooms during the day, particularly if they are overtired, simply so 'they can know day from night'. If your baby is waking multiple times through each day sleep cycle or can only catnap, then knowing day from night is not the problem and you need to consider darkening your baby's room to assist in melatonin production.

If, on the other hand, you have one of those rare babies who takes two or three excessively long day sleeps of between two and four hours, and then struggles to sleep at night, then you do need to teach her day from night, so having her sleep in a slightly lighter environment during the day helps ensure she doesn't fall into a pattern of big day sleeps and poor night sleeps from excessive daytime melatonin production. This is where you could get into a pattern of upside-down days and nights which results in either full wakefulness or brief sleep periods through the night and massive quantities of sleep during the day. This pattern is more common in babies under four months of age.

High caloric/fluid intake at night

If your baby takes the bulk of her calorie consumption or fluid intake during the night, it will impact on her ability to eat solid foods or drink milk or water during the day, as well as affecting her sleep patterns. An appropriate day meal plan is important to ensure you discourage your baby from waking for feeds at night, before you entirely eliminate them.

Signs of sleep imbalance

Once you lock in the night sleep (11–11½ hours of your baby's full sleep-requirement quota), you need to balance her *remaining* sleep requirement between 7 a.m. and 7 p.m. You do this by working within two distinct sleep windows during the day to correct any sleep-time imbalances. Morning sleeps should occur between 7 a.m. and 12 p.m. and afternoon sleeps should occur between 2 and 7 p.m. Morning sleeps will impact on how long your child can sleep during the next daytime sleep window as well as her waking time between 6 and 7 a.m. the *following* morning. Afternoon sleeps will impact on your child's settling time between 7 and 8 p.m. and if your child is a low sleep requirement baby on a midday sleep, it may affect the length of time she can stay asleep in the middle of the day (12 to 2 p.m.) of the *following* day. Sleep taken between 12 and 2 p.m., however, will generally not affect a baby's 7 p.m. settling time on the same day or their 6 to 7 a.m. waking time the *following* morning.

If your child has a higher sleep requirement, she'll generally be able to sleep for longer periods during both her morning and afternoon sleep sections (7 a.m. to 12 p.m. and 2 to 7 p.m.) without it affecting the other sleep window of the day or her 7 to 8 p.m. settling time that night, or her 6 to 7 a.m. waking time the following morning. This is *not* the case for lower-sleep-requirement babies (who require 14 hours sleep in 24 hours). Hence, what works for one baby won't necessarily work for another, which is why you cannot apply the same routine to every child.

A mismatch between your child's sleep requirement and the times she sleeps during the day are the most common cause of reoccurring sleep inconsistencies. Once the night cycle of 11½ hours is achieved by a lower-sleep-requirement child you only have two and a half hours of sleep to work with through the day, which needs to be either divided up between the two windows of the day (7 a.m. to 12 p.m. and 2 to 7 p.m.), or provided in the midsection of the day (12 to 2.30 p.m.). A typical routine miscalculation for a lower-sleep-requirement baby occurs when her 24-hour sleep requirement is achieved between 7 p.m. at night and 11 a.m. the next morning. For example if, after a full night's sleep of 11½ hours, you try to get her to have one large morning sleep between 7 a.m. and 12 p.m. she will typically have only a brief catnap or not sleep at all during the second daytime sleep window.

Once this miscalculation cycle starts, babies get very overtired by the end of the day. This is when parents with a lower-sleep-requirement baby can easily fall into the cycle of teaching their baby dependent associations for the sensation of feeling tired, and why some children find it so hard to self-settle at night compared with the rest of the day. After a poor night's sleep due to the need for regular assistance to resettle, a child will naturally be more prone to needing a longer sleep in the morning to compensate, which perpetuates the cycle of poor afternoon sleep and an overtired baby needing assistance to go to sleep again at 7 p.m.

You should also ensure a lower-sleep-requirement baby doesn't oversleep during the day time, leaving her struggling to achieve a full night's sleep. Never steal a baby's sleep from the nights to achieve a daytime quota of sleep. If you allow her to have only nine hours sleep at night to achieve longer day sleeps, you risk shifting her body clock and damaging her full-night sleep quota of 11 to 11½ hours. This often happens when a low-sleep-requirement baby is expected to take a big sleep in the morning and a big sleep in the afternoon despite it not suiting her sleep needs.

So, always establish a baby's night sleeps (11 to 11½ hours) first, and if she cannot take the routine amount of sleep suggested after a full night's sleep, it is likely to be too high for her so she will need a different routine during the day.

The biological clock

There are many stages of brain activity while a child is asleep which each have a different function. However, there are really only four basic stages during sleep that you need to be concerned with. They are:

- Stage 1: surface sleep
- Stage 2: power sleep
- Stage 3: healthy sleep
- Stage 4: dreamy sleep.

Understanding these stages will help you correctly assess your child's need for intervention at sleep time to ensure as few crying sessions as possible during the night and day while your baby is learning to sleep undisturbed. But first, let's start with a baby who is fully conscious.

Fully conscious

Fully conscious is being wide awake and alert and is the state your baby needs to be in when you leave her to go to sleep. If you'd like her to be able to self-resettle when she stirs during the transitional stages of sleep without calling out (crying), you need to remember she has no concept of sleep or time lapsing so she must go to sleep initially in the same environment she'll encounter in the middle of the night or in the middle of her sleep cycle. If she has her own room, this sleep will occur in her cot, in her room, on her own after you've said goodnight and left, and when she is relaxed about the sensation of being tired independently. For this reason I always aim to keep a child fully conscious throughout the entire settling routine until I say goodnight and leave her in her room to drift off to sleep peacefully.

During her settling routine, despite her obvious alertness, her tired body is preparing her for sleep. The normal body reactions aiding your child's natural progression into the stages of sleep will occur when she starts to relax. She will close her mouth and start breathing predominantly through her nose. One nostril will close, lessening the oxygen supply to the brain, and she will begin to breathe shallowly. This triggers a drop in body temperature and hormones, which helps prepare her for the process of going to sleep.

Once your baby begins to fall asleep she enters the realm of the four sleep stages first introduced in Chapter 2 and now outlined in more detail.

Stage 1: Surface sleep

Surface sleep is the transitional stage between being awake and being asleep, or being asleep and waking up again, or being asleep, rolling over and getting comfy and going back to sleep. Surface sleep lasts for between three and eight minutes, during which short dream snippets may occur, usually involving recall memory and depicting images from the day. The brain's electrical activity slows as exhibited by a beta brainwave rhythm known as a k-complex brainwave pattern.

I am careful about attending to a child during surface-sleep windows, either when she first starts to fall asleep or when she first wakes up from being asleep, particularly in the middle of the night. To not give your child the vital sleep her body needs does not help her.

Stage 2: Power sleep

Power sleep occurs when you've fully drifted into a sleep cycle and are well on the way to the deeper stages of sleep, after which you're likely to stay asleep for a prolonged period. It occurs about five to ten minutes into a sleep cycle when your breathing slows down and your heart rate drops. If you're holding your baby, this is when she becomes limp and heavy in your arms and you're safe to move her if you need to because she's less likely to stir. This is when the brain shows slow beta rhythms interspersed with periods of fast alpha rhythms, called 'sleep spindles', and some delta rhythms. This stage lasts for about half a baby's night sleep.

Stage 3: Healthy sleep

After around 20 to 30 minutes in the first two stages of sleep, the body drops into what I call 'healthy sleep', which is the deepest level of sleep and is when the brain measures its slowest waves, its theta and delta rhythms. During this stage of sleep the body maintains and restores itself and growth hormone secretions are at their highest. After a baby first goes to bed at night, this stage of sleep is at its longest but it gradually shortens as the night progresses. This appears to be why the first sleep of the night is generally the best.

Stage 4: Dreamy sleep

Dreamy sleep occurs when the body and brain become active during sleep, with heart rates increasing and eyes fluttering back and forth. Scientists call this 'REM' (rapid eye movement) sleep and children have more REM sleep than adults. Research suggests that a baby's brain is as active, if not more so, during dreamy sleep as when she is awake. In stark contrast to the fluctuations in body metabolism that occur in dreamy sleep, muscle activity is almost non-existent, and the body is virtually in a paralysed state.

Researchers believe REM sleep is associated with the inner workings of the brain, with information learnt during the day processed by our brains during REM sleep. Other brain functions, such as problem solving, memory consolidation and creativity, are also mediated during REM sleep. REM or dreamy sleep forms the last stage of a full sleep cycle before the brain goes back to the start. This is when your baby comes back to a surface sleep, and the whole sleep cycle begins again.

How long do these sleep cycles last in children?

Each complete sleep cycle lasts around 40 to 45 minutes in total but can be as short as 20 and, more commonly, 30 minutes. The reason the shorter length cycles occur is unclear, but the impact these brief sleep cycles have on a baby's day is quite profound. At the point where a baby's sleep cycle completes its four stages before beginning the new cycle with surface sleep, your baby or toddler needs the environment to be the same as it was when she first started the sleep cycle to be able to go back to sleep in this second surface sleep.

While there's a need for the same environment each time a child transitions from one full sleep cycle into the next full sleep cycle, this is only one aspect of what may affect a child's ability to sleep. Also consider sleep requirement, distance between naps, the amount and frequency of food intake, and physical factors like warmth, comfort, light, noise and movement. And as already discussed it's essential to look at how you communicate your need for her to go to sleep independently on the first few days of your new sleeping journey while everything corrects itself.

What causes catnapping?

After observing and analysing many babies – including their sleep times and length, environmental factors, communication, physical needs and emotional factors – I've found there are four main reasons children under two adopt the pattern of sleeping known as catnapping. These relate to:

1. them being overtired or overstimulated
2. a sleep debt or routine miscalculation
3. physical comfort factors such as being cold or moving excessively
4. associations and communication difficulties.

Some babies simply need a routine that suits them to eliminate catnapping. However, if you've already tried to establish a routine and your baby continues to catnap you will need to look elsewhere to help you work through the problem.

Catnaps can actually be useful for babies with lower sleep requirements, who may need as little as 13½–14 hours sleep in a 24-hour cycle, with 11–11½ hours during the night and up to two to three hours during the day. However, some lower-sleep-requirement babies who have three 30-minute catnaps during the day remain tired and can be grumpy. If your lower-sleep-requirement child is only taking a 30-minute catnap two or three times a day and you'd like to increase and balance the amount of daytime sleep she's having, you can use catnap cycles, or what I call 'bridging naps', to your advantage. To do this allow her only the shortest possible sleep-cycle length of 20 rather than 30 minutes because it can result in a dramatically improved sleep pattern during the next sleep, and a well-rested and far happier baby.

Catnappers who wake naturally will usually cycle through the day with a 30-minute sleep in the morning, a 30-minute sleep in the middle of the day and a 30-minute sleep in the late afternoon, achieving a total of one and a half hours day sleep.

By contrast, catnappers who are taught to wake after 20 minutes usually cycle through the day with a 20-minute bridging nap in the morning, a one-and-a-half to two-and-a-half hours sleep in the middle of the day and a 20-minute bridging nap in the late afternoon. This comes to a total of between two hours, ten minutes and three hours, ten minutes, which is a gain of between 40 minutes and one hour, 40 minutes' sleep during the day.

Your baby's sleep requirement may also increase with this new sleep routine and though the sleep is not taken in the conventional 'two big sleeps a day' format, she is still able to achieve almost an identical amount of sleep, if not more in some cases, just by you providing it in a different way.

There is no way every baby will suit the same routine suggestion. Do away with the one-size-fits-all mentality, which actually causes sleep problems, and look at all the options available to your baby for her sleep needs.

The psychology of sleep

The first thing a child needs to be comfortable with while going to sleep and going back to sleep is the feeling of being awake in her cot. The second thing she requires is feeling comfortable with you leaving the room. So whenever you set out to repair any sleep-time issues, work on these basic skills first.

To do this you need to teach your baby how to play in her cot and develop short-term absence cues to use with her through the day and night. To address associations and deliver the right messages to empower your baby to go to sleep and go back to sleep, you need to develop a new settling, resettling and waking routine. Before you ask her to sleep under the new routine conditions you will need to ensure she's able to understand you by providing language-rich opportunities during daytime non-sleep activities; for example, nappy change time provides an opportunity for you to guide your baby and help her understand you, so she feels comfortable with you guiding her at sleep time.

Your child will then need to be given opportunities to get to know the new sleep-time routines through role playing before you introduce her to conditions and expectations at sleep time. Even once this is done, you may still need to provide temporary physical comfort until she feels autonomous with the task of self-settling and self-resettling without the need to be held, rocked or breastfed. This temporary physical comfort often takes the form of a wrap or tuck-in technique for a baby under the age of 12 months, or a Safe T Sleep for older children. Once you've catered for these needs, make sure you take her sleep requirement into consideration before choosing your routine or implementing a sleep adjustment. Only then should you try to correct any learnt, behavioural or habit issues.

Signs of association problems triggering sleep disruptions

Unlike the sleep imbalances discussed in 'The biology of sleep', sleep disruptions caused by an association dependent upon a parent's intervention will follow a fairly predictable timetable during the night. If a child goes to sleep at 7 p.m., she will stir and require you to provide those same conditions or a different set of typical resettling conditions between 10 and 11 p.m., around 2 a.m., and again between 4 and 5 a.m. They will then wake between 6 and 7 a.m., ready for the day – that's if you were able to settle them at their 4 to 5 a.m. waking, which can often be a challenge after ten hours of sleep. If your child goes to bed earlier or later than 7 p.m., then simply adjust the time windows to see if your baby's sleep-time dramas are the result of an association requiring your intervention to resettle.

The other clear sign is when your child cannot settle or go back to sleep without your presence, even if it's only for a moment to touch her tummy, pop a dummy in her mouth, or quickly lie her down. You need to help your child develop independent settling and resettling associations to resolve this problem.

Communication and the psychology of sleep

Without the ability to guide your baby or toddler during the day at non-sleep times, you will have no possible chance of guiding your baby at sleep time. This need to have experienced, balanced, guiding lines of communication through the day once a child reaches six months of age is high, but absolutely essential by 12 months of age. It is most common to experience some difficulties in managing your baby during the day if you haven't developed consistent, respectful, guiding lines of communication for them by the time they're around eight months old.

Going to sleep independently is a skill your child develops through listening to you and trusting you at all times of the day, not just at sleep time. If you haven't exposed your child to being guided using parent-governed lines of communication while she's awake and at her best, starting a sleep-training exercise using this line for the first time while she is tired is likely to be stressful for her and result in tears. For example, if you can't ask your baby, 'Lie down and wait for Mummy' while you change her nappy, then how can you ask her to lie down when you put her in her cot and wait patiently while you leave the room and then drift off to sleep?

Other examples of communication problems that can affect your ability to settle your child to sleep could occur when you ask her to do things for you like:

- getting dressed
- getting in the pram, high chair or car seat
- staying in the pram, high chair or car seat
- getting her to wait on your hip or lap without fussing
- feeding her
- playing on the floor without always demanding you pick her up
- coming inside from outside.

If you're experiencing these common daytime communication difficulties, reread the first part of this book to understand the importance of respectful communication and how it affects a baby's ability to sleep.

Once you've established the ability to guide your child through the day you should be able to teach her to go to sleep on her own using your new, correctly 'defined' routines and cues. There are many times in the day when your child needs to be guided from one event to the next – which is called 'a transition'. Babies under two often find this difficult because even the slightest change in routine can represent unpredictability for them, resulting in stress. When this happens they may start crying in an attempt to create a predictable set of conditions that they are governing, such as you picking them up so they feel less vulnerable.

In order for your baby to learn how to cope with a parent-governed line of communication at sleep time, however, you need to take the time during the day when she's not tired and depleted to practise guiding her respectfully. To do this use the flow of communication to give her an emotional tool kit with vital life skills that will help her in every area of her life, not just sleep.

When you practise your flow of communication and define your statements and expectations of behaviour, you help your child work through the sensations associated with being guided, and build her trust through predictable cues and reassuring feedback. Your baby then learns that while her short-term demands may not always be met, you will always keep her informed while you guide her through certain events. By remaining confident and following through you teach your child to trust and cope with the sensation of being guided, while also indirectly teaching her the vital skills required for learning how to go to sleep with your guidance.

Predictability and the psychology of sleep

If your baby is having a hard time in the area of sleep, it's time to fully guide her to a better way. You cannot look to your child for guidance about how to put her to bed, because she just doesn't know. It's your role to take that stress away from her.

Assuming control of a situation does not, however, mean being controlling. It is about balance, so you always need to look at how to re-establish a better way of doing things, correcting a situation lovingly, and then returning control of that new healthy set of conditions back to the child. This is where your wisdom and her need for freedom to become autonomous and confident come together.

We do this in a four-step process:

1. Plan the new settling, resettling and waking routines you'd like for your baby.
2. Role play those routines with your baby to help her become familiar with the process before you use them on her.
3. Begin the new routines and confidently define them with their desired outcome, i.e. going to sleep and back to sleep independently.
4. Reinstate the feeling of governing sleep-time routines back to the baby through the predictability of those events, allowing her to start guiding the new appropriate parent-established flow of sleep time.

By doing this you establish the new conditions of sleep, yet your baby feels in control because she knows exactly what to expect.

Mikaela and her sleep-time blues

I met Mikaela when she was nine months old. Sleep time for her and her parents was extremely stressful and unpleasant. At night Mikaela's mother would rock her for hours before she fell asleep, then carefully put her in her cot and leave her to sleep. Mikaela would wake up shortly after, discover her mother had vanished and she was in her cot by herself and cry out.

Mikaela's mother would then return to Mikaela's room, pick her up and either attempt to rock her back to sleep or take her back to the master bedroom to sleep with her and her husband. By now Mikaela was nervous her mother would disappear again, so it often took hours to rock her back to sleep. And if she took Mikaela to the master bedroom she would crawl all over them, play, poke their eyes and, eventually, lie over her mother's head (to make sure her mother didn't disappear when Mikaela had that sleepy feeling again) and fall asleep for brief periods. As a result, Mikaela was overtired and only took three 30-minute catnaps during the day. Her mum, unable to settle her, was utterly exhausted and questioning her ability as a mother.

Mikaela clearly had a lower sleep requirement so we created a new sleep routine and role played it for Mikaela. From then on, she would always go to sleep with the same set of conditions: having two books read to her, wrapped with one arm out so she could get her dummy, then a final snuggle and sing-song before being tucked into bed with a 'nigh' nigh'' from her mother as she left Mikaela in her cot still awake.

On the first day Mikaela was not impressed. It was all very new for her to be in her cot alone. We kept reassuring her. It took her 20 minutes to go to sleep, but her new wrap and the new timing of her routine meant she could sleep for over two hours during her day sleep. We were making progress.

On the second day, Mikaela complained about going to bed while we read the stories, because she was now able to understand the sequence of events that told her it was almost sleep time. But by sleep time, she was ready to go to sleep by herself after crying for a minute or two. She was learning the sequence of events perfectly.

On the third day it was her mum's turn to put her to bed for the first time in the routine, without me in the room with her. She followed the new routine and Mikaela loved it because it was Mummy and she knew the sequence of events. Mikaela didn't cry at all but her mother was crying when she walked back to where I was waiting. I assumed it was the relief of being able to put her baby down so peacefully but she told me it was not only her relief that Mikaela felt so empowered by her new routine but that she had actually pre-empted the whole thing.

At just nine months of age Mikaela looked towards the room she was usually wrapped in, tried to lie herself down on the bed to be wrapped, and after the singing portion of the routine, gave her mother a sloppy kiss on the cheek then reached in towards the cot to be put to bed. As her mother tucked her in firmly Mikaela got her dummy and put it in her mouth, then turned her head to the side and closed her eyes. This was Mikaela being in control of a routine that we had established, and highlights the importance of developing a parent-directed flow of communication within a routine-based predictable format, and sticking with it until you achieve your results.

12

Solving sleep-time blues/ troubleshooting

In this chapter I provide a broad selection of problem-solving tools to help you resolve some of your child's sleep-time issues. After reading this section, you can decide the best course of action to help you overcome any hurdles. Hopefully the information will empower you with a deeper understanding of your child's sleep to help you avoid running into any of the typical troubles while helping him and any children you may be blessed to have in the years to come.

The reason I'm giving you these lists of dilemmas and resolutions in this book and on my website is because I don't believe every child should be on a strict daily routine. Only the more unsettled children or exhausted or stressed parents will need the guaranteed relief that comes with having a strict routine. I also believe a lot of sleep-time problems and unsettled behaviour can be solved through investigation and appropriate adjustments to routine and daytime communication to *remove the reason* for it, rather than adopt a crying-management-only approach to the tears once they appear. It's better to avoid unsettled behaviour, than try to manage it once it begins.

I advocate a balanced approach first and foremost, and believe that armed with the right information there is a good proportion of parents whose children have relatively simple sleep miscalculations or basic association problems that can be corrected quickly with just a little sleep-time tweaking and a more consistent approach to managing the baby's daytimes and teary or protesting wakeful times. While some sleep-time issues are simple to work through, any changes should be incorporated with basic and respectful communication strategies to ensure children are able to cope with requests to sleep, and the changes being made. No matter how simple sleep-time miscalculations appear, children need:

- a consistent settling, resettling and waking routine
- the opportunity to experience these new conditions through role play first
- to learn how to be awake in their cot and playing happily
- to be able to trust their parents' movements and be comfortable with them leaving the room
- a *fair* amount of sleep – they should not be expected to take a quantity of sleep that is just too much for them
- good clear communication throughout the day so they're used to guidance.

These basic, respectful tools and adjustments should provide tremendous improvements in your child's and family's sleep within a short period. However, once you've used this information to try to work through his sleep-time problems and feel you haven't been able to strike the right balance for your baby within three days, you should stop and adopt one of the balanced, pre-designed and well-refined PRM routines provided in Chapter 13.

No particular problem-solving strategy suits everyone. The needs of children and their families vary, with some requiring a looser framework and others a precise daily routine in order for their baby to be happy and content and for the family to recover from problems they've been experiencing. Assess your child's and family's needs before planning a course of action. If a parent or child is experiencing the following issues, whether mild or severe, resolve the problems quickly with the correct PRM routine to reduce stress as soon as possible:

- A child needs assistance to go to sleep and go back to sleep all the time.
- A child is not sleeping adequately during the day or night or both.
- A child requires hours of combined breastfeeding or bottle feeding each day to go to and stay asleep.

- A parent with a six month old plus is feeling their life is out of control.
- A parent with a six month old plus is feeling as though they or their child can't enjoy their day because the baby is so unsettled.
- A parent has completely lost their confidence, or can't even think about where to start to correct their child's sleep-time problem.
- A child is showing signs of being particularly unsettled at sleep time or during their waking time, or both.
- A mother has been diagnosed with postnatal depression.
- A child has previously been to sleep school and it hasn't resolved his sleep-time problem.
- Parents have previously tried control crying or other routines or other 'sleep time only' solutions and their child hasn't achieved long-term sleep.
- A parent is too tired to even think about trying to work it all out.

If this is you, and your child is over six months, don't try to work out what's wrong, go immediately to the corrective routine for your child's age group in Chapter 13 and then, once sleeping well, if appropriate or necessary, build up his sleep intake once harmony has been established in your house again.

When working through any sleep-time imbalance, read Chapter 2, 'Sleep: Understanding the basics' first to understand sleep from your child's perspective, and the many elements that make sleep achievable for him. You should also take note of:

- assessing your baby's sleep requirement
- signs of sleep imbalance
- crying interpretation
- crying support and repair.

What's normal and common

Before I talk about what could be causing your child's sleep-time problems, let's look at what's fairly normal so you can ensure you're not expecting too much of him. Compensation patterns of sleeping or eating will perpetuate poor sleeping or eating. For example, if he doesn't eat breakfast, then snacks on biscuits, fruit juice and crackers through the morning, he'll continue to refuse breakfast. If he sleeps poorly at night and you allow him to sleep in until 9 a.m., he'll continue to have unsettled nights. The pages that follow provide an idea of the sorts of things that can affect your child's sleeping patterns and need adjustment to find a solution.

When and how sleep times affect overall ability to sleep

Sleep intake per 24 hours is set per child, though it appears you can increase their need by providing more stimulation (not just physical). Day sleep affects night sleep and night sleep affects day sleep. Too much accumulated day sleep can cause prolonged wakings through the night. Too much accumulated night sleep can cause prolonged wakings through the day. A child can be tired but unable to sleep if you've used up his sleep requirement in one chunk, that is 13½ hours between 7 p.m. and 11 a.m.

From six months on, night sleeps should be between 11 and 12 hours long. Babies can get in the habit of sleeping shorter times (nine to ten hours) at nights but will then need more sleep during the day. The nights can be reset by limiting the amount of sleep offered during the day. If your baby has been very unsettled and needed to be attended to several times during the night, his need to sleep in later in the morning or have a big morning sleep may disappear when you correct his sleep patterns and he begins sleeping solidly through the night. If he sleeps peacefully all night don't expect him to need as much day sleep as he needed when he was waking frequently and exhausted after an unsettled night.

Some babies don't sleep well for the rest of the day if they're given the chance to take a longer nap or have too much sleep between 7 a.m. and noon, even if they have a moderate sleep requirement. A large morning sleep may encourage early morning wakings and/or discourage a significant second sleep during the day. Some babies over 12 months only need one large sleep of two to two and a half hours a day, rather than two sleeps of one to one and a half hours, to be able to maintain good night sleep. A late afternoon nap (past 5 p.m.) will cause late settling times at night.

An overtired child who is in a pattern of catnapping will show tired signs more frequently. Often parents report their seven, nine, 12 or 18 month old can't stay awake for more than one and a half hours in the morning. A five-minute power nap on the breast or in the car is equivalent to a 20- or 40-minute bridging sleep. This could keep your baby awake for an additional two to three hours.

Babies come to several brief windows of semi-consciousness during sleep sessions as they naturally progress from one sleep cycle to the next. These semi-conscious stages of sleep are called surface sleeps and typically last for between three to eight minutes. If you intervene and assist a child to sleep within this eight-minute window, you can teach him to need your intervention on a subconscious level, or trigger a session in which he is inconsolable for up to 20 to 40 minutes.

Babies/toddlers will generally only sleep half to three-quarters of their normal at-home, in-cot sleep when sleeping in a pram, in another sleeping environment, or at daycare. Babies and toddlers can also suddenly lose sleep and become unsettled when there's significant changes in their life that make it unpredictable and difficult to trust that they can predict further changes. These include the arrival of a new baby, moving house, separation of parents, someone moving in or temporary house guests, holidays, grief in the family, Mum/Dad or both going away for work/holiday.

How and when you feed your baby affects his sleep

Calorie intake is set per child, and your child's calorie intake can be consumed either through the night or through the day. You can deliberately or inadvertently:

- increase a child's calorie intake need by providing less sleep
- decrease a child's calorie intake need by providing more sleep.

The need for night feeds beyond six months once solids have been introduced has two causes: hunger (not enough food, not enough protein, not enough solids through the day) and association (learnt pattern of dependence feeding/suckling to go to, or go back to sleep). Children also have growth spurts that impact on their need to sleep for up to five to ten days at a time. This pattern usually follows a sudden decrease in sleep need (and elevated hunger), followed closely by a sudden increase in sleep need (and decreased hunger).

Your baby may or may not need one or two night feeds until he's six months old. After that age, babies who are hungry during the night need to start solids. Once you introduce solids to your baby's diet, he should be able to sleep through the night. If you don't introduce meat into his diet by seven to eight months, he may go back to requiring one night feed between 11.30 p.m. and 1.30 a.m. until the protein source is introduced. Often the only way to encourage the intake of solids during the day is by reducing or eliminating milk feeds through the night.

If a baby or toddler needs multiple feeds during the night it may only be a sleep association, and not have anything to do with hunger (though it will affect his ability to eat during the day). Associations are more likely to be the problem if he's going to bed around 7 p.m. and waking between 10 and 11 p.m., around 2 a.m. and again between 4 and 5 a.m., requiring your help to go back to sleep.

If babies over six months have a feed after 4 a.m. and then go back to sleep, this is considered the beginning of their day and the time will be stolen from their day sleep and food intake opportunities. Forty minutes before the day's usual first feed a baby's body may start to prepare for that feed. If he is fed at 6 a.m., he may start to stir from 5.20 the next morning. Then, if he's fed at 5.20, he is likely to stir at 4.40 a.m. the next day, and so on.

Hunger signs look very similar to tired signs (yawning, red eyes, irritability) after six months. Babies can appear to need more sleep if their calorie and food fuel intake is too low, or can appear to need less sleep if their calorie and food fuel intake is too high. Excessive milk feeds create poor solid intake and affect sleep, and excessive solid intake creates poor milk intake and affects sleep. Excessive night calorie intake will detract from daytime calorie intake causing cycles of night wakings for food. Snacking too often on whole foods (solids and milk are seen as whole foods) in the morning can have the same impact on sleep as excess sleep in the morning (encouraging early wakings and a short second sleep of the day).

The associations your baby has affect his sleep

Babies can have a set of associations that require intervention (patting, rocking, feeding, your bed, cuddles) to go to sleep or a set of associations that don't require intervention (babbling, moving head from side to side, playing with ear, sucking thumb) to go to sleep. Even if babies can put themselves to sleep with a set of associations that *don't* require your intervention, they may still have a set of associations involving your intervention to go 'back to' sleep.

As we know, babies don't understand the concept of sleep or time lapsing. They only know feelings, and have associations attached to those feelings. If you stay in the room with a baby when he's going to sleep, and then sneak off, he'll start to fight the feeling of being tired because it's become associated with you disappearing. This is what causes a tired baby to fight sleep. If a baby has had severe reflux, and has associated the sensation of lying down with pain, this is a 'learnt' loss of trust in the process of lying down beyond the actual experience of pain, and you need to teach a new association and trust through your loving encouragement.

The environment in which your baby sleeps affects his sleep

Babies who are cold will often try to roll onto their tummy and tuck their arms under their bodies to stay warm or lie against the side of a cot for comfort.

Sudden night wakings

Babies often experience a phenomenon called a 'sudden partial waking', where they wake suddenly and scream a frightening cry. Many parents report this sounding like their baby has been bitten by a spider or ant and strip their baby and cot to check. During sudden partial wakings babies can sit or stand up or cry, and still be asleep. This brief waking passes quickly if you don't rush in and disturb your baby in the first five to ten minutes, which disorientates him. It's more common in overtired babies. Males are more prone to becoming overtired as they have a lower sleep requirement.

Routine miscalculations: signs, symptoms and solutions

As you've read in Chapters 2 and 11, the origins of sleep problems in children between six and 24 months are very varied. Most sleep solutions, however, deal exclusively with sleeping and feeding times and neglect the actual cognitive, emotional and communication needs of babies. While some of these strategies may produce results, to truly help a baby learn how to sleep independently with less confusion or stress to him, and in a way that will empower him with the ability to understand, learn and feel confident with the skills needed to go to sleep and back to sleep, you must take *all* needs into consideration.

In 'Signs of sleep imbalance' in the previous chapter and in this following section I'll explore some classic sleep-time imbalances that are predominantly timing based, which I call 'routine miscalculations'. You need to always lock in the night sleep first, then work in the two distinct portions of the daylight hours – the morning and the afternoon – to assess sleep-time imbalance.

The morning sleep is between 7 a.m. and 12 p.m. and impacts on your child's:

- subsequent sleeping potential for the remainder of the current day
- ability to sleep solidly between 4 and 7 a.m. the following morning.

The afternoon sleep, between 2 and 7 p.m., impacts on your child's:

- settling time that night between 7 and 9 p.m.
- sleep needs during the previous sleep session (as in, is the big mid-afternoon sleep compensating for a poor mid-morning sleep and, if so, is this a regular pattern?)
- ability to sleep well that night between 7 p.m. and 12 a.m.

It's important to balance your baby's day sleeps so you can make the most of the long 12 to 13 hours ahead of him in which he's mainly awake. If you use up his entire day-sleep requirement by 11 a.m. with a single two-and-a-half-hour mid-morning sleep, he has an eight- to nine-hour day ahead of him, during which he can only possibly take a brief catnap if his sleep requirement is low. This will leave him exhausted and overtired by the end of the day, and he's more likely to require intervention to go to sleep at night. This can be the beginning of a cycle of a learnt pattern of dependent associations to go to sleep, which will make it difficult for him to sleep through the night without crying out for your help. An overtired child has a higher potential of waking multiple times between 7 and 10 p.m.

Shifted body clock

When your baby goes down too late at night (say, between 9 and 10 p.m.) and wakes up late (between 8 and 9 a.m.), his day sleeps are shifted to later in the morning and later in the afternoon. This shift perpetuates a cycle of late settlings at night.

When your baby goes down too early at night (say at 5 to 6 p.m.), and wakes up too early the next day (between 4 and 5 a.m.), his day sleeps are shifted forward to earlier in the morning and earlier in the afternoon, perpetuating a cycle of early settling at night time.

The late shift

Wake him at 6.30 a.m. and balance your day sleeps either by copying the timings of his existing sleep routine but in a new time zone (e.g. if he always went back to sleep after three hours of being awake and slept for one and a half hours, then wake him at 6.30 a.m. and don't put him down until 9.30 a.m., and allow only one and a half hours sleep), or as described in the PRM routines, after you've assessed his sleep requirement. This encourages daytime sleeps at appropriate times, and promotes a healthy 7 p.m. bedtime.

The early shift

From six months onwards keep him up until the first appropriate nap time of the day, which is never before 8.45 a.m., and move forward with your day as per your PRM routine. This encourages daytime sleeps at appropriate times, and promotes a healthy 7 p.m. bedtime, which promotes a healthy 6 to 7 a.m. rising.

Stolen partial night time sleep cycles

Stolen partial night time sleep cycles occur when a portion of a child's 11- to 11½-hour night sleep between 7 p.m. and 6.30 a.m. is stolen and used as a day sleep. Here are three typical examples:

1. Morning sleep cycle thief: when your baby wakes at 5 a.m. and stays awake for two hours until 7 a.m. and then sleeps between 7 and 9 a.m. This is two hours of sleep shifted from the night into later in the morning.
2. Afternoon sleep cycle thief: shifted sleep can happen in the evening when your child goes to sleep at 5 p.m. and sleeps until 7 p.m. then wakes and plays until 10 p.m. before settling for the night. This is two hours of sleep shifted from the night into earlier in the afternoon.
3. Evening sleep cycle thief: this happens in the middle of the night, when your baby wakes for two hours between 12 and 2 a.m., for example, and then goes back to sleep for the remainder of the night. The following day your child needs longer day sleeps to compensate for the broken sleep he experienced the night before. Excessive accumulated daytime sleep steals sleep at night.

To correct *major* sleep imbalances quickly a child should be put onto a defined age-appropriate PRM daily routine (see Chapter 13). Below I highlight the structure of the routine changes needed to correct such problems. In all cases, assess your child's sleep requirement and make adjustments to his sleep times.

Morning sleep cycle thief

For the morning sleep cycle thief, don't provide a 7 a.m. nap even if he wakes at 5 a.m. Put him down no earlier than 8.45 a.m. and don't let him oversleep. Maintain this for a few days and his shifted night pattern will return to its rightful place of 4 to 6 a.m. rather than 7 to 9 a.m. In cases of a well-established pattern of early waking and early feeding you may need to provide a temporary sleeping swaddle or firm tuck-in at all sleep times in addition to the settling routines to help him go back to sleep during his surface sleep to prevent him from sitting or standing up, which makes resettling hard. If he stirs at that time but remains still, you have much better chance of him self-resettling without the need for your intervention.

Afternoon sleep cycle thief

For the afternoon sleep cycle thief, don't provide any naps after 5 p.m. and carefully assess the length of his afternoon sleeps. A late afternoon bridging nap closer to 4 p.m. should be a brief sleep, rarely exceeding 20 to 30 minutes. This is a case where your child may be better suited to a different routine.

Evening sleep cycle thief

People who have babies taking a couple of pretty decent-sized sleeps during the day often say to me, 'He's a great sleeper through the day, but terrible at night'. If you have a night sleep thief, you've got the amount of sleep he needs through the day wrong and he's oversleeping during the day. If your child were to sleep the solid 11 to 11½ hours required through the night cycle, you'll find he would no longer sleep as long during the day. You can't have your cake and eat it too.

Assess your child's sleep requirement for day sleeps carefully, and correct the amount he's allowed to take through the day and your nights will be quickly restored. When I suggest this, the response is usually 'I'm so tired, I need him to sleep that much through the day', or 'He's so tired, he needs to sleep that much during the day'. There are two important factors to adjusting day sleep. They are:

1. you and he won't be so exhausted when he's sleeping right through the night
2. the day sleeps are going to dwindle eventually as he gets older, but prolonged wakings at night will remain because you have nothing to work with through the days.

Correct your days now, and your peaceful nights will make the slightly more active days more fun and less exhausting.

Catnapping

Catnapping is when your baby takes multiple 20- to 40-minute sleeps through the day and resettling is impossible. To correct this sleep imbalance quickly, a child should be put onto a PRM routine (see Chapter 13). While the suggestions below may not be the complete resolution for catnapping, I will highlight the general structure of the routine changes needed to correct such problems.

Keep him awake for longer periods between sleep. He's already overtired, so the fear of him becoming overtired is null and void over the age of six months. You need to take measures to correct the situation quickly and looking for tired signs or being concerned about him becoming overtired isn't a worthwhile way to deal with the problem. This is also a sign of a potential environmental imbalance. Perhaps he's not warm enough – being cold will always wake a baby sooner. Perhaps you've inadvertently broken his trust by changing the environment once he's gone to sleep – maybe holding or feeding him to sleep then putting him down. Perhaps he's in an overstimulating environment with, for example, too much light or noise, which will impact on his ability to recover from catnapping.

Upside down days

Upside down days occur when your baby takes two or three excessively long sleeps of between two and four hours through the day. This results in only brief sleep periods or full wakefulness through the night. You need to wake him up from a daytime sleep after an appropriate amount of time. To do this he will have to make a quick transition and you'll need the assistance of routine. He will almost certainly be 'jetlagged' as you reset his body clock, but it will only last for one to three days and then he'll only experience the same level of tiredness as any baby in the first three days of establishing a new pattern to his circadian rhythm.

High caloric/fluid intake at night

This occurs when your child consumes more calories (via milk or food) or fluids through the night than during the day. Using a routine will help fix this problem. On the day of commencing your PRM, don't give the baby any food at all from 2 a.m. on the morning you're due to start until the first designated feed time of 7 a.m. You then get a head start on feeding for the next two days. Stick to the routine for your feeding and sleeping windows through the day and your baby's body's need for food will automatically shift to the daytime.

You need to act quickly when a baby's circadian rhythm is imbalanced. Don't increase daily food intake without first decreasing, or eliminating, night food intake. Even if his calorie intake is low on the first day, maintain your evening cycle of resettling without offering food and your child's calorie intake imbalance will correct by the next day. Ensure you offer more food than normal at each meal, because he needs to eat more through the day to stop his hunger pattern continuing through the night.

You can't increase daily fluid intake without decreasing, then eliminating, night fluid intake. This means no fluids from 2 a.m. on the morning the new routine starts. Introduce lots of opportunities to drink water through the day and remember milk is a whole food, not just a drink, so assess his needs correctly.

False sleep

If your child has a milk feed every morning at 5 a.m., sleeps till 6.30/7 a.m., and then sleeps well through the day, your ability to maintain this level of sleep without the milk feed at 5 a.m. is reduced. This early morning sleep is a false sleep because without the milk his body wouldn't be able to take this sleep, so please don't count it in his general daily sleep quota. For example, if he slept from 7 p.m. to 5 a.m. and you had to feed him to achieve a one-hour sleep to 6.30/7 a.m., and then you added that one hour to a second day sleep of two hours, his sleep requirement, if averaged over seven days of consistent sleep, would be 13 hours a day. If you then corrected his sleep patterns so he no longer needed a 5 a.m. milk feed to sleep till 6.30/7 a.m., his average daily sleep intake may drop down a little as the extra sleep he used to achieve between 5 and 6.30 was not a naturally occurring sleep needed in his sleep requirement.

Progressive decline in sleep

Progressive decline in sleep occurs when your child peaks in sleep requirement one day, sleeping between 16 and 17 hours, then drops down to only 11 hours of sleep intake the next day. Gradually over a couple of days, he tries to recover from the very low sleep intake by increasing his intake to between 13 and 14 hours one day, then 14 and 15 the next day before peaking to 16 to 17 hours sleep again. Sadly, the next day his sleep consumption may plummet to a miserable 11 hours again.

This progressive decline in sleep is a clear sign of an imbalance, and can manifest in many ways. Sometimes your baby will have one good day of 15 hours then one poor day of 13 hours, before going back to 15 hours one day and 13 hours the next. Other times he will sleep a consistently higher amount each day for a four-day window, then a consistently lower amount each day for a four-day window. By allowing your baby to take however much sleep he likes the day after a very poor sleep, you perpetuate a cycle of poor sleep, rather than balance it.

Keep a sleep diary for seven days and calculate his daily intake each day, excluding any prolonged wakings of 20 minutes he has during the day or night sleeps. Add the seven-day totals up and divide that total by seven to work out your baby's average 24-hour sleep requirement. You will then need to put your child on a routine and fix in his true 24-hour sleep requirement to that routine.

Taking the time to keep a diary may feel frustrating, but if you want to do this correctly, you need to know your baby's true intake rather than just an assumption or relying on wishful thinking. Not every baby is the same. I always say to parents, 'You've been doing without sleep for this long, you may as well invest a full week or two into developing a resolution that is permanent so it no longer has to consume another moment of your child's or your energy'.

Classic sleep-time blues: signs, symptoms and solutions

The following section is full of typical sleep-time problems and is designed to help you assess your own stumbling blocks so you can decide on the best way to help your baby/toddler learn how to sleep better. Some of these questions will be of interest to you, some won't as they aren't applicable to your situation, but I hope they're all enlightening and help you think a little more about the way you and your child communicate and your relationship grows.

While finding a solution to your child's possible routine miscalculation, we are going to break it down into two clear areas:

1. Basic sleep miscalculations.
2. Solutions.

Q1: My baby wakes at 5 a.m. How do I get him to sleep longer?

POSSIBLE CAUSES

- Too early or too long a morning nap time the day before, for example before 8.45 a.m. for a six to 12 month old with low sleep requirement, or before 9.30 or 10.00 a.m. for a 12 month old plus with average to high sleep requirement.
- The first feed of the day is too early or too big.
- He went to bed too early the night before, such as 6 p.m.
- Environmental reasons such as daylight, birds and traffic or other household members disturbing them.
- Learnt hunger pattern: false sleep.

TO FIX

- When you base a six- to 12-month-old baby's first sleep of the day on his waking time, you can perpetuate an early morning waking every day by putting him down too early the evening before to compensate. The only way to correct this pattern is to have a 'no sleep before 8.45 a.m.' policy for a LSR baby 6 to 12 months old, or a 'no sleep before 12 p.m.' policy for a LSR baby 12 months plus. Equally, have a 'no sleep before 9/9.30 a.m.' policy for a HSR baby six to 12 months, or a 'no sleep before 10/10.30 a.m.' policy for a HSR baby 12 months plus.

- If your baby wakes very early, and is then allowed to have a big sleep because he's tired from his early waking, he will wake early every morning and have a big mid-morning nap instead of sleeping in to 6 to 7 a.m. and having an appropriate sleep based on that good waking time mid-morning. The only way to balance this is to work out his sleep requirement and taper his morning sleep down to an appropriate length while still maintaining your 'no sleep before ______' policy, depending on your child's sleep needs.
- The time of the first feed of the day is important. One of the most noticeable triggers for a baby's morning waking time is the first feed time registered by his body's biological clock. If you usually give him his first milk feed of the day at 7 a.m., his body will anticipate that feed and start to prepare for it 40 minutes before. An early milk feed at 6 a.m., for instance, may promote stirring and possibly even a bowel movement by 5.20 a.m. If you then feed him at 5.20, he may become unsettled at 4.40 the next morning. Stick to a 'no feeds before 7 a.m.' policy for six month olds plus. Excessive food intake can often replace good sleep as a form of energy, so providing extra feeds or snacks because he's tired and grouchy will continue to promote wakefulness.
- Put your baby to bed at 7 p.m. Don't put him down earlier, for obvious reasons, or later. Later will cause shorter night sleep patterns, promoting a long day (for example, ten-hour nights mean 14-hour days) which makes a baby or toddler overtired and promotes early morning wakings.
- If the problem is noise, light or someone disturbing him, then eliminate light by blacking out the room until the sleep repairs itself, close the door and don't disturb him by turning on lights or rattling around if you get up early, and consider getting a white noise machine if you don't want to worry about what noise you or others in the house are making.
- If it's none of the above environmental reasons (as in, it's still dark and quiet) check if the room is too cold. Your child should be wearing appropriate clothing. Try to regulate the room temperature before changing the amount of layers a sleeping baby is wearing.
- Re-read the section about false sleep.
- If you've worked through the above points and you're still experiencing problems, your baby is likely to have a low sleep requirement and you may need to go onto a routine to resolve the sleep problems.

Q2: My baby has 30- or 40-minute catnaps several times throughout the day. Can I do something to fix this?

POSSIBLE CAUSES

- Routine miscalculation.
- Being put down too early in the morning if he's six to 12 months old.
- Napping too often if in the six to 24 months plus age range.
- Milk feeds too close together.
- Any possible 5 a.m. feed is creating false sleep. This means your baby is only sleeping due to digestion, therefore throwing out his sleep requirement.
- Too long a night sleep pattern because you're compensating for his frequent wakings – for instance 6 p.m. to bed, then five to ten wakings during the night, making him and you tired and causing him to wake naturally at 8.30 a.m.
- Dependent associations.
- Environment.

TO FIX

- Ensure he's ready for a good sleep when you put him down. Putting a catnapper down when he shows tired signs will mean he'll continue only taking catnaps because he'll constantly feel tired sooner because his naps are too short. Pushing past this to find an appropriate length of time to keep him awake *before* you put him down to sleep will encourage better sleep. This is where looking for tired signs only as a way of resolving sleep problems can be ineffective from six months of age.
- Place him on a modified routine (LSR or ASR) if over 12 months old and it will quickly correct the problem and encourage up to 2½ hours sleep through the day and 11 to 11½ hours at night.
- Correctly assessing his sleep requirement will encourage a catnapper to double the length of his day sleep with a simple routine adjustment. He may only need one sleep a day or no nap before 8.45 or 9.30 a.m., depending on sleep requirement, or no nap before 12 p.m. if he's 12 months plus.
- Ensure the night sleeps are no longer than 11 to 11½ hours long until you resolve the sleep disruption. To allow a night sleep session to go for longer than this could be eating into your baby's valuable day sleep allocation.
- Ensure he's not cold and that other environmental conditions aren't causing problems.
- Implement a full repair PRM Routine 1 (see page 262).

Q3: How can I stop my baby waking early on his second sleep of the day (mid-afternoon), after having just one big sleep in the morning, or not taking another sleep all day or, when he does, it's short? He's grumpy and ready for bed by 5 p.m.

POSSIBLE CAUSE

A classic symptom of a low-sleep-requirement child.

TO FIX

Put him on a routine to suit his sleep requirement and age group.

Q4: My baby/toddler barely naps or doesn't take any sleep all day but seems to be really happy and full of energy. Is it possible that she doesn't need sleep?

- Even if your baby is really happy and full of energy, he'll most likely be overtired and running on excessive adrenalin and hormones. Sometimes overtired, wired children are labelled as hyperactive, or incorrectly tagged as ADD or ADHD. While they may appear really energetic and super happy, these babies are highly strung, overstimulated, have trouble sitting still and taking information in, or concentrating. They are happy but can have a short fuse and can become suddenly unsettled late afternoon, only to pep right up to the point of frenetic after dinner. This can manifest in hysterical laughter at even the most simple things, and while it's beautiful to see a child so full of beans and energy, it's not balanced if there are no shades of tired or placid moments to his day. You don't, in most cases, want to stop that buzzy, super-energetic element of his nature, but you do need to find harmony and some middle ground for his health and wellbeing.
- Excessive food intake to compensate for poor sleep can promote no sleep as well.
- Vacant staring episodes (glassy or glazed over eyes) or five-minute power dozes in the car, pram or during a breastfeed could prevent an extremely overtired child taking any sleep during the day.
- Use a low-sleep-requirement routine (see page 260) based on the age group suggestions. There's no need to assess his sleep requirement if your child is this overtired. Just concentrate on getting him to sleep better. The low-sleep-requirement routine provides opportunities to take great sleep (14 hours plus in a 24-hour day), and can increase sleep intake by as much as five hours a day.
- Implementing a full recovery program is very important in these cases.
- You'll need to work hard on communication and positioning and the wait game through the day first to help him stop and accept the feeling of tired in an appropriate way.

Q5: I can't resettle my baby when he wakes up after a short sleep?

- If he's only sleeping 30 to 40 minutes before you experience failed attempts at resettling, please see question 2.
- You may be asking him to take a long sleep and his body doesn't need it because of too short a time between sleeps or having a low sleep requirement.
- If an overtired baby is overstimulated during a natural peak in a sleep cycle (every 20, 30 or 40 minutes) he can come to a full waking and be physically unable to resettle. A classic example would be excess light hitting the back of the retina, halting his melatonin production. This will cause him to wake up and be extremely difficult to resettle.
- Excessive movement startling him to a full waking, or a baby standing/sitting under 12 months before he's even awake, and subsequently being unable to lie himself down without your intervention, may make resettling difficult.
- Some babies over 12 months still need two to two and a half hours sleep a day in one large sleep cycle rather than two shorter sleeps. These are typically LSR and ASR babies.
- You may have established a set of confusing environment-based getting up routines. Sometimes you pick up your baby straight away when you come in, sometimes he has to cry before you pick him up, and sometimes he has to go back to sleep. This ultimately encourages crying and confusion upon waking because he can't predict you and this can trigger early wakings and difficult resettling efforts.
- You may not have established the ability to guide your child respectfully yet, making asking him to lie down and try to go to sleep for you a difficult task. Look at your communication.
- Catnappers generally require a full PRM Routine 1 (see page 262).
- For confusing messages, it's important to establish a language-based set of routines around sleep-time events such as settling, resettling and waking routines plus playtime in the cot and the up cue before you pick him up, so when you don't pick him up, it doesn't seem unusual.
- Manage the transition in sleep cycles and interpret his crying correctly.

Q6: My baby wakes up at 8 p.m. every night and is happily awake until 10, then goes down for the night. How can I get him to sleep through this time?

- If six to 12 months old, his late afternoon sleep pattern is excessive or too late. No napping past 4 p.m. for babies on two larger sleeps per day, and not past 5 p.m. for LSR babies on bridging sleeps.

- Too much day sleep for a six-month-old, high-sleep-requirement baby still taking a third brief late afternoon nap in addition to two larger daytime sleeps. This may be a sign that he no longer needs a late afternoon nap.
- If 12 to 24 months old, any sleep after 4 p.m. for children taking two one- to one-and-a-half-hour sleeps a day or any sleep taken after 2.30 p.m. for those taking a single larger two- to two-and-a-half-hour sleep.
- It could be a shifted night pattern.
- Feed snoozing? Don't allow him to doze on any feeds through the day.

Q7: My baby wakes several times during the night but only needs me to attend quickly (often only a minute or less) to go back to sleep. What can I do to change this pattern?

POSSIBLE CAUSES

- Sleep association (see page 16).
- Subconscious (surface sleep wakings: see page 195).
- He may be cold.
- If he's under 12 months of age his need to feel secure may not be being met.
- Lost dummy.

TO FIX

- Make sure he's warm enough and feels secure if he's under 12 months, particularly if he's asking to be held to go back to sleep. He may need to be wrapped while you establish a new self-resettling association with going to sleep, and staying asleep.
- Establish new settling, resettling and waking cues through role play and communication, and manage environmental factors for the transition.
- If you're feeding briefly, assess meal-time intake during the day by looking at his meal-time windows and food intake to remove the night feeds.
- Be sure to look closely at and correct your settling, resettling and waking routines before you attempt any form of change.
- Manage any crying confidently and remain reassuring, while being 100 per cent consistent with the definitions you give the cues.
- Stop using the dummy or teach him the dummy pot game.

Q8: My baby will sleep through the night and have two sleeps of up to one and a half to two hours each during the day, but I then need to resettle him multiple times via patting, rocking or dummies during these sleeps. How can I correct this?

POSSIBLE CAUSES

- Associations are making settling and resettling impossible without you.
- Possible loss of trust because the sleep environment changes from when you put him to sleep and when he wakes up. Babies naturally become partially aware of their environment multiple times each sleep session (typically at the 20-, 30- or 40-minute mark). If you don't plan on being there when he becomes partially aware of his sleep environment, you shouldn't be there when he first goes to sleep. This is about being honest, and maintaining the delicate balance of trust a baby needs to be able to go to sleep and stay asleep without stress.

TO FIX

- For multiple wakings you will need a full routine management for a high-sleep-requirement child appropriate for his age group.
- Use balanced parent-governed lines of communication during the day. Incorporate sleep-time routines like settling, resettling and waking cues. Role play to develop your baby's trust in the process, and assess possible environmental conditions, particularly if he's asking to be held to either go to sleep or go back to sleep. He may be cold or need the extra comfort of a firm wrap while he learns how to sleep through the surface sleeps he will naturally cycle through. Make sure you follow the normal surface sleep pause before attending to crying so you don't startle him, wake him or trigger episodes of 'thrashing'.
- Manage the transition for a couple of days.

Q9: My baby will sleep through the night and take two day sleeps (up to one and a half to two hours each), but I need to resettle him multiple times through his day sleeps via feeding. What do I do?

POSSIBLE CAUSES

- His surface sleep associations, generally environmental needs, are not being catered for, including the need to feel held.
- Possible loss of trust because the sleep environment changes once he goes to sleep, so you put him to sleep, and then he requires this to go back to sleep. Babies naturally wake multiple times through the night.
- Possible false sleep as the result of breastfeeds, causing routine miscalculation because he's only staying asleep due to the sedating effect of the hormones during breastfeeding.

TO FIX

- Assess daily sleep requirement.
- Full routine management.

Q10: Could it be possible that my baby only needs 30 minutes sleep all day?
No, I believe it's impossible for a baby to only need 30 minutes sleep all day. In a very long career with babies I've *never* not been able to help a baby who appears to sleep next to nothing each day to learn how to sleep effectively. The smallest amount of daytime sleep I've seen a child from the six- to 24-month age bracket take after being put on a PRM and having 11 to 11½ hours night sleep is between one and a half to two hours through the day. The cause of low sleep here is a combination of unassessed sleep requirement, overtired body responses and a need to refine environment, routines and communication strategies a little.

Full repair PRM Routine 1 (see page 262) will have your child sleeping right through the night, and up to two to three hours during the day in as little as one to three days, even if he's never previously been able to sleep. In this latter case, when you've tried many other sleep training strategies or tried other routines and he's just wide awake and wired all day after one 30-minute sleep during the day, you should bypass the sleep requirement section of this book and lock him straight into the low-sleep-requirement routine suggestion for his age group. I promise you, it will change your life.

Q11: My baby will only sleep lying on me. What do I do to get him to sleep in his cot?
The cause of this is probably a combination of a few key things:

- Associations: he's learnt he can't go to sleep without you there.
- Trust: he is wanting to make sure you don't disappear which makes him very unsettled if you try to move him.
- Positioning: learning to sleep on his tummy, and upright on your body can make lying on his back a difficult task.
- Communication: allowing your child to govern sleep-time suggestions, even when he's not in a healthy sleeping routine, is not the right balance of communication. As parents, there are times when you need to be confident and help your child find a better way.
- Independence: not feeling comfortable being on his own, or in his own space, or not being able to trust that your absences are predictable in length and frequency makes it very hard for a child to feel comfortable about his parents being out of his sight. So he can experience

just being in his own space or feeling confident enough to explore the world around him, let him alone to be able to go to sleep on his own.

This is a significant sleep situation to resolve if you want to achieve consistent, stress-free sleep for your child and regain a healthy balance in your life. There's nothing healthy about an adult being stationary for the amount of hours a baby needs to sleep in a 24-hour day. There's nothing healthy about neglecting your dietary and fitness needs, or your marriage. If you're in this situation, whatever school of parenting appealed to you to get you in this situation is not appropriate for your baby or your needs and is not sustainable. You'll need to embark on a PRM, paying close attention to:

- the environmental needs of your child. I strongly recommend wrapping any child under 12 months of age until he is comfortable with and used to his new sleeping environment as this acts as a surrogate cuddle and helps him transition off you with less stress.
- adopting a confident parent-directed daily routine to take the burden of running your family off your child. It's important you learn about your child and understand his motivation for occasional crying. If you've adopted the approach of not letting him cry with the loving intention of sparing him any upset, while I admire your intentions, you have a mighty job on your hands. You're essentially stopping your child from feeling anything but happy, which is not always possible or healthy. It's best to introduce your child to a normal range of daily events and guide him through them with patience and compassion so that when it comes time for him to step out into the big wide world without you around to make everything better, he knows how to cope. Mummy and Daddy have told him it's okay and normal to feel a little uncomfortable with change, but trust that it always gets better in time, or to feel a little grumpy when he is tired is normal, and it can be resolved with some quiet relaxing, some healthy food, or a good old-fashion snuggle in his bed and a big sleep.

Q12: My partner can settle my baby but I cannot. Why? And how can I help my baby be comfortable with both of us?

When it comes to babies I find this tends to be because of one of the following:

- Mum does not attempt to settle the baby without feeding him, making it hard for Dad to settle him.
- Fathers naturally tend to hold their child a little more firmly in their arms or in the cot, which stops fussing and enables the baby to drift off more quickly. This becomes a comforter for the baby and he happily accepts this as a normal settling routine and goes to sleep more quickly. Once a dad realises his baby will settle quickly when he holds him firmly, he becomes more patient and follows through until he's asleep. This means the baby knows Daddy means business and he should sleep and nothing else. When Daddy is confident, going to sleep for him is associated with feelings of reassurance and confidence in the baby.
- One parent unknowingly undermines the other's attempts because they know the baby goes to sleep quicker for them. This is often done inadvertently by the baby's primary carer (the person who stays home with the baby during the day), traditionally the mum. The message it sends to the baby affects the other parent's ability to settle her and the primary carer becomes the only one who can do it. Some fathers then don't attempt to settle the baby to sleep, assuming that unless the baby is fed, he will be unsuccessful.
- Environmental comforters.
- Positioning.
- Communication.
- Trust.
- Independence.
- Settling, resettling and waking routines.

As parents may have inconsistent styles of settling, you'll need to establish full settling, resettling and waking routines, as well as look at environmental comforters like wrapping, in the case of an under-12 month old, and firm tucking in. You will also need to role play. When you need to incorporate this many changes, it's easier to just follow the positive routine management plan for your child's sleep requirement.

Q13: My baby will not go to sleep in the morning at all. What do I do?

POSSIBLE CAUSES

- Too long a night sleep session.
- Shifted body clock/false sleep after early morning feed.
- No longer needs a morning sleep once over 12 months of age.

TO FIX

- This is very rare in a baby under 12 months if he's waking at a reasonable time, like 6 to 6.30 a.m. If he is under 12 months and you're experiencing significant sleep problems in the morning, use positive routine management with an emphasis on eliminating environmental factors that could be making it difficult for him to sleep, such as light, noise and movement.
- If your baby is over 12 months of age, take a peek at my 12 months plus LSR routine (see page 272) and you may find he's doing what is natural for his body's needs. You can still achieve a HSR sleep routine of two sleeps per day but each sleep is generally around one to one and a half hours long, a format that clearly suits his needs. If you've tried to encourage sleep in the morning and he's just not interested, shift him into the 12 months plus LSR routine.

Q14: My baby will only sleep in the car, pram, or in a sling or hammock. How do I get him to sleep in the cot?

POSSIBLE CAUSES

- Motion associations with sleep.
- Positioning.

TO FIX

- Address positioning issues.
- Wrap and use Safe T Sleep for an under-12 month old to emulate the security of the cot environment for mobile sleep environments.
- Use a sleeping bag and tuck-in for an over-12 month old.

Q15: My baby sleeps well during the day, but not at night. What do I do?

POSSIBLE CAUSE

This is a classic case of sleep debt common in lower-sleep-requirement babies. Your baby sleeps well during the day (in the same routine as a higher-sleep-requirement baby does with two large sleeps) *only* because he's sleeping poorly at night. Once a child starts to sleep effectively through the night, he can't sustain longer sleeps during the day. Your baby is far better suited to either the LSR routine or modified HSR routine with ASR sleep-time suggestions (see Chapter 13).

TO FIX

Correctly assess your child's sleep requirement based on his age and implement an appropriate daytime routine to suit his daytime sleep needs. Keep in mind that he should have 11 to 11½ hours of sleep through the night.

Q16: My baby sleeps well at night, but not during the day. Can this be fixed?

POSSIBLE CAUSES

- Classic low-sleep-requirement symptom.
- Possibly different settling routine used for day sleep.
- The sleeping environment is too stimulating.

TO FIX

- Assess your child's daily sleep requirement and choose the best routine for him. When a child's day sleeps are very short (40 minutes or less all day) he almost always has a low or average sleep requirement and responds quickly to the new daily plan.
- A PRM will ensure you have consistent day and night routines so your baby is able to sleep effectively at all sleep times.
- Carefully assess your child's sleep environment to consider what short-term aids you can put in place and/or what overstimulating conditions (light, noise, movement) you can temporarily remove to help make the learning process much faster. Once his sleep is resolved, you can gradually eliminate the aids, and reintroduce the usual conditions of light and noise.

Q17: My baby goes to sleep in his cot but always ends up in our bed. I'd like to get him to sleep in his bed all night. Can you help?

POSSIBLE CAUSES

- This is a resettling association which happens when a child has been taught on a subconscious level that during his brief surface sleep, to go back to sleep he needs a different set of conditions to the ones he has for settling.
- He may be cold.

TO FIX

- Carefully re-establish consistent settling, resettling and waking routines, and role play them.
- Learn how to manage the surface sleep phase of sleep.
- Learn how to manage his crying carefully.
- Assess his room temperature.

Because of all these possibilities, I suggest you establish an appropriate routine to ensure there are no other reasons for the night waking.

Q18: We tried to get our little boy to sleep in our bed, but he just doesn't sleep. How can we achieve this?

POSSIBLE CAUSE

It either doesn't suit him or you need to work on your communication skills and, in particular, your positioning requests through the day. This means you need to set fairly clear boundaries around the task of going to sleep in your bed.

TO FIX

If it's clear sleep is a significant problem for your baby you may need to consider another method. Alternatively, work on positioning him through the day for nappy changes, sitting while reading stories and lying down for milk feeds, etc. Establish settling, resettling and waking routines and set similar boundaries in your bed as you would for a cot. For example, once you start your settling routine he cannot sit up or stand up and don't talk to him other than to say your cues. Once your settling routine is complete, set boundaries around his positioning and what he's allowed to do, for example, he can roll but he cannot poke you, etc. Develop cues for each boundary – 'no touch eyes', etc. – and define those statements. If he cries, pause and lie still with your eyes closed and repeat your resettling cues periodically. Repeat management for resettling routine and use a waking routine when he's allowed to sit up after your waking cue, 'Good sleep, time to sit up'.

Sleeping arrangements need to suit your baby's requirements as much as yours. If he's trying to sleep but whimpers or excessively wrestles through the night, it's possible he doesn't find it comfortable or peaceful to try to sleep between two grown-ups who move a lot and make noise. In this case, adopt a settling routine for his cot and move on. Co-sleeping doesn't suit every baby, even if it's what you want.

Q19: My baby sleeps in his cot at night, but will only sleep in my arms during the day. So how can I get him to not do this?

POSSIBLE CAUSES

- A daytime settling association. This occurs often when a child has been taught that during the daylight hours he needs an entirely different set of conditions to the ones he has for settling after a bath at night.
- He may be overtired, causing him to become easily overstimulated by light and noise through the day. If he's unsettled about sleeping in his cot, the change of conditions will cause him to open his eyes, which triggers a chemical reaction in his brain that affects the hormones that facilitate sleep.

TO FIX

- Assess his sleep requirement and adopt a routine that suits his needs.
- Re-establish consistent settling, resettling and waking routines, and role play them. Learn how to manage both the surface sleep part of his sleep cycle and his crying while he learns to self-settle.
- Eliminate light in his room during the day until you've repaired his sleep. Once he's sleeping, and is no longer overtired, slowly reintroduce light into his daytime home sleep environment.

Q20: My baby will only sleep in his pram during the day. I'd like to get him to sleep in his cot. How can I do this?

The same causes and fixes as for Question 19 apply here. If you cannot guide him successfully through the day with events like nappy changes, feeding or asking him to sit still on your lap or in the pram, read through the communication sections to learn about the three lines of communication.

Q21: My baby has reflux. Can this affect his sleeping?

Reflux most certainly affects sleeping if it isn't treated. If medication has been prescribed by his doctor and hasn't alleviated the symptoms within three weeks of starting treatment, you need to go back to the doctor. When a baby lies down, stomach acid tracks back up his oesophagus and irritates the tissue. When this happens repeatedly the tissues of the oesophagus become inflamed and lying down becomes a painful ordeal. This makes going to sleep very difficult for the baby because he's experiencing pain. Also, as children rely heavily on associations with going to bed, he may learn to fear lying down, anticipating the pain.

TO FIX

This should be dealt with in two ways:

1. Make sure his symptoms are relieved by seeking medical advice from your doctor or paediatrician.
2. Once the discomfort has been dealt with, be sure to move him past the learnt pattern of fear of lying down by resolving the sleep-time issues with a full positive routine management.

You need to be patient and consistent to help him learn as quickly as possible that sleep is no longer painful. Some parents might not want to expose their child to a situation that their baby is so fretful about, but it's best not to leave a child burdened with a fear he no longer needs to be concerned about. Show him that Mummy and Daddy have helped him feel better so sleep time doesn't have to evoke unpleasant feelings unnecessarily.

Q22: My baby/toddler seems to be cutting teeth. Could this be impacting on his sleep?

Cutting teeth could definitely be impacting on his ability to go to sleep or to stay asleep. Regardless of what anyone tells you, teething is clearly uncomfortable and in some cases very distressing for babies. When he's in a good routine, the bulk of his growing should occur while he sleeps, but when he's having higgledy-piggledy days, where sleep is difficult, then teething will impact on him entire day.

TO FIX

If you know your baby is suffering from very sore or uncomfortable teeth, offer eight-hour pain relief close to sleep times if possible rather than when he's awake. Your baby's ability to cope with discomfort will be higher when he's awake and with you than when he's tired and on his own during sleep time. I reserve (whenever possible) the use of these pain relievers to around 30 minutes before bedtime. Maintain pain relief through the night as discomfort windows are often between 11.30 p.m. and 3.30 a.m.

For those children on a PRM, it is very common for any typical sleep-time teething symptoms to either appear for the first time or reappear between 11.30 p.m. and 1.30 a.m. In this case, offer another dose of medication (as per instructions) and then follow through with your crying management (see pages 398–399 for appropriate ways to help him through the night when he's not feeling well or is experiencing discomfort).

Q23: My baby needs to burp before he goes to sleep. How can I help him and could this be causing problems?

I occasionally hear about babies needing to burp before sleep, but rarely when they're over six months, unless they suffer severe reflux. I've dealt with thousands of extremely unsettled babies and one of the first things many parents tell me is that their infant needs to either burp or break wind before he can settle off to sleep. When babies cry and fuss because they're protesting or upset they have a tendency to gulp air and this makes their tummy rumble and move about. When you pick them up, air naturally rises and shifts and they have a tendency to burp and break wind. They often settle because they were asking to be picked up at this time and you've obliged, so the cycle of winding starts at sleep time. This in itself becomes a routine or an association of sorts governed by your baby.

TO FIX

Look at assessing his true need versus his short-term demand to be picked up and burped. Don't be frightened of a transitional window as this will never free him of this disruptive sleep routine. Teach him a whole new enjoyable settling routine that doesn't involve this cycle of crying, being picked up, and burping. When you establish your new routine management, don't perpetuate the cycle of picking up and winding your baby to sleep, or this will need to be done over and over again through the night.

Q24: My baby snuffles and vocalises a lot during the night, but doesn't really cry. Can I do something to help him sleep more soundly?

If he's vocalising a lot but not crying leave him be, and turn down your monitor. Most of the time babies are oblivious to their own snuffling and movement and, even if aware of it, they're not bothered by it. Infrared imaging of babies sleeping through the night shows them cycling through different stages of sleep and, on some occasions, waking, happily snuffling and squirming around their cot for up to 40 minutes, then drifting back off to sleep.

TO FIX

- The best thing you can do is to leave him alone. Imagine if every time you rolled over during the night someone came and patted you and asked if you were okay. It would disrupt you, and you would likely wake up.
- If your child making noise makes it difficult for you to sleep yourself, place the receiving end of the monitor outside his door so you only hear if he cries. If he's close enough to your room, and you can hear him crying without the monitor, ditch the monitor altogether. If he's in the next room, then it's very unlikely you need a monitor.

Q25: My baby always wakes up when we go to bed. How can I stop this?

POSSIBLE CAUSES

- Change in sleep conditions.
- Sensitivity to noise.
- You're going to bed at a time when he hits a surface sleep phase, which is typically between 10 and 11 p.m.

TO FIX

- Close his door.
- Get a white noise machine or white noise CD.
- Be conscious of the time you go to bed. Read about the 'Sleep Bus' (see page 354) and 'The physiology of sleep'.
- Check the environmental conditions near his room: lights, noise, etc.
- Consider your resettling associations: do you pause before you attend to him?

Q26: Is it possible for my baby to have nightmares?

Under-two year olds rarely have nightmares unless they are exposed to frightening or confusing concepts on TV, or there's significant unrest in your house with parental fighting or grief or divorce, for instance. A baby's capacity to have nightmares, as we know them, is reduced by the lack of development in his imagination. Nightmares are more prevalent in children over two and it is common for pre-schoolers to experience clear instances of nightmares.

When a child under two wakes screaming at night, it's more likely to be due to a phenomenon called a sudden partial waking. These screaming wake-up calls should cease if you adhere to the surface sleep pause and don't accidentally disturb him before he's in a full state of consciousness from sleep. If you disturb him before this you can cause what is sometimes called 'wild thrashing'.

Behavioural patterns which are described in sleep clinics as *true* night terror phenomena, are far more prevalent after the child has reached around two and a half years of age. Even in these instances, the episodes of night terrors appear to completely vanish when a routine is established. By three years of age, I see children who have developed an imagination start to have what appear to be nightmares with clear dream recall immediately after the event in some cases.

TO FIX

Adhere to your surface sleep pause before attending to him if he's under two to be certain you're not disorientating him by attending to him while he's not fully awake.

Q27: When my baby wakes up during the night he's not hungry. What could be causing this?

POSSIBLE CAUSES

There are two reasons for your baby's consistent night waking that don't include a need for feeding. Both are environmental factors. They are:

1. Temperature/comfort.
2. Associations.

- Night wakings that are not feed related are generally always about the environment. There are obvious problems like temperature, and it is usually because he is too hot when he first goes to bed between 7 and 10 p.m., or too cold as his body temperature and the night temperature drops. During day sleep sessions it appears babies are prone to becoming particularly cold, even on a mild to warm day.

- The associations your child initially went to sleep with may have changed, or he's developed a set of resettling associations requiring your intervention in order for him to go back to sleep. You will know it is an association because you'll consistently have to help him go back to sleep. Being too cold may be what originally caused him to call out to you for a cuddle to warm up, so make sure he isn't getting cold and consider wrapping him until he's older.

TO FIX

- You may need to wrap him and regulate his room temperature.
- Check his clothing is appropriate, and consider a tuck-in if he's over 12 months old.
- If he's expecting you to repeatedly help him back to sleep, read the information contained in 'The psychology of sleep' and about associations to understand the origins of his sleep problem.
- Seriously consider a full PRM routine (see page 262).

Q28: **My baby goes to bed at 10 p.m. and wakes around 8 or 9 a.m. Is this okay?**

POSSIBLE CAUSE

Your baby has a shifted body clock which I refer to as the 'late shift'.

TO FIX

It's simple to repair this sleep pattern in this age group. If your baby can self-settle and self-resettle and the only problem you have is the times she chooses to sleep, read about the late shift and the body's circadian rhythms.

Q29: **I want my baby, who is under 12 months, to sleep in as I'm not much of an early person. If I put him down later in the evening will I achieve a later waking time?**

Sleeping in is an unrealistic expectation of a baby in the six- to 12-month age group, though not for a child over a year old. Babies rise with the world; 6 to 6.30 a.m. is a pretty good sleep-in for a baby who goes to bed at 7 p.m., as they should. Perhaps you're going to bed too late, or you need to give your body a chance to recover from the terrible sleep disruption you've experienced over the last few months since your baby graced your life with his presence. You need to correct your baby's sleep-time problems so you're not so exhausted in the morning.

TO FIX

- You can encourage a child 12 months old plus to sleep in a little later if he's on a solid midday sleep from the LSR routine, but be sure he's taking adequate sleep during the day to help him enjoy the second half of the day and cope well until he's due to go to sleep at 7 p.m. Once these children are taking a minimum of two hours of solid sleep at lunch and sleeping right through the night from 7 p.m., they can gradually, in 20-minute windows, a week at a time per increase, be offered a later sleep in. Stop increasing the windows when your baby starts to wake naturally either in the morning or at the lunch sleep. If he stops sleeping so well at lunch, then you're altering his sleep need to suit your sleep-in desires. While this is tempting, he'll be overtired by 7 p.m., which may cause him to wake through the night.

- Be aware, putting a baby or toddler to bed later will generally encourage an earlier wake-up time. Read 'The biology of sleep' for more.

Q30: My child fights sleep and I can't work out why. What do I do?

POSSIBLE CAUSES

- The most common reason babies fight sleep is because of changes in their sleeping conditions. If a parent or carer puts a baby to sleep a certain way – be it in their arms, or by staying in the room with a hand on the baby's back – and then sneaks off; when the baby wakes up, having no concept of sleep or time lapsing, he will startle and call out to his parent. This leads him to associate the sensation of feeling tired with his loved one disappearing, creating a situation where he fights the feelings associated with going to sleep because he's concerned you may disappear.
- Other reasons can be through failed attempts at control crying or 'pick up/put down' strategies, and he's unable to understand the inconsistent conditions of sleep and doesn't have the skills he needs to cope with that request. These inconsistent approaches, with no predictable strategies incorporated around resettling *and*, most importantly, waking-up time, result in either short-term success, or no success and a loss of trust. The child then becomes fretful about his sleeping environment and the process of sleep.

TO FIX

- Read Chapter 2.
- Assess the most appropriate routine for your baby.
- Implement the environmental changes he may need in order to learn how to sleep.

Q31: My baby seems to be sleeping fine and I don't want to lose that. Do you think I should shift him to a routine just in case?

If you're in a good routine, and by that I mean a consistent 24-hour cycle in which your baby is sleeping well at night and in the daytime, regardless of whether it fits with other people's suggestions or not, don't try to fix something that isn't broken. In your case, a new daily routine will *not* help maintain your baby's good sleep, *but* consistent settling, resettling and waking routines and excellent, balanced communication will help him maintain sleep. Be aware of your child's changing sleep needs as he grows. Don't expect him to need as much sleep at ten, 12 or 18 months as he needed at seven months (if he's been sleeping well). Be prepared to change and adapt if he shows signs that a regular sleep time is starting to make it hard for him to sleep at another time.

Q32: My baby sleeps well some days, and badly on others. Why?

POSSIBLE CAUSE

This is a common problem that comes down to sleep requirement. Parents often *want* their baby to sleep their 'best' day sleep every day, when the reality is their baby's sleep requirement means they actually need to sleep the average between their best and worst days to lock in a realistic and consistent daily routine.

TO FIX

- You need to keep a sleep diary to work out your child's average daily sleep requirement.
- Please read about progressive sleep decline.

Q33: I'm really worried about waking my partner and other children when my baby cries in the middle of the night. Can you advise me how to best handle this?

This is most people's biggest concern when they have other children. If you've been rushing into your baby's room as soon as he cries you may have created patterns of subconscious sleep associations during his surface sleep, meaning he'll cry out for you to recreate those associations.

TO FIX

The only true solution to this is to eliminate the crying out by putting your baby's needs first. There are a couple of ways you can do this:

- Send the older children and your partner off for the weekend and resolve the problem over this two-day window, when you don't have to be concerned about disrupting the others; or

- Consider a white noise machine for your older child.

Talk with your partner about investing a weekend to help your baby learn to sleep through without the need to call out. Start at a time when you can all rest more during the day. While I usually suggest you start any routine management on a Monday so you can focus on having calm quiet days, if you're very concerned about others becoming tired for the two days it takes to correct the sleep patterns start on Saturday. Establish your new routine and follow it carefully.

Q34: Are music CDs just as helpful as white noise?

If your baby is sleeping well with a music CD playing in his room, there's no problem using it. Music CDs can be very soothing for some babies, and some parents have established a lovely sleep-time association using CDs. However, if you need to go in during the night to switch the CD back on when he wakes, then you've developed a resettling association that will require your intervention.

TO FIX ANY POSSIBLE PROBLEMS:

- Consider putting the CD on repeat so the conditions you've made available to your baby when he first went to sleep don't suddenly change. While some babies will love their lullaby CD at sleep time, there can be inherent problems when you create an environment-based association around sleep, which is what a music CD does. Some babies will then be unable to sleep without it forever more. If this occurs, he's limited to sleeping in a room in the house where he can hear the CD playing. If this isn't possible, as it generally isn't, you'll need to re-establish a new association with sleep.
- If you want to correct a significant sleep-time problem, work with products that either don't cause sleep associations or can be used everywhere. I'm a big fan of white noise CDs for settling. White noise is essentially 'silence', and you don't run the risk of establishing an association, and you still get the added benefits of eliminating the noises that wake up babies.

Q35: My older child is accidentally waking my baby during the day when he's a little loud during play. I don't want to ask him to be quiet. Is there anything else I can do?

It's hardly fair, with all the changes that have happened in your older child's life, to ask him to be really quiet while their new baby brother or sister sleeps.

TO FIX

- Playing and chatting happily at a normal everyday volume is something every toddler should be able to do. However, it's reasonable to set appropriate boundaries for older children, like no banging on the baby's door, or shouting the baby's name to deliberately wake him up, and no wandering into the baby's room whenever it suits him.
- As mentioned, I'm a big fan of white noise CDs and it might eliminate the noises that wake your baby up. By placing the CD player in your baby's room, your older child can play and chat freely, you can relax and stop feeling tense about your older child being a normal chatty, noisy kid, and your baby can sleep on oblivious to the ruckus his big brother or sister is causing.

Q36: My baby was sleeping fine until two months ago and now he's not coping at all. What happened?

POSSIBLE CAUSES

There are generally a few typical triggers for sudden changes in sleeping habits:

- You may be holding on to a sleeping routine he's grown out of instead of keeping up with his changing sleep needs. While it's not unusual to want an extra hour in the day to complete things on your 'to do' list, staying a step ahead of him changing sleep needs ensures you don't suddenly have to deal with significant sleep disruptions that lead you to losing a large portion of your day and subsequent night's sleep. Even if he no longer needs to sleep the old pattern of two one- to one-and-a-half-hour sleep sessions during the day, it doesn't mean he can't still achieve up to two and a half hours sleep either at one session, or with supporting bridges, regardless of his age group.
- Your communication may have become a little imbalanced. This can happen if a child starts to develop a confident child-directed line of communication and you don't sustain your parent-governed line. When this occurs your child starts to create predictable sets of conditions around environments to feel a little more in control of a day that is always changing without warning. You then find he resists your guidance through the day at times like nappy change, getting dressed, getting into the high chair, car seat or pram, resists you feeding him and resists your guidance at sleep time.
- Conditions in the sleeping environment may have changed.

- Emotional changes, such as a sudden loss of trust in his world, can happen when changes make things feel unpredictable. These changes could include a new sister or brother arriving in his life, moving house, going on a holiday or someone moving in or moving out. Perhaps there is a divorce, sudden bickering, a change in nanny or teacher in his daycare, or there is a grief in the family. During these changes a child has every right to feel uncertain.

TO FIX

- Assess your child's sleep needs and re-establish your daily routine.
- Read about communication to understand the importance of respectfully establishing a balanced line of communication.
- Try to observe his behaviour in response to any environmental changes. If you introduced a light, remove it. If you eliminated a wrap, introduce a sleeping bag and firm tuck-in (if he's over 12 months old) or a wrap again until he's ready to get rid of it. Consider the change in temperature and adjust accordingly.
- When emotional changes occur, support your baby, keep him close, and communicate with him during the day using your flow of communication to keep him informed of any impending changes to help him settle down. Avoid fighting in front of him, and try to have an air of reassurance around you so he can feel confident that while things are different they are still safe. Always have consistent predictable settling, resettling and waking routines (at sleep time so he feels in control of the event, but if there are major traumas occurring in his or your world, you may need to keep him close and just get through it before asking him to sleep away from you.

Q37: We've tried everything but my baby has never been a good sleeper. Can you help me?

If your baby has always been an unsettled sleeper, don't despair, even the most unsettled baby has been able to learn how to sleep. In full recovery, they can be sleeping within 12 to 36 hours.

TO FIX

Put him on the full recovery program (see page 262).

Q38: Can my baby have a cup or bottle in his bed?

I don't recommend a cup or a bottle in bed for children under 24 months old. It's important to provide fluid intake in the form of water regularly during the day when he's *not* in his bed. Only once have I felt there was a genuine thirst during the night in a boy who was 21 months of age, so

I provided him with a spill-proof cup in the dummy pot, and treated it in the same way I did the dummy by showing him the cup and reminding him to 'get your cup' when I attended to him when he called out during the first night of his new self-settling sleep routine. By the following day he was entirely self-sufficient with his cup through the night and no longer needed to call out. If you do need to offer him a drink at night, and this would be a rare occasion, only ever offer water in his cup.

Q39: My baby was premature. Does this make a difference to his sleeping ability?

Premature babies may have different settling abilities until they reach around eight to ten months of age if they were born more than four to six weeks premature; otherwise, by twelve months of age, there is no need to keep adjusting a baby born four weeks premature for sleep purposes. If your baby is only six to seven months old when his age is adjusted, follow the normal routine suggestion for positive routine management for his adjusted age, not his birth age.

Q40: I have a baby with profound hearing impairment. What adjustments do I need to make to help him sleep well?

Hearing impairments make a significant difference to settling routines. In the case of deaf children, their ability to predict their environment is very dependent on watching those around them. Be careful and be sure to introduce full visual cues, much the same as signing, about leaving his room with the intention of allowing him to go to sleep. This 'signing' could be both visual and contact/physical, in much the same way you would sign directly onto a child's hand if he was visually and hearing impaired. So, in the middle of the night when your baby is needing to go back to sleep, you can use your sign on his hand to tell him you'd like him to go to sleep and you're about to leave and he'll be able to understand. The same principle applies for his waking routine.

TO HELP

- I would certainly encourage him to develop an attachment to a comfort item for sleep time only.
- In a child six to eight months of age, pursuing sleep *should* be easier if you wrap him firmly and pop him in the comfort of a Safe T Sleep. If he's just having a little grumble and protest on those first few days, leave him be.
- If he's having a more difficult time, or he's older, take more time when helping him sleep. Always keep doors open, come in and out

of his room regularly without fussing with him, and tidy clothes or toys away to tell him you're nearby and he can relax.

- Use a visual hand gesture and physical on-hand signing cue each time you plan to step out of the room for a moment to tell him you'd like him to sleep on those first few days. It may take him a while to go to sleep but if you always make the outcome of your little sleep-time ritual the same, the time it takes for him to go to sleep will become shorter and shorter.
- Take it very slowly when encouraging him to try to self-settle. Work hard on cot playtime strategies, and a visual short-term absence cue to build his confidence in that environment and help him become comfortable with you leaving the room.
- Pursuing sleep should be maintained as should clear boundaries around not standing in his cot while you're in the room. Ask him to remain lying down and follow your bedtime ritual, which should be in the same format as my settling, resettling and waking routines (bearing in mind that a hearing impaired child should be able to clearly see you and your face while you're reading her books). If you need to stay near him room and potter in and out as you put washing away, keep asking him to lie down until he falls asleep.
- Leave a night light on in the hall and him door open if it's stressful for him to have it closed so she becomes comfortable with this consistent environment.
- For more information, talk in more detail with staff of organisations dealing with these questions. They will have many practical suggestions.

Q41: My baby has profound sight impairment. I know I need to do things differently, but how and what?

Because this book is about a language-based framework, it should be helpful for you and your baby. Many researchers believe that when one of the five senses is lacking or missing entirely, the other senses strengthen to compensate. It would be great to think that given your child's world is predominantly auditory based it encourages the language centre of his brain to develop and adapt quickly to new routine styles of communication, so the use of routine styles of settling, resettling and waking routines should be quickly adjusted to, particularly if you role play.

TO HELP

- Encourage him to develop an attachment to a comfort item for sleep time only.

- Ensure strong smell association with Mummy and Daddy in his cot by placing a well-used pillowcase (unwashed) under his fitted cot sheet. Rub his comfort item on your hair, neck and even down Mum's top if he's still being breastfed. Pursue the PRM suited to his age and sleep requirement.
- For more information, talk with staff of organisations which deal with these impairments for more detailed suggestions about helping your baby sleep.

Q42: I don't think my toddler, who is over 18 months, wants his day sleep any more. How can I tell?

POSSIBLE CAUSE

I've never met a 12 to 24 month old who hasn't been able to take a day sleep on my LSR Routine 1 – 12 months-plus age variation repair plan (see page 272). A 13- to 14-hour night sleep could be causing problems with his ability to take a day sleep, even if he regularly wakes through the night. I never recommend such long nights when it takes away from the ability to take a daytime nap because these children are too young and are growing and learning too rapidly to successfully get through an 11-hour day when they're only 12 to 24 months old and need to be in their best form to learn, grow and enjoy the last half of their day without a daytime sleep.

TO FIX

- If your toddler is sleeping too long at night, follow the PRM Routine 1 suggestion for age variation 12 months plus (see page 272) and he will start to sleep again during the day.
- If, on the other hand, he's not sleeping for a long time at night, and is full of beans and excited all day, then he's likely to be overtired, and you'll need to look carefully at the meal plan in the above-mentioned routine. Adopt the full recovery program, paying careful attention to the meal-time windows to correct his sleep-time problems.
- If your toddler truly doesn't need a daytime sleep under the age of two years, the signs of this are as follows:
  - A solid night's sleep with no fussing upon going to bed each night. Hours of fussing at a 7 p.m. bedtime can indicate your child is over-tired, and is having trouble winding down, so needs a day sleep.
  - Willing to go into his cot for a midday rest, and chat quietly through the day nap time for up to an hour without going to sleep. If your child is fighting going in his cot, his reluctance

to take a daytime sleep is actually a communication-based problem rather than a true need for no sleep. Develop balanced, respectful, two-way communication flow with your toddler through the day.
– Able to cope at 5 p.m. and isn't having a tantrum or being hard to manage leading up to this meal, and equally doesn't become *too* overexcited after dinner. A normal level of elevated energy is always present after the last meal of the day, but excessive frenetic behaviour after 5.30 p.m. is indicative of overtiredness.

If it's clear your baby isn't tired, based on the above list of signs, maintain his quiet rest time in his cot so he can have a period of between one and two hours where there's reduced stimulation (NB: television is a poor option for quiet time). This will give him a chance to have a quiet wind down, and will refresh him for the second portion of the day. It also ensures you and your partner stay well rested and have a little wind-down time, too, so you can have a healthy lunch and recharge your batteries so you can be in top form for the second half of the day.

Q43: My little boy (over 18 months) talks for up to an hour when I first put him to bed at 7 p.m. Is it time to drop his daytime nap?

No. It's quite a common situation for toddlers to have a little debrief about their day. You'll hear him rattle off all his experiences almost systematically, and process all the different expressions and emotions he felt and witnessed during the day. This is a healthy part of early childhood and it's perfectly fine to allow it to run its course without interference. However, it shouldn't go for more than an hour, and doesn't change the routine waking time you provide each morning, or for each day sleep. To allow him to sleep in the next morning will cause a shifted sleep cycle, and perpetuate the pattern. If he chats for an hour and finally goes to sleep at 8 p.m. and you compensate by letting him sleep in till 7 or 7.30 a.m., it means he can't fall asleep until 1 p.m. after lunch, which impacts on his settling time that night. This makes getting him into bed before 8 p.m. difficult, and he then still needs to have his little debrief. A later debrief will obviously stop him from dozing off to sleep until closer to 9 p.m., and so a vicious cycle begins.

TO FIX IF CAUSING A PROBLEM

- If he's having difficulties going to sleep beyond the age of 12 months, either at night or during the day, he'll need to be on the PRM Routine 1 with the 12-month variation.

- Don't allow any daytime sleep to be over two hours if this is common at night-time, and his midday sleep should be from 12 to 2 p.m. and no later.

By allowing him to have a little debrief every night, and still working within your timeframe, you'll avoid routine miscalculations and encourage better sleep. If he's chatting, there's no need to interfere with that natural healthy settling process. We spend a lot of time encouraging confidence and independence in babies' cot environments, and chatting busily to himself about his day is a lovely sign of this being established.

Q44: At what age can I give my toddler a pillow to sleep on?
If he's under two years, don't introduce pillows to the cot for any reason. Pillows are unsafe for babies under two, and he's perfectly capable of sleeping flat without one. Babies' bodies are designed to sleep flat to keep their airway clear. If anyone suggests the use of pillows or cushions in the cot for any other purpose (to cuddle for instance), be very careful about the choices you make. I would be extremely reluctant to consider a pillow as an option for any reason until he is two years of age or older.

Q45: When can I transfer my toddler to a bed?
I don't recommend introducing a bed for a child under two years old. It's the kind of milestone you want him to achieve around his second birthday having prepared him for it carefully. Moving from a cot to a bed can be the trigger for some troubling episodes of settling problems and night wanderings, so prepare him for the excitement of the situation, and the boundaries of being in a bed.

If a child under two has a tendency to find settling or resettling challenging, he won't be able to cope with the responsibility of a big bed just yet. To move him into a bed too soon may be a negative process and therefore make it a less than pleasant experience rather than an exciting new opportunity that is pleasing to both him and you, and gives him a sense of achievement rather than anxiety or confusion.

13

Daily sleep requirements

In this section I provide complete, almost minute-by-minute daily routines to help babies settle into their new PRM quickly. You *shouldn't* even consider starting any daily routine or sleep repair until you've done your homework and taught your baby the skills for your new expectations of sleep time. Until now I've concentrated on preparing your baby and the *event* routines around parent-governed lines of communication and play; that is, nappy changing, playing in a cot, sitting happily in a high chair, and so on.

The chapters in this section outline more of these event routines and, most importantly, provide you with new settling, resettling and waking cues and routines. These new routines shouldn't be used for anything except sleep, so please read the entire section *before* starting any new sleep routine. Once you've read the book and done your homework and are ready to repair your baby's sleep, it's time to see how all these event routines fit together in a 24-hour cycle so you and your baby can have happy days and peaceful nights.

You can't hope to repair sleep until you've established good communication, independence and role played event routines. Remember there are two kinds of routine: environmental and language based. You need to develop a language-based routine you can use anywhere, making your baby's sleep transportable from one place to another and sleep routines transferable from one person to the next. Because your child's comfort with her event routines is not dependent on a particular room or person you can take the routines anywhere and ask anyone to follow your plan. You can wake up in the morning, pack a bag and drop your baby at her grandparents' house for the day, or go on a holiday with her, or sleep elsewhere. You can even change times zones with ease.

There is, however, a hitch, which is that you need to invest three solid weeks into locking the daily routine in place first, during which you need to remain consistent with your flow of communication and daily-routine management at home in order to permanently repair your baby's sleep and make her happy. After you've given your child the time to become completely familiar with, and therefore in control of and trust, the entire daily routine you can slowly become more adventurous about where you take her.

This strategy is designed to provide predictability for your child and you, so neither of you becomes a prisoner of a routine. But when you first start her new routine and she begins sleeping well for the first time, be careful about working *with* her body clock. Do things bang on the time suggested in the program, so you can actually work with her body rather than just her temperament. Eventually these times will be ball-park because the language and skills will be set, so asking her to go to sleep will be a simple task. Until then you may want to take advantage of a locked-in need for sleep or food at certain windows to achieve your goals more quickly. If your child doesn't respond rapidly to the shift in the timetable and takes a little bit longer to settle in, then tone down the amount of movement you're making within the routine times until you find your baby's comfort zones.

For babies under six months of age

You may wonder why I don't provide specific routines for babies under six months in this section. The reason I focus on routines for six month to two year olds is that there isn't enough space in one book to put all the standard-routine suggestions that a rapidly changing baby's little body needs. Since the 1960s there have been standard high and average routine suggestions available for babies in the nought to six months group which can be found in most books and sourced from most early childhood clinics, so I won't repeat them. It is when parents don't fall into a natural flow with their baby, or those standard routines don't fit their baby's sleep needs that I suggest you investigate their sleep requirement further and adopt an appropriate routine to cater for their true sleep requirement. That usually needs to happen at about six months of age but it's difficult to find anyone who doesn't use a one-size-fits-all approach, which is where positive routine management comes in.

Babies are also so extremely precious when they are under six months that the communication style needs to be carefully examined before implementing any form of solid routine for this age group so you don't confuse them. I am predominantly in the business of sleep repair and establishing communication. So although a good proportion of new families will find their way by using the communication, independence and play event routines I outline, as well as incorporating the settling, resettling and waking routines, there will be a large group who, having tried the standard suggestions and found no significant flow, will need to adopt a more solid routine to find sleep repair.

You can find your way for a newborn by either adopting a casual flow, such as the loose suggestions highlighted below which will suit many babies or, in the case of a fussy, unsettled baby, by following a more specific routine suggestion from your local baby health care centre or clinic. This will give your baby time to settle into the world, and give you time to identify and resolve any issues such as reflux before they reach six months. If at that point, however, you're still unable to find resolution to sleep-time difficulties using the tools in this book, then you will need to adopt my PRM routine to end any ongoing fussiness and settle your baby into her new world of peaceful nights and happy days. Remember: it's okay to have a little 'getting to know your baby' stage when she is first born without rushing frantically into a one-size-fits-all feeding and sleeping regime. Many babies find their way naturally when a parent understands communication and the need for predictability and sleep associations.

My casual flow suggestion for new babies

At this very early stage of development, just being awake and feeding are hugely exhausting tasks for a baby. Add to that nappy changes, getting dressed, being picked up and put down, and having very important conversations with Mummy, Daddy and Granny, and it's a bit overwhelming for the little possum. I have a few standard things I'm always conscious of when I meet a baby having a tricky time.

Firstly, please don't feel you need to stop breastfeeding. This is often a mother's first area of doubt but it's rarely the actual issue. If you're concerned about your milk supply or the effectiveness of your feeding I highly recommend you see a good lactation specialist who can come to your home and help you develop a good breastfeeding strategy and plan.

Good solid breastfeeds need good solid winding. Go out of your way to ensure your baby has no wind at all after her feed. After that initial burp keep going until you can get another burp. I do this each side of a breastfeed just to make sure a baby doesn't develop layers of milk and air trapped in her tummy.

Try not to allow your baby to break her feeds too often because the more she detaches, the more likely she is to throw up after the feed is finished.

When your baby is very little be conscious of not allowing her to nap too heavily during her feed because it may impact on her ability to sleep solidly at her next in-cot nap time.

Watch out also for little snacking feeds affecting her ability to feed well enough at a regular feed time, as this can affect her ability to stay asleep for a prolonged period. This is an area of great debate so do what you feel is right for your baby based on your observations of her needs because no one knows your baby as well as you do. However, if she is having several little feeds between big feeds it can definitely affect her ability to have a full feed later.

For some babies, this doesn't seem to matter and they still manage to sleep well. However, for other babies, it really does matter and they don't sleep well because they get hungry sooner. If your baby doesn't respond well to this style of snacking demand feeding, it will tire her out to feed too frequently. Feeding every 40 minutes to an hour will affect the length of time she'll be able to sleep. Try to find a way to soothe her without always relying on a breastfeed as this will only perpetuate a cycle of shorter sleeps, which will create an unsettled baby who needs help to calm down, which in turn perpetuates the cycle of snacking demand feeding.

Watch for early positioning issues

Many new parents say to me, 'My baby won't sleep anywhere but on me.' Sometimes this means they're appealing to a baby's natural desire to sleep on their belly. This ensures the baby stays warm, and limits stimulants like light and movement. However, apart from being a dangerous practice, it also means your baby isn't learning how to cope with the positioning required to settle in her cot on her own, which is on her back, flat and still.

The other problem that can occur early on is when a baby won't lie down anywhere, whether it is in your arms, on the floor or in her cot, and you have to hold her upright the whole time. This is problematic for obvious reasons:

1. If you want your baby to be able to go to sleep in her cot, she needs to be comfortable with lying down. Some parents need to work on this more than others, but it is an important skill for your baby to gain. If she refuses to be in any position other than upright on your shoulder then I'd discourage any upright positioning for two full weeks. The first couple of days can be challenging but as she becomes used to the new position she will settle quickly and her sleep will start to improve immediately. Always check for reflux first, however, if your baby appears to be in discomfort when lying down.
2. If you want your baby to be able to resettle at a waking, the conditions she encounters at the 40-minute mark should be the same as the conditions she fell asleep in. This is called a 'sleeping association'. If your baby is falling asleep on the breast or falling asleep in your arms, you're destined to need to recreate those associations at each 40-minute mark so she can go back to sleep. This results in a tired baby and tired parents. Tired babies wake more often, and tired parents becomes stressed. The parents' stress is transferred and the baby becomes even more unsettled. So don't fall into the trap of assisted settles in your arms or on your breast only to then put her in her cot and leave.

Making a sleep environment that caters for your baby's needs right now

If your baby is clearly overwhelmed, you need to cater for that. Some experts believe a child needs to get used to noise and light and movement. While I agree with this, when your baby is very tiny and just getting used to her new surroundings you should make things as calm, quiet and dimly lit as possible. I would advise you to close blinds in the house 20 minutes before sleep for a week or two until she settles down. Make her room as dark as possible until good sleep is established, and after that you can think about introducing light back into her sleep environment. Avoid using overhead downlights because babies' eyes are naturally drawn to these bright lights, and use lamps instead.

Your baby needs to be swaddled well so her arms and legs don't move at all. If she has her hands up by her face, and it's confusing her to nuzzle her fist like she's about to be fed, wrap her with her arms firmly by her side or across her body. Get a sheet and cotton blanket and firmly tuck-in down the sides of the crib so she feels snuggled and warm. If it is a cool day babies can get cold quickly during their day sleeps so if your baby has multiple wakings and you need to snuggle her or she needs to cry to warm up before she can fall asleep again you probably need to add an extra layer or two of blankets.

Create a predictable, safe cycle of routine-based behaviour so your baby can settle into a flow. She will find this comforting and relaxing. An example would be:

- Baby wakes for a feed.
- Go in, turn on the lamp and unwrap her, let her have a little stretch and some quiet time in her cot while you prepare her change table and room for the next part of her day. Get cloths and wraps out ready for her next sleep, put any washing away, get her nappy ready, etc.
- Get her up and change her nappy.
- Take her to your feeding couch, sit down to feed her and try to keep her awake during the feed.
- Wind well at the end of feeding on one breast or mid feed, then feed her the other breast or complete feed, then wind after that.
- Have a little quiet one-on-one focus time, chat quietly to her, touch her, massage her tummy while you chat, stroke her face, hold her hands.
- Offer a little quiet playtime on the floor on a soft base like a sheepskin.
- Look for tired signs, and wait for a couple of clear ones – for a newborn these usually occur about one or one and a half hours after waking up.
- Be careful not to misread a dislike for lying down, or light in her eyes, or a loud and active sibling unsettling him as tired signs; keep an eye on what is going on around her to ensure you're spotting true tired signs
- Tell her 'It's time for sleep, Mummy loves you'.
- Take her to her room, change her nappy as needed.
- Wrap her firmly and turn off lights while cradling her in your arms.
- Close the door and sing 'Twinkle Twinkle Little Star' slowly and quietly while rocking her in your arms as she accepts the sensation of feeling tired.
- If she is fighting the feeling of being tired hold her tight until she calms.
- Ensure she isn't thinking you're about to feed her; watch her face and make sure she isn't nuzzling into you as this may frustrate her and create tears.
- Give her a little kiss and say, 'Lie down'.
- Slowly lower her into her crib and tuck her in firmly.
- Stop to stroke her face from the crown downwards so you brush over her eyes, and your fingers meet under her chin; repeat this action as you quietly repeat, 'Time for sleep, Mummy loves you, nigh', nigh'',

but try to stay out of her line of sight so you aren't giving her mixed messages – stand side on to the cot, one hand in, bent over. Repeat three or four times then step back.

Your baby should sleep till the next feed. Once she wakes, repeat this pattern.

General flow with most babies

After a full night's sleep a lot of babies don't last terribly well during the first waking of the day and need to go back to bed sooner rather than later. After the first daytime sleep the next two waking periods will be your baby's longest before you need to put her down in her cot. As the afternoon approaches I tend to do the second-last sleep in the pram while out shopping or on a walk (good for fitness and to keep those baby blues at bay). When a baby is little and unsettled I often suggest she has the final sleep of the day in a baby sling on you. She is overtired by now and a doze will help her not become so overtired she screams at night.

After the final feed of the day, give your baby a bath, then a massage, then a final top-up feed before putting her down at around 8 p.m. I always suggest a rollover feed, and perhaps two more night feeds at, say, 2 a.m. and between 4 and 5 a.m. if needed. Between these feeds assist her to settle using your resettling stroking and cues and an occasional cuddle to calm her before trying again.

No matter how long a baby sleeps or how many feeds she has at night, I start every day at the same time, including waking time and feeding time, because this creates a consistent pattern for you and your baby each day. This may mean you need to wake your baby. If she is sleeping poorly at night and sleeping longer in the morning to make up for it, it will only perpetuate a cycle of poor sleep the following night. Hence, the idea of not waking sleeping babies is flawed because not waking them often leads to unsettled babies who can't sleep any more anyway.

A note on settling and resettling

Always put your baby in the cot awake, and let her know you've left so she can self-settle, otherwise she will wake regularly because her sleep environment has changed. If you choose to stay in the room make sure she thinks you've left and can't see you so she can focus on going to sleep rather than what you're going to do next.

Give her a minute to try to calm herself. Listen to what she's trying to tell you via a cry, and give her the chance to have that natural little cry as she first falls asleep (which enables her body to release endorphins that help her go into a deeper sleep). If, however, she is having a hard time and not able to calm down a little, repeat your pattern of cues and strokes, ensuring you sound reassuring and calm.

Step back out of her line of sight again and allow her to try to settle. Repeat these steps until she settles. If she's becoming very upset and you've tried several times to calm her with gentle stroking and cues, give her a cuddle to reassure her before you try again. Don't allow her to go to sleep in your arms, however, unless you're willing to continue holding her while she sleeps. If you disappear after she falls asleep she may try to fight sleep. Your baby needs to trust you and be able to predict you. Changing the conditions of how she goes to sleep does the opposite.

I don't recommend leaving infants of under six months to cry without assistance. They may cry a little more if you attend to them, but you're ensuring trust isn't compromised during this vital stage of psycho-social development when she's learning to trust her needs will or won't be met by a carer. I would prefer to attend and resettle young babies regularly until they settle than leave them without attendance. A young baby shouldn't be left feeling overwhelmed.

That said, some settling cries are normal and shouldn't be interfered with. A baby crying with breaks of 30 seconds or more between cries should be either left or given more time to settle down. If she continues to have longer breaks and starts to settle, you should leave her be. Just being awake and having the odd callout cry between settling cycles, like 'cry cry hic . . . cry cry hic' or 'cry hic, cry hic, cry hic,' is a baby's way of creating a rhythmic settling pattern and she may fall asleep within a three- to eight-minute window of these cries beginning without intervention.

It's important to listen carefully to what your baby is saying when she cries. Is she saying, 'Help, Mummy, I can't cope', or 'Boy oh boy I'm tired and it feels a bit uncomfortable'? If it's the latter, give her a chance to try to calm herself down and settle off to sleep with as little intervention as possible. If it's more serious, then go back to your cues and stroking and occasional hugs until she moves into that settling cry, then step back for longer until she settles.

As far as routines go for this age, babies don't even have circadian rhythms to speak of until they're four months old, so you can't necessarily lock in a strict routine, though working to a loose schedule is great for many mums and babies. Over the coming five to six months, feeding should become more efficient, and the amount of milk consumed by your baby at each feed will naturally increase. Your baby's ability to consume larger amounts in more efficient timeframes will have a flow-on effect to how long she can stay awake and stay asleep. The number of feeds needed to sustain your child through the night will gradually decrease as will the number of sleeps she needs during daylight hours.

Initially, your baby will have roughly eight feeds over a 24-hour period. During the next five months, as her intake per feed increases and the amount of time it takes her to drink it decreases, the number of feeds she needs will go down to five or six feeds per day. The feeds that increase in volume consumed will be the ones during daylight hours, with the feeds after her 10 to 10.30 p.m. feed becoming increasingly redundant for nutritional and hydration needs. Your baby health clinic can supply you with the recommended consumption levels for both breast- and bottle-fed babies to help you ensure your baby's intake is adequate.

As the quantity and efficiency of the feeds increases, your baby will start to stay awake for longer periods between feeds during the day, progressing from up to four sleeps during daylight hours over the first month to roughly three sleeps during daylight hours over the second month. Between the second and the third month, it will become more apparent what her sleep requirement is. For example:

- An average- to high-sleep-requirement baby will need roughly two longer sleeps a day – one midmorning and one early afternoon (both up to two hours long) as well as a late afternoon bridging nap (between 4 and 5 p.m.) of between 40 minutes to an hour. This requirement will kick in by around three months of age and last until around five months. After that her late afternoon bridging nap will become, or need to be made, a little shorter (between 20 and 40 minutes) to sustain a healthy 7 p.m. bedtime.
- A low-sleep-requirement baby will have one short mid-morning bridging nap (gradually decreasing from one hour to 30 to 40 minutes by around five months of age), one long midday sleep (of about two hours, depending on the amount of sleep she's allowed to have, or naturally has, during her mid-morning and late-afternoon bridging naps), followed by a short afternoon bridging nap (gradually decreasing from one hour to 30 to 40 minutes by around five months of age).

Locking in times to prevent poor sleep cycles

During your baby's first few months it's worth locking in some basic times in your routine. The most important times are her night sleep settling time and morning wake-up time, and the start and end times for the first and last sleeps during daylight hours. Each of these times will complement the other and lock in good sleeping for both the early morning waking time and 7 p.m. settling time.

Nights and mornings first

The nights are the foundation of all your baby's daytime sleeping and feeding patterns. A realistic expectation in the first month would be to settle her between 7 and 8 p.m. and always wake her, regardless of the progress of her night, to start her day by 7 a.m. All day sleeps can then be worked into the routine around this basic framework. By the fourth week, aim to always settle her by 7 p.m., monitoring the time she goes to sleep in the late afternoon and how long she sleeps for. Never offer any additional day sleeps if it detracts from night sleep.

First day sleep

The first sleep of the day helps you manage the remainder of the day, so be mindful of the time you put your baby down. For the first one to two months this should be roughly an hour and 15 to 30 minutes after your target wake-up time of 7 a.m. Even on the days she wakes a little earlier, always aim to settle her no earlier than 8.15 to 8.30 a.m. to discourage a cycle of early morning wakings. From the eighth to tenth week and onwards, try to keep her up until around 8.30 a.m. each morning and gradually, by the twelfth week, push that out to:

- 8.45 to 9 a.m. for high-sleep-requirement babies, who go down again for their second day sleep a little later than low-sleep-requirement babies and so go down a little later on this first sleep, and for a longer period of time
- 8.30 to 8.45 a.m. for low-sleep-requirement babies, who will go down again for their second day sleep sooner than high-sleep-requirement babies and thus go down a little sooner on this first sleep, and for a shorter time.

Encourage efficient feeding with no dozing and a long alert period before putting her down for her second sleep of the day and space the day well.

Final sleep time of the day

The last sleep or nap your baby takes during the daylight portion of the 24-hour cycle should be monitored to ensure she doesn't sleep so late or for so long she can't fall asleep again by 7 p.m. She's supposed to be tired enough at the end of the day to need to sleep for 11 or 12 consecutive hours (with or without the need for feeds), so it's normal for her to be fairly tired and grouchy after her bath. In the first precious six to eight weeks this last nap of the day will usually need to be assisted (with a sling, etc.) and be shorter than her normal day sleeps. The latest wake-up time is 5.30 p.m. in those first few weeks. Eventually, her late afternoon sleeps will be one and a half hours and then two hours prior to the 7 p.m. night sleep.

By the time your baby shows a propensity towards having a higher or lower sleep requirement during the day, the late afternoon sleep will begin to vary between the two groups. High-sleep-requirement babies will tend to sleep a little longer and need to be put down and woken earlier in order to maintain their 7 p.m. settling time. Low-sleep-requirement babies will sleep a little less and will need to be settled and woken a little later in the day. Experiment with your child's wake-up times and lengths of sleep to meet her needs while aiming for a 7 p.m. settling time at night. It's okay to be strategic about the timing and length of this last daytime sleep, so you can wake your baby to reduce or eliminate tears at the 7 p.m. settling time.

Night feeds

Over their first six months babies move from needing regular three-hourly feeds in a 24-hour period to only needing a dream feed at around 10 p.m. before sleeping through and not feeding until 7 a.m. the next morning. (A dream feed is where you wake and feed your baby between 10 p.m. and 11 a.m.) Initially, the dream feed will be at around 9.30 p.m. and will slowly progress to 10.30 over the next eight weeks. During the first few weeks of life, babies wake roughly every three hours after this dream feed for more feeds, so there'll be two late-night feeds after a dream feed until the 7 a.m. morning feed. As babies grow, the dream feed remains between 10 and 10.30 p.m. and they start to sleep through till 2, then 3, then 4 and eventually 5 to 7 a.m. before requiring another feed. This is safe and healthy as long as there's no difficulty with a mother's milk supply (in which case you may need to see a lactation consultant for help). Once in a pattern of your baby sleeping to a certain time for three or more days in a row, try to maintain the night feed schedule and resettle her without feeding between her feed windows whenever possible.

It's fairly common for a baby who was once sleeping through the night from her dream feed to 7 a.m. to suddenly develop a hunger at night again around the fifth month, when her body's need for higher calorie intake encourages her to source solids. Until solids are introduced, your baby may start to show genuine hunger through the night again and require an additional night feed until both solids and an iron source have been introduced into her diet.

Remember that babies' circadian rhythms don't develop until around the fourth month, so you need to rely on the sleep and feeding you provide during the day to keep her regulated and balanced, well slept and well fed. Once she's five months old, you can begin to use the more detailed tools outlined in the sleep section of this book to tweak her routine, develop her sleep skills, or adopt a healthy routine.

Reflux

Finally, if your baby is suffering from reflux, and has needed medication, I generally provide a dummy for short-term relief. With severe reflux, the stomach acid tracking back up a baby's oesophagus can often irritate and inflame the area. The more this happens, the more inflamed the area becomes until eventually any reflux causes significant pain. A dummy in the interim can help your baby keep the peristaltic action flowing downwards, which often prevents too much reflux and stops the acid from burning the oesophagus. Therefore, if you feel the short-term use of a dummy is necessary, that's fine, but be conscious of saving its use for when she is lying down, and only use it if she's having a tricky time.

Once your doctor is happy with the medication, your baby's discomfort will pass and you may need to re-establish a more positive association with lying down. If a baby has had bad reflux, she may associate lying on her back with the sensation of pain because this is when reflux is most noticeable. Once her reflux is under control, she may still be nervous of the impending discomfort and cry in anticipation of an event that will no longer happen. This is when it's important to get rid of the dummy, and gently work through it with her until she regains trust in lying down.

It's best not to avoid something that used to be a problem or your baby won't learn it's no longer a problem. When your baby develops a learnt pattern of response to an event, help her past it even if you're nervous about her crying. Crying is normal while your baby learns to trust her new environment with your guidance and reassurance. Help her through it gently with assistance in cot settling until she feels better about that environment again, then quickly transition to my systematic approach to sleep and settling.

Too many parents find themselves attending centres or seeking advice from strategists who only use control crying to resolve a sleep issue. I'm personall[...]bout how a completely unfamiliar carer can use contr[...] baby in a completely unfamiliar environment to hel[...].

[...] your child compassionately and consistently until she's [...]y always being reassuring and your baby will settle down quickly.

Before you begin your new routine for babies over the age of six months

Once you've read the book, follow the structure outlined on page 8 carefully. When you've done your homework and your baby is skilled and prepared for her new routine and sleep-time repair to begin, choose a time to start your PRM carefully. The following will help you do that:

- For one to three weeks leading up to beginning your new daily routine and sleep strategies, keep your baby away from places likely to cause illness, like public swimming pools and parties.
- Make sure she is physically well, and all medical issues (reflux, eczema, etc.) are under control before you begin.
- Go for a final medical check-up to make sure her lungs and ears are clear.
- Do the grocery shopping with easy meal plans in mind to take pressure off yourself and ensure you continue to eat well on those first few busy days.
- Pre-cook and freeze food for your baby so you're not trying to cook or you may feel overwhelmed and run behind during the first few days.
- Make sure all environmental changes to your baby's room are ready at least a day before you begin.
- Do not immunise your baby within three weeks of starting your program, or for three weeks after the program has commenced.
- Ensure your baby's nutritional needs (iron, vitamins and minerals) are catered for before you start and she is well hydrated in the days leading up to beginning, particularly if she drinks a lot of milk during the night.
- The night before you begin, for example on Sunday night if you plan to start your program on Monday morning at 6.30 a.m., stop all feeds from 2 a.m. onwards until 6.30 to 7 a.m. the next day and resettle her any way you can (nil by mouth though) to try to get her to have more sleep (though don't use your new resettling routine until tomorrow).
- She must be awake by 6.30 a.m. on the day you begin, no matter what kind of a night she's had.

- Once 6.30 a.m. arrives, follow your routine exactly and keep your baby awake until her designated sleep time. Don't offer sleep early and don't allow more sleep than is suggested.
- Only one person should manage your baby's routine for the first five days of the new plan so don't play tag team. Whoever puts the baby down should manage the baby and get her up after sleep time is completed so they are trustworthy for the baby.
- For the first few days, stay close to home and 100 per cent available to your baby's new needs. Don't have friends over or be distracted. Don't go too far in a car if she is prone to tiredness outside her sleep routines until she's recovered her sleep (usually about five days).
- You may need to temporarily or permanently reshuffle some of her activities to fit in with her sleep and meal-time needs.
- Don't use your settling or resettling routine and cues without starting your corrected daily routine and defining what your cues mean. Only begin when you're completely ready to repair your baby's sleep quickly and permanently by maintaining everything for three weeks from the morning you start.
- Try to start on a Monday so there isn't too much movement in or around the house.
- Try to have older siblings cared for, and see if people can help you out with school drop-offs for the first few days.

Once you've determined you need a daily routine, you will need to work out what routine is best for your child. There are a few simple steps to do this:

- Assess whether your child is an urgent repair case or not.
- Assess your child's sleep requirements.
- Choose the routine that suits your child's needs based on whether she is an urgent repair case or based on her individual sleep requirement.

Children who I classify as urgent repair cases are profoundly overtired or unsettled babies and toddlers and need the full recovery program. The aim is to take the pressure off exhausted parents by providing a well-established, refined daily routine and PRM program to ensure a very speedy resolution to their child's sleep problems through balanced and respectful communication. Each plan is designed to minimise the need for crying during sleep time and achieve dramatic results within 12 to 56 hours. It ensures a child can achieve upwards of 14 hours sleep a day, even if she's previously been taking as little as eight hours per 24-hour cycle. Once trust in the routine is established and sleep is repaired, these children can move on to a new routine based on their new recovered sleep requirement.

To take advantage of all the strategies outlined in this book you need to record the results of your child's sleeping pattern to work out whether she has a low, average or high sleep requirement. Keeping a seven-day sleep diary will help you calculate her sleep requirement so you can implement the best routine for her. If you have older children you can take advantage of a 'modified' routine. School runs and extracurricular activities don't always fit in with the standard 'one longer morning nap and one longer afternoon nap' routine of other programs. So my routines are designed for you to adjust to suit your family needs while still providing the right amount of sleep.

As already outlined, the daily routine comprises your communication, meal-time, playtime and independence event routines. In Chapter 15 I give you settling, resettling and waking routines, which form a vital part of your new daily routine. The chapters in this part of the book all relate to sleep-time issues, including the typical triggers for a baby waking during the night and solutions to those triggers.

Urgent repair cases

When I'm repairing sleep problems I need to identify the children and families experiencing the greatest difficulties and help repair their situation as soon as I can with as little fuss as possible. If sleep is very messy in your house, continue reading this section. However, if you and your baby are generally coping pretty well but you'd like things to run a little smoother, bypass this full recovery section and begin reading the section on sleep requirement assessment.

Once I've identified a family as an urgent repair case, I place the baby/toddler on a full recovery program. You need to read the whole book and do your homework before implementing the new routine so you don't have the stress of trying to fix something when you don't know what's wrong. I've provided a checklist (see page 346) for those who think their entire days are out of control so you can assess whether you need to be fast-tracked to a full recovery routine within the next few days (assuming you've read the book up to here and are making progress with communication, independence and playtime strategies).

To make this as easy as possible, the fail-safe full recovery program allows you to offer a sensible amount of sleep to help a profoundly unsettled baby/toddler recover quickly without having to assess her sleep requirement. I've refined this routine over many years, so please don't vary it. If you fit into the categories on the checklist, please move to the PRM 1 suggestions for your child's age group in the full recovery program and follow the instructions carefully. You should see an almost complete recovery within one to three days of starting the routine and a full recovery from sleep-time issues within around five days.

As mentioned, you need to allow a three-week settling window in which you lock in your new solid sleep by maintaining all the environmental aids and following your routine carefully. Once your child's trust in the process of sleep has been repaired you can then move on to the next phase with ease, if it is necessary, to maintain healthy sleep for everyone. During the next phase of the recovery process you can *consider* putting your child on to the average/high-sleep-requirement routine, which comprises two large day sleeps if it's appropriate for your child's individual sleep requirements. Or you can look at how you can reintroduce normal levels of stimulation in her room during sleep time and be confident she will become more flexible with sleep when you're out or away from home. Remember, though, don't rush to make changes when things are working because they're working for a reason. Feel free to sit pretty for as long as your baby is happy.

Sleep requirement assessment

To assess your baby's actual sleep requirement, keep a sleep diary of your child's sleep intake for a full seven days in the following manner:

- Choose a day to start and record her sleep times per 24 hours from her wake-up time on day one to her wake-up time on day two, and so on.
- Note the exact time she goes to sleep and wakes up again. If she wakes during the day or night and you need to resettle her, note the time she wakes and when she goes back to sleep again.
- Add up your child's sleep requirement over the full 24 hours, being sure to calculate only the sleep she's actually had. If she wakes for 10 minutes or more during the night or day, deduct that time from her total sleep intake.
- If she has any milk after 5 a.m. before going back to sleep, deduct all sleep taken after that milk feed until her day begins again, from her daily sleep needs.
- Calculate the sleep she has from her waking time in the morning on the first day (less false sleep), to her waking time in the morning on the second day.

An example of a sleep diary would be:
7.15 a.m.: Awake (NB: the hours prior to this waking are added to the previous day's total)
10.12: Asleep (2 hours, 10 minutes)
12.22 p.m.: Awake
3.54: Asleep (31 minutes)
4.25: Awake
7.15: Asleep (3 hours, 39 minutes)
10.54: Awake
11.35: Asleep (7 hours, 40 minutes)
Next day
7.15 a.m.: Awake
Total daytime sleep: 2 hours, 41 minutes (calculated up to 7 p.m.)
Total night-time sleep: 11 hours, 19 minutes
Total 24-hour sleep: 14 hours.

Keep this sleep diary for a week, then add together the totals of all seven days and divide by seven to give you your child's average daily sleep requirement.

If your sleep diary shows that your child's average daily sleep intake over a seven-day week is:

- 8 to 14½ hours, you have a lower-sleep-requirement (LSR) baby
- 14½ to 15½ hours, you have an average-sleep-requirement (ASR) baby
- 15½ to 16½+ hours, you have a higher-sleep-requirement (HSR) baby.

Understanding your child's sleep requirement

If your child has a low sleep requirement (LSR) it generally means one of two things. Firstly, she is extremely overtired from getting such a poor quantity of sleep, and secondly, that you need to repair her sleep as quickly as possible with a fail-safe routine, providing a minimum 14 hours sleep in a 24-hour period.

Once you've done this, you can reassess her response to the LSR routine to see if it's appropriate for her to remain on or not. The answer will either be a clear 'yes' or 'no' and, if needs be, whether she is coping and sleeping or not you can shift her on to the ASR routine with ease if she seems to need more sleep. Just because your child initially presents with a low sleep requirement, it doesn't mean she's a true LSR baby, it just means you need to adjust her sleep promptly and reassess within three weeks. That said, a good proportion of babies who present with LSR thrive on their new LSR routine and still achieve the same amount of daily sleep that many babies on the ASR routines achieve.

If your baby presents with an average sleep requirement (ASR) you're lucky because you can choose which routine suits both your child's individual needs and your family's needs. You can either slot your baby into the LSR routine to achieve up to 14½ hours sleep or more in a 24-hour period, or you can choose the adapted sleep on the HSR routine. Not all ASR babies respond well to the typical 'two longer sleeps a day' routine offered for higher-sleep-requirement children. Your baby may respond better to the LSR routine if she has a tendency to be an early riser, or a tendency to only take one good day sleep, and only a poor or no second day sleep.

The LSR routine is also suitable for ASR babies who are second children and have to be part of the kindergarten run or have a sibling who has a midday nap. Adapting to this LSR routine creates a daytime flow with all the children going down at the same time during the day. Alternatively, you can place your baby on the HSR routine (modified to accommodate her *slightly* lower sleep need), which is good for babies who like taking two big day sleeps. It's a favourite with many parents because it gives them two breaks in the day and allows them some free time at lunch time. It's also a very common routine style and a lot of mums like sharing a similar routine to their friends' and mothers' group families. Either way, your choice will promote the same amount of sleep, just using slightly different timetables. Please note, if your baby is ASR but in need of full recovery, then you should follow the full recovery routine suggestion for her age group.

If your child has a high sleep requirement (HSR), and is having trouble sleeping it's usually because of an association problem rather than miscalculation. While her behavioural difficulties may be due to communication and environmental miscalculations and independence skills being a little under-explored, I often find these HSR babies just need some time and space to find their way at sleep time.

Follow the routine suggestions for your baby's age group and transition to one sleep a day anywhere from 18 months to two years of age. Once you've done your homework, simply set a date and create harmony by implementing your program and assisting her while she adjusts to your new requests and guidance. Within a couple of days she will be sleeping like a dream right through the night.

About the PRM routines

There are two basic routines for babies in the six- to 24-month age bracket. PRM Routine 1 is designed:

- for babies who need the full recovery program
- for LSR babies
- as an option for ASR babies
- as a HSR-single-sleep routine for children from 16 to 18 months or older.

PRM Routine 2 is designed:

- as an option for ASR babies aged six to 14 or 16 months
- for HSR babies aged six to 16 or 18 months.

You should read through all the information relating to your chosen routine before embarking on your sleep repair PRM, so start your sleep diary today but keep reading on to learn more about your baby's sleep repair.

Before you start reading about the routines . . .

When you're following your daily routine plan for your baby's age group, it's best to type or write up the routine in a brief, time-layout form and pop it on your fridge or bench-top as a quick reference guide. You can then refer to the detailed timetable and management suggestions in this book for clearer directions if you have any issues. As variations are made to the timing of events as your child grows older or to fit in with family commitments (while being sensitive to your baby's ability to make these adjustments) or to tighten up the lunch-time sleep (from two hours, 30 minutes to two hours, ten minutes to encourage the afternoon bridging nap), insert the new sleep- and meal-time variations into your written/typed framework. This is how it becomes a personalised routine management, tailored to your baby's needs.

During the day, refer to the box on foods appropriate for your baby's age (see page 460). This list is good for all the routines, tailored or otherwise, as it meets every baby's dietary-intake requirements. You will also find those foods that may cause a reaction in your child in the box so you can carefully monitor her intake of these items, and those foods to avoid in her diet altogether. This is not a definitive list. It goes without saying that children under two years should not be offered foods with no nutritional value, such as lollies, chocolates, chips, or sweetened drinks. Nor should your child have too much of one single kind of food because this can lead to fussy feeders. At this age you need to be responsible about what you feed your child because you're creating eating habits for your child on both a behavioural and neurological level and she will learn to *crave* certain types of food and fluids to respond to her hunger and thirst needs.

A note about premature babies

If your baby was born *four or more* weeks prematurely and is currently six to seven months old, adjust her age to reflect what would have been her actual due date, rather than her premature birth day. After ten months, it is unnecessary to adjust back to due date unless she was eight or more weeks premature, in which case adjust her age to her due date until the age of 12 months.

PRM Routine 1

This positive routine management is for children who:

- need full recovery
- are six to 24 months old and have a LSR
- have ASR, offered as a choice (see Routine 2 as an alternative).

The routine covers all ages up to two years, though for simplicity it's written as a single broad document, with meal and sleep variations for babies aged six to nine months and ten to 12 months. Changes to the routine for children older than 12 months have been added as a reference guide. You can adjust your written/typed version according to your baby's age and needs. As you're aiming for 'full recovery' here, which means ensuring your baby understands and follows the routine and is happy during the day and night, stick to the timetable rigorously for the first three weeks. Once your baby is successfully following the routine and sleeping to her natural sleep requirement you can introduce adjustments to fit in with your family needs so long as they don't cause confusion for your baby.

6.00–6.30 a.m.: Natural waking. Any wakings before 5.30 a.m. should be managed with crying interpretation and support.

Waking routine and playtime in cot for 15 to 20 minutes. Throughout the day remember your wait game and cue.

6.30–7.00: Breast/bottle feed (don't let your baby snooze). By nine months you should aim to have this feed no earlier than 7 a.m.

Change nappy, then free playtime.

7.15: Prepare baby's breakfast. Use pre-emptive and forewarning language such as 'Nearly time for breakfast', 'Nearly time to sit down and wait for Mummy', 'Yummy apple and oatmeal'.

7.20–7.40: Baby's breakfast. If your baby is hard to feed, use the meal-time routine.

7.50: Dress for day and then free playtime (she may want to help you but allow her freedom to venture off if she wants). Prepare cot room for morning bridge, if necessary. Use flow of communication: 'Nearly time for stories', 'Nearly time for nigh' nigh's'.

8.30: Nappy change, if necessary, then sitting room for settling routine.

By 12 months the morning-bridging nap will have naturally been phased out, so use this as a quiet time for the baby until 9.30 and don't do the settling routine.

8.45: Bridging nap (strictly 19–20 minutes only) until 12 months old. Waking routine, then cot play until 9.30 while you set up play stations.

For children 12 months and older, at 9.10 allow ten minutes of quiet time for her in her high chair with either books, toys or a favourite DVD or to watch you do your final morning-tea preparations if she's grizzly.

9.30: Latest time for waking from bridging nap, even if under 20 minutes.

Morning tea. By nine months you can add fruit puree to this feed.

9.45: Independent playtime at play stations. This is a baby's most active, energy-burning session, so try to avoid the car or pram at this time. This is also the time to help her become comfortable with being put down to play independently, a skill she'll need for sleep – think of it as sleep-earning play. It is also the best opportunity for you to do housework and/or cooking (if you do the whole day's cooking during this time you get it out of the way). The busier you are the happier your baby will be to play independently. If she's not settling down to play use your flow of communication and follow through. If you leave the room, use the short-term absence cue, 'I'll be back'.

10.30: Be prepared: this is a typical ten-minute tired window for LSR babies and in the early days (maybe five to ten days) of your new routine if your baby is getting weary and showing it, a play outside or a little cuddle time while you play with her favourite toy for a few minutes will help. Put her down again once she calms down.

10.45: Focus one-on-one play for 15 minutes. Give her your undivided attention and don't answer phones. Use your cue, 'Nearly time to pack away'.

11.00: Pack away toys completely, prepare cot room and swaddle for your baby's lunch sleep while she keeps you company and 'helps'. Allow ten minutes' quiet time for her in her high chair with either books, toys or a favourite DVD or to watch you prepare lunch. She may have a little blood-sugar drop here and her hunger signs might look like tired signs but don't be fooled: she needs to eat here. Use your cue, 'Nearly time for lunch, yummy chicken and vegetables'.

11.20: Lunch of vegetables with a protein every day; by eight to nine months she can be offered a dessert such as fruit puree. Follow your routine when feeding her and use your cues if there are problems.

11.40: Wait game and cue while you clean up. Change nappy using cue for sleep: 'Nearly time for sleep, let's go find our books'.

11.45: Begin settling routine.

11.55: Final page and pack away, using sleep cues.

12.00 p.m.: Sleep (one and a half to two and a half hours).

1.30–2.10: Natural waking time. Leave your baby in the cot for as long as you can, allowing her to self-resettle if need be. If she wakes before 1 p.m., use your resettling routine until 2.30. Once she's had a minimum of one-and-a-half hours' sleep and is fully awake, use your waking routine and cues. Allow her to have independent play in the cot for 20 minutes or until 2.30.

Hint: If you weren't able to cook during your baby's independent playtime, cook and freeze a large batch of food during sleep time once or twice a week. By 5 p.m. children are tired and hungry, making it a bad time to cook which is why I don't include it in the routine.

2.30: Breast/bottle feed plus snack by nine months.

This milk feed will naturally go between 12 and 15 months of age and your child will just have the snack, but you can offer milk in a cup if she's interested.

Adventure. Time to enjoy the great outdoors in a car or pram. No napping allowed unless it's within the afternoon bridging-nap time. Use your cues for bridging nap.

4.15: Bridging nap (20 minutes) in pram or car for six to nine month olds only.

4.45–5.00: Latest time to wake from bridging nap, using waking cues, regardless of how long it took her to fall asleep. At six months she could take her 20 minutes right up to 5 p.m., but as she gets older tighten the afternoon bridge window to close at 4.45 p.m. so you're not offering sleep if it isn't needed because it can cause problems at other sleep times. This afternoon bridge phases itself out by the ninth to tenth month.

5.00–5.10: For the first three weeks of recovery you need to be at home at this time. Use it to do your final pack away for the day, using cues, 'Time to pack away', 'Nearly time for dinner . . .'

5.10: While you warm dinner allow ten minutes' quiet time in the high chair with books, toys or a DVD, or watching you, depending on her mood. This is another blood-sugar drop window so you may see hunger signs that look like tired signs. Don't be fooled: babies need to eat here, not sleep.

5.20: Dinner then playtime in high chair as you prepare her bedroom, tidy the kitchen and organise your own evening meal for when she goes to bed at 7 p.m. (NB: Eat a healthy meal to stave off depression and poor sleep, and to connect with other members of your family.)

6.00: Nudie playtime, using pre-emptive cues for bath.

6.10: Bath time. Make sure you watch your baby throughout the whole bath. Use pre-emptive cues as you head towards 6.30, 'Nearly time to pack away', 'Nearly time to get out of the bath'.

6.30: Take her out of the bath. Dim lights in preparation for bed. Dry and dress her quickly but calmly. As she will be tired, you might need to reassure her, 'It's okay, bubba, you're just tired. Nearly time for milk and nigh' nigh's.' Be patient; she should be tired enough to sleep for 11 to 12 hours.

6.35: Breast/bottle feed, ten minutes only. Don't allow her to doze here as it will interrupt your settling routine. Even a five minute doze during this feed can lead to 40 minutes' crying on settling.

6.45–6.50: Begin settling routine at 6.50 at the latest. Use pre-emptive language during book reading.

6.55: Final cue, 'Last page, then nigh' nigh's', and pack away. Enjoy a last cuddle and complete settling routine.

7.00: Bed. If your baby cries, interpret the cries using an adult perspective before you go in to resettle. Remember your cues and resettling routines.

Milk and food intake per day

There should be no night feeding once a baby is on solids. Some six month olds won't have started solids, though usually they'll have been introduced to some by now, so they may require a single parent-guided night feed at around 10 p.m. Teach your baby not to mistake the night feed for waking-up time or playtime. Go in and offer her the feed rather than her waking and demanding it. Don't confuse your cues and definitions. By six months, I recommend you adopt the routine and food suggestions and drop all night feeds unless directed otherwise by a doctor.

A six to nine month old has four breast/bottle feeds of milk and three solid meals a day. By nine months the need for the morning-tea breastfeed decreases as she approaches the natural weaning process at ten months.

At around eight to nine months, children are introduced to pureed fruit after their 9.30 a.m. milk feed. After ten months children should have three solid meals, two snacks and three breast/bottle feeds. By 12 months a child will start to drop the afternoon breast/bottle feed, so she will have two to three breast/bottle feeds of milk, three solid feeds and two snacks. It is best to offer the solids and snacks before the breast/bottle feed to encourage healthy eating. The three solid meals should consist of:

breakfast: rice cereal and fruit; lunch: vegetable and protein plus dessert (fruit or yoghurt); dinner: vegetable and carbohydrate, or similar.

Give your child extra water during morning playtime, from 9.45 to 11 a.m., and in the afternoon, between 2.30 and 5 p.m. Don't give her water 30 minutes before breakfast, lunch or dinner as it will make her feel full and she'll eat less.

For those on full recovery, LSR or ASR variation Routine 1

Children who fall into the low-sleep-requirement (LSR) group need a very specific routine to encourage more sleep. Many babies who need this corrective or alternative routine won't be able to sleep for more than an hour at midday if you allow them to sleep even a minute over their 20-minute bridging sleep at 8.45 a.m. The lunch sleep success depends on you being vigilant with that bridge sleep. If your child does wake from her lunch sleep in less than an hour and 20 minutes, always attempt to resettle her using the resettling routine along with careful interpretation and support of crying until 2.30 p.m. If she doesn't resettle, enter the room using your waking cues and routine and carry on as normal with playtime in the cot.

If your attempts to resettle her when she wakes early are unsuccessful within the first couple of days, only try to resettle her if she wakes up under an hour. There's no point trying to resettle her if it's not working because it will just teach her to cry for prolonged periods before you get her up. For sleep to be a positive experience for your baby during those first few days don't pursue it too rigorously but just follow the routine sleep times to encourage better sleeping. The problem usually sorts itself out after the first two to three days and she'll start sleeping soundly. I'm preparing you for the possibility of more difficult scenarios here in case you're anxious if she doesn't sleep the required time at first.

If you have to resettle your child be consistent and don't confuse her by giving up and getting her up when she demands it. Your main aim is to help her understand the cue rather than taint it by changing its definition. On that first resettling attempt, it may not even be about the amount of sleep she has but about ensuring she's not confused about the definition of the cues. Be aware of the Sleep Bus (see page 354) and listen to what your child is saying while you help her go back to sleep. Once she's gone to sleep, if she wakes a second time after accepting your guidance once, it signifies the end of sleep time so don't try to resettle her at this point.

Regardless of the progress of the day, don't alter the times in your daily routine-time framework because doing so can lead to prolonged tiredness and more days of early waking and crying. Start the next stage of the routine when required. You'll get stunning results if you adhere to the timeframes. Don't allow extra sleep or adjust her routine if she's not taking the sleep as suggested in the routine. Just wait for the cyclic effect of tiredness to encourage better sleep next time. If one sleep doesn't work out, the next sleep window should remain the same as on her routine. Be confident and provide clear direction rather than procrastinating and stressing through doubt and fear.

Also note that LSR babies and those on a modified routine will naturally have a higher need for calorie intake, thus there will be a difference in frequency of feeding and the amount of food consumed per age group between low- and high-sleep-requirement routines.

LSR variation for six to nine month olds

Breakfast: Rice, barley or oat cereal and pureed fruit.

Morning bridge: Bridging-nap length is 19 to 20 minutes in total and you shouldn't allow even a minute more sleep to ensure success for the rest of the day using this routine. Excess sleep here will result in crying and short sleeps elsewhere during the day. Set an alarm clock to ensure your baby is woken before she drops into too deep a sleep cycle beyond this 20-minute power zone. It's best to enter her room at 19 minutes and give her a minute to wake up. This will ensure you enter the room when she would naturally be in a light phase, which prevents her from being grizzly when she wakes up. If you miss your 20-minute window, she could be grizzly for a further 20 minutes while her system tries to take a full 40-minute REM cycle even once woken. Enter the room using your waking routine and stay happy and confident even if she's not impressed at being woken on the first couple of days of your new plan. Establish playtime in the cot and allow her to play until 9.25 a.m. While she's taking her nap and playing in her cot, set up her play stations in the main living area, and make morning tea ready for a fun morning of exploring her world. At 9.25 a.m. pack toys away in the cot and take her out for the morning-tea feed.

Morning tea: For six to eight month olds: breast/bottle feed only. This feeding window should be 15 to 20 minutes maximum and designed so she has a lovely snuggle and drink of milk before starting a busy play session. On the first day she may not be used to this frequency of feeds and only need a little feed, but her intake will increase within a week of starting the program. Once the allocated time has passed, end the feed if it is not already ended, and carry on with your routine.

For nine month olds: after her milk feed offer her some pureed fruit. Between the ninth and tenth month she may not be interested in her milk feed. This is natural and she will start to transition from four milk feeds a day to three by around the age of ten months. This is why you start to add fruit and water for morning tea. By ten months, she will only have fruit and water for morning tea.

Lunch: Vegetables, rice cereal, rice, meat and dessert.

Lunch sleep: This sleep can be up to two hours and 30 minutes long. For babies whose sleep requirement is lowest, which is often indicated by an inability to take the afternoon bridge after a two-and-a-half-hour lunch sleep, you'll need to cap his midday sleep at 2–2.10 p.m. until her afternoon bridge is dropped at nine to ten months. Only then should you allow her to take the full allocation of sleep.

When a baby has a well-established, existing catnap cycle of ten to 30 minutes for her day sleeps before she starts the new routine, she *may* need assistance to resettle past this on the first three days though if you swaddle her this will be rare. Avoid resettling if she's had a reasonable amount of sleep.

The ideal outcome on the first couple of days is a minimum of one hour, 20 minutes. If that occurs, be satisfied and try to leave her for as long as you can before going in and doing your waking routine and encourage her to have a longer playtime in the cot. Her need to pick up the sleep the next day will occur if you're consistent with your routine times. It's a waste of your and your baby's energy if you know you won't succeed at resettling her. You could also inadvertently teach her to cry until you pick her up. I try to avoid resettling during the day and wait for the cyclic effect of the routine to work rather than battle with a baby. Only if her main sleep is too short would I resettle on those first few days.

Afternoon tea: For a six to eight month old: breast/bottle feed. This milk feed will remain for some time, well beyond her first birthday. Some children opt to keep this feed until you decide it's time to have milk in a cup with their afternoon tea.

For nine month olds: offer breast/bottle feed and a snuggle, then pop her into her high chair for a little snack. It is a long time between her solid lunch feed at 11.20 a.m. and her solid dinner feed at 5.20 p.m. so she will need a substantial snack in addition to milk to sustain her. This can be fruit plus yoghurt or finger foods like a Cruskit with avocado, cream cheese or ricotta (watch for dairy reactions), or cheese or homemade smoothies or a biscuit.

Afternoon bridge: A six to seven month old has a sleep window from 4.10 to 5 p.m.; an eight month old from 4.15 to 4.45 p.m. but the nap should only be 19 to 20 minutes long. Keep peeping at her every three to five minutes so you know the time she drifts off to sleep, and then wake her either when her allocated nap time ends, or when her sleep window ends, whichever comes first. If she doesn't fall asleep early enough and doesn't nap the whole allocated time, wake her by 4.45 or 5 p.m. depending on her age and carry on with your routine.

This is a good sleep for her to have in the pram whenever possible because most babies have had enough of their cot by this time, and though they need this sleep they may require some assistance to take it. As you can't assist her in her cot, you should only help her in an honest assisting environment like the pram. So get it out and go for a stroll. If it's warm, stay in the shade. If it's hot, raining or blowing a gale, head to a shopping mall. If you can't do either, then push her in the pram at home briefly until she drifts off to sleep. This is also a good sleep for her to have in the car if you need to pick up older children.

If your six- to seven-month-old baby has difficulty going to sleep at 7 p.m. on the first and second day of your new routine, and she's taking her bridge sleep right up until 5 p.m., then you'll need to taper it back to 4.45 to ensure she doesn't have difficulty falling asleep at 7 p.m. on subsequent nights. This may mean you need to tighten her midday sleep back a little (to 2/2.10 p.m.) so she falls asleep earlier during the bridging sleep. Her night sleep is the most important sleep to lock in first, and then you adjust the days depending on just how much sleep she has left to take. Never steal from the nights to achieve better days.

By the ninth or tenth month, your child's need to take this sleep may diminish. Before making decisions about day sleeps, wait two to three days in a row to see if there's a pattern. Continue to swaddle her and lie her down. If she lies there happily looking around contently snuggled in her swaddle but is unable to drift off, it is clear she's transitioning out of the afternoon bridge. Continue to offer it until she's ten months if you like. As her need for the afternoon nap lessens, let her sleep as long as she likes at the midday sleep, providing at night she still sleeps through till 6.30 a.m. This way, if she no longer wants to have her late afternoon bridging nap she's still had a good amount of daytime sleep and a solid night's sleep, around 13½ to 15 hours in all. This is adequate and for many babies who have been very poor sleepers, it is possibly more sleep than they've ever been able to achieve before.

If after a few days of good sleep and no afternoon bridge your baby goes to sleep at 7 p.m. with no problems, but wakes 40 minutes later and needs help to go back to sleep, it may mean she's overtired and you'll need to encourage the afternoon sleep. To do this, tighten up her midday sleep again (back to two hours) so she can take the afternoon bridge. Keep to the afternoon-bridge routine and wake her when the window comes to an end or she reaches the 19-minute mark. If after encouraging this afternoon-bridge sleep for a couple of days you're unsuccessful, don't wake her from the lunch sleep anymore. Allow her to sleep until she wakes up and continue the routine. The evening overtired, partial-waking cycle will resolve over the next day or so. Don't alter your routine.

Dinner: Vegetables, rice cereal/rice: this meal is similar to lunch but does not include meat. No dessert.

LSR/ASR variation for ten to 12 month olds

Breakfast: Rice, barley, Oat/Weet-Bix, oats, semolina or baby's muesli cereal and stewed or mashed fruit or toast fingers.

Morning bridge: See information in six to nine month olds' section. Bridging-nap length is 19 to 20 minutes only. Don't allow even a minute more sleep. I'd prefer 18 minutes to 21 or you risk compromising her lunch sleep.

Morning tea: Between the ninth and tenth month, your baby may no longer be interested in her milk feed. This is natural and she'll start to transition from four milk feeds a day to three by around the age of ten months. This is why you started to add fruit and water for morning tea. By ten months, unless she's still very keen on milk, she'll have fruit and water only for morning tea. This can be pureed fruit or some finger-food pieces of banana, peach and pear, etc.

Lunch: Vegetables, pasta/rice/couscous, meat.

Lunch sleep: This sleep can be up to two hours, 30 minutes long if she wishes, even three hours if she's sleeping up to and beyond 6 a.m. each morning and settling well at 7 p.m. Start out at just two hours, ten minutes if she's been a troubled sleeper though. In a few weeks you can start to build on the solid framework of good sleep, if she indicates she may want to sleep longer, by allowing her to sleep until 2.30 p.m. Some children don't have that requirement and don't mind if they wake at 1.30 or 2 p.m. A good indication she's satisfied with the quantity of sleep is if she's happy and coping during the afternoon. It's normal for babies to have a little blood-sugar drop around 5 p.m. as their bodies prepare for dinner, which is why a quiet time then is good as you prepare their meal to prevent tantrums and tears from a hungry baby. However, if she copes well at all other times of the afternoon and goes to bed tired but sleeps solidly, then she's not overtired and has met her natural lunch-time sleep requirement. This isn't about fixing a baby to make her take a spectacular amount of sleep, it's about finding a way to have a happy baby all day who sleeps beautifully all night.

Avoid resettling if she's had a reasonable amount of sleep. The ideal outcome on the first couple of days would be a minimum of one hour, 20 minutes. If that occurs be satisfied and encourage him with your waking routine and have a longer playtime in the cot. Her body's need to pick up on sleep the next day will happen if you remain consistent with your routine times. It's a waste of your baby's energy and yours if you know you'll be unsuccessful at resettling her and could inadvertently teach her to cry until you pick her up.

If she does wake within one hour, then always attempt to resettle her using the resettling routine and careful management of crying until 2.30 p.m. If she doesn't resettle by 2.30, enter the room using your waking cues and routine and carry on as normal with playtime in the cot. If she does go back to sleep, even if it takes her quite some time to fall asleep on those first few days, the next waking, no matter how soon, signifies the end of this sleep time. The latest waking time is 2.30 p.m. It's important not to confuse the language at this point, as you will perpetuate a cycle of poor sleep the next day if you allow compensation sleep beyond the designated sleep repair windows.

If you remain unsuccessful at resettling her after a few days of her waking before 1.20 p.m., you might decide to only try to resettle her if she wakes in under an hour. This isn't usually a problem after the first two to three days as she'll sleep soundly after this time. If lunch sleeps continue to be a problem, adjust to the six to ten months' variation.

Before I enter a baby's room and use my waking cue and routine, I encourage lying by themselves for as long as possible after they wake up, even if they are calling out or protesting a bit, as long as there are pauses in the crying. Lying happily in their cot is such an important thing for babies to become comfortable with because all of us have nights in our lives where we wake up and it takes a little time and work to go back to sleep.

So leave her to chat and play in her cot for as long as you can before you go in, even if she's wrapped. It is ideal for your little one to have a restful, reduced stimulation time for up to two hours to be in her best form for the rest of the day. Once you go in and use your waking routine, then establish her usual playtime in the cot to lead her up to as close to 2.30 p.m. as possible.

Afternoon tea: Offer breast/bottle milk feed and a cuddle, then give her a snack in his high chair. It's a long time between her solid lunch feed at 11.20 a.m. and her solid dinner feed at 5.20 p.m. so she'll need a snack and some milk to sustain him. The snack can be fruit, yoghurt or finger foods like a Cruskit with avocado, cream cheese or ricotta. She can eat this while you're out and about for your afternoon adventure but only in the suggested afternoon-tea window until 3.00 p.m., and not as comfort food as a way of managing behaviour.

Afternoon bridge: Usually after ten months this sleep peters out if she's sleeping well at her lunch sleep. This bridge shouldn't be offered to babies over 11 months old when starting your repair routine. I only occasionally offer it to ten month olds for the first two to three days of implementing a new routine to help them settle into the new pattern, particularly if they're having problems with the length of sleep they're taking at lunch. The sleep window is from 4.15 to 4.45 p.m. and is strictly only 19 to 20 minutes long.

Lie her down and keep peeping in to see when she goes to sleep. Wake her after 19 minutes or when her sleep window ends, whichever comes first. Even if she doesn't take the whole allocated nap time, wake her and carry on with the routine. If the afternoon bridge doesn't lengthen in those first two to three days, don't offer it any longer. Stopping it will encourage a better lunch sleep over the next few days.

Dinner: Vegetables, pasta/rice/couscous – this meal is similar to lunch but doesn't include meat.

LSR variation for 12 to 24 month olds

Breakfast: Rice, barley, Oat/Weet-Bix, oats, semolina or baby muesli cereal and stewed or mashed fruit or toast fingers.

Morning tea: Snack of fruit and water.

Lunch: Vegetables, pasta/rice/couscous, meat and dessert.

Lunch sleep: This sleep is as per ten to 12 month olds.

Afternoon tea: Between the 12th and 15th month your baby will still be enjoying this breastfeed, though it will no longer be a primary dietary need as solids start to occupy most of her daily calorie intake. If she chooses to take it or not, it will not impact on her sleep or happiness. Offer the breast/bottle milk feed and a cuddle, and if she says 'Yes please', then go right ahead, but if she says 'No thank you', don't force it. If she doesn't want it she shouldn't have to have it. She'll need to have an afternoon tea solid snack first, however, and it should be more than just fruit as it's a long time between her solid lunch feed at 11.20 a.m. and her solid dinner feed at 5.20 p.m. Include yoghurt or finger foods like a Cruskit with avocado, cream cheese or ricotta. She can eat this while you're out and about on your afternoon adventure but it should only be eaten in the afternoon-tea window.

If the milk feed stops her from eating some solids at afternoon tea, she should have some solids before milk is offered because she will not be sustained by milk alone between lunch and dinner. Remember this is about balance, so ensure she has a good snack to get her through. Don't feed her outside the meal-time windows on the recovery plan. Food and sleep intake are closely linked and these plans are carefully refined to make sure sleep is achieved as easily as possible.

Dinner: Vegetables, pasta/rice/couscous – this meal is similar to lunch but doesn't include meat. No dessert.

Typical triggers for night wakings

Once your child is established on PRM Routine 1, she should have few night wakings. However, any imbalance in a baby's day will show up in the night-time sleep cycle of babies on a solid routine. They also have common time windows indicating behavioural wakings, discomfort, illness, hunger, dehydration, and routine miscalculations. These occur so consistently I've adopted a method to help me fine-tune routines, which has helped me determine what's happening in the most challenging, unsolvable cases.

There are many possible triggers for night-time waking, including depression and anxiety in one or both parents. If you have difficulty with your child's sleeping during particular times, these suggestions will help you work through the problem to eliminate the cause of the waking. This information should only be used for a baby who is on PRM 1, whose sleep issues have been solved, and who is generally sleeping well. It's designed to determine why a child might suddenly experience a disruption at night. You can then work on it the next day to avoid it occurring again, rather than thinking 'if she cries, this is how I have to manage it'. My strategies encourage you to work out why your baby wakes and resolve it so it doesn't reoccur, and only then to deal with any communication or confusion issues that remain after such episodes.

At night, babies should only come to significant partial wakings between 10 and 11 p.m., at around 2 a.m., and between 4 and 5 a.m. All other wakings between these windows are caused by a disruption that pulls them out of their sleep cycle, and their normal, solid three-to-four-hour window of block sleep is disrupted. The most common triggers of disruption to each solid block of night sleep are:

Trouble going to sleep initially at 7 p.m.

This is a classic behavioural/association window. She may be having too much or too late an afternoon sleep. Shorten or start the afternoon sleep earlier. If it continues, it's one of two things:

1. Wrong daily routine: reassess her daily sleep-routine needs and adopt a routine that suits her *actual* needs, and not your desire for her to sleep at certain times.
2. Daytime communication is not balanced: if you know she's usually able to self-settle, it may be that you haven't been using balanced lines of communication during the day to ensure she's comfortable with you guiding her.

Wakings between 7 and 10/11 p.m.

If she's having trouble after initially going to sleep:

- She was already asleep when you left: which means you weren't honest with her and she was startled when she woke to find you gone. Always let her know by leaving the room before she falls asleep.
- She is too hot: as this is the hottest time in her 24-hour day, it's important to keep her cooler though the first part of her night. A fan or air conditioning may help but there's no need to cool her after 10 or 11 p.m. It's important to be aware of this for babies who are swaddled. Babies who are uncomfortably warm during this first portion of the night are likely to fall asleep and then wake up for short periods of time frequently (around every 40 minutes) between 7 and 10 p.m. Babies who are extremely hot are more likely to wake and stay awake for prolonged periods between 7 and 10 p.m.
- She is non-symptomatic but may be starting to get ill: it's common for babies to feel unwell and feel uncomfortable before they show symptoms of an illness. Often, they wake momentarily, frequently, without needing intervention. This is when whatever illness they've caught is taking hold at the end of the day when their resistance is lower. If you offer a paracetamol-based analgesic designed for her age group and she settles within 20 minutes, or stops waking, she's probably feeling unwell and you should look into the cause further. Always ensure her ears are clear when she's on sleep training.

After the initial settling-in period of any PRM is over (after the first three weeks) it's unlikely your baby will continue to wake for prolonged periods at night without it being a routine miscalculation (if she's able to self-settle and self-resettle ordinarily). In this case you should reconsider your sleep-routine times and, in particular, look closely at her afternoon sleep, and the length of sleep she's taking through the entire day. When her afternoon sleeps are the cause of prolonged waking in this first window of the night, they are either too long, and may need to be a bridging nap only, suggesting the low or modified routine may be more appropriate or, in rarer cases, the afternoon sleep may be too short and she's become overtired. If she's overtired she's more likely to wake frequently for short periods of time. If you suspect she may be overtired, offer more sleep during the afternoon sleep for ASR and HSR babies, or try to encourage an afternoon bridge for a LSR baby.

Wakings between 10 and 11 p.m.
This is a behavioural/association window indicating the daytime communication between you and your child isn't balanced. If you know she's able to self-settle ordinarily, you may not have been using balanced lines of communication during the day to ensure she's comfortable with you guiding her.

Wakings between 11.30 p.m. and 1.30 a.m.
This is a classic illness or discomfort window so a prolonged waking in it may indicate your child is experiencing symptoms of an illness, unlike the 7-to-10 p.m. sign of an impending illness. If you've seen she's teething during the day, or she has a cold or ear infection, tummy bug, etc., she's more likely to run a temperature at this time and be clearly uncomfortable, if not in pain. If so try to pre-empt the discomfort she starts to feel at this window when the body is working to fight the illness by offering pain relief at 10 p.m. so she can sleep peacefully.

If she has a food intolerance, as far as gut response to wheat, dairy, etc., it will show up around this time. If you introduced a new food the day before or that day and she is unsettled here, remove the food from her diet and trial it again in another week's time. If it occurs again, remove that food from her diet for six months before trying again. If it occurs again at your next trial, don't reintroduce it until she's two.

If she is low in iron or, in a more subtle way, not eating enough meat, then she's more likely to have prolonged wakings. If her food intake is unbalanced, her body will wake her to feed here, to supplement the poor nutritional balance from the day. If she's not drinking enough water through the day from six months of age and onwards, then she will wake here. You need to ensure you balance his diet, incorporating meat once a day until his prolonged wakings settle down, and make sure she's getting a good blend of vegetables and fruit. Don't replace solid feeds with milk as her body won't be sustained by it at night during this growth window and she'll continue to have prolonged wakings.

If you know she's physically well, and have catered for his dietary and hydration needs, a clear pattern of prolonged wakings at night at this time (three times or more is a pattern) is a sign of excessive accumulated day sleep. Reassess your child's daily sleep requirement over a five-day window, removing the lost sleep from the middle of the night to determine her true sleep need.

Wakings at or near 2 a.m.

This is a classic behavioural/association window of time suggesting daytime communication isn't balanced. If you know your baby is usually able to self-settle, you may not have been using balanced lines of communication during the day to ensure she's comfortable with you guiding her.

Wakings between 2.30 and 3.30 a.m.

This is another classic illness or discomfort continuation window, although it seems to indicate a lesser level of discomfort or dietary imbalance: the tail end of an illness, or the last days of teething or ear aches will commonly lead to wakings here, as opposed to wakings at the 11.30 p.m. to 1.30 a.m. window suggesting a child may still be unwell. See 11.30 p.m. to 1.30 a.m. wakings for guidance. Provide her with discomfort relief to cover her from 11.30 p.m. to 3.30 a.m. if you know she's been unwell and prone to waking for a few days.

Wakings between 4 and 5 a.m. (more commonly 5 a.m.)

This is a classical behavioural/association window suggesting that daytime communication isn't balanced. If you know your child is able to self-settle ordinarily, then it may be that you haven't been using balanced lines of communication during the day to ensure she's comfortable with you guiding her.

Wakings between 5 and 6.30 a.m.

This is when she's waking early and is unable to go back to sleep. There are a number of possible reasons for this, including:

- Her morning sleep the day before was either too early or too long.
- If your baby is hungry her food intake the day before was too low. Increase the overall quantity and quality of food you offer at the three main meals of the day. If she is fussy at meal times, reduce the morning and afternoon snacks so you're not overfeeding her then. Never give snacks of low nutritional value outside the meal-time windows suggested because she won't eat foods of a higher nutritional value at meal times.
- She may have missed out on enough balanced independent playtime the day before, leaving her challenged across the board and prone to tiredness.
- The first feed of the day the previous day was given too early, or was too long, too big or a combination of all three.

- She's overeating in the morning in general but, in particular, the food taken the previous morning between 7 a.m. and 12 p.m. could be impacting on her ability to sleep in. She doesn't need three breakfasts, or a large morning tea, and you should follow age suggestions for dropping feeds.

Moving forward and maintaining your LSR or ASR routines

Slight adjustments to any routine are necessary as your child grows and her daily sleep requirement increases then decreases. For example, she may still need two to two and a half hours' sleep during the day but only in one solid block. So the 19- to 20-minute bridging naps transition into one longer sleep in the day. The afternoon nap will naturally phase itself out by the time she's nine to ten months old. You will lie her down for their sleep and she will lie there happily, but not fall asleep.

Eventually she'll take maybe three afternoon bridges out of seven, or only the odd bridge here and there. If this happens you may decide to discontinue the routine of lying her down, knowing that if her body needs it she will drift off independently. If she does fall asleep naturally during an afternoon-bridge window, even if you haven't put her down, only allow it to be a 19- to 20-minute sleep or wake her by 4.45 and 5.00 p.m. (depending on her age group), whichever comes first. This can only happen in the set afternoon-bridge window until your child is ten months old. After that she's not allowed to drift off as it will cause tears at bedtime at 7 p.m.

It may be slightly more challenging to identify when the morning nap is no longer useful. Your child will not naturally drop this sleep but it should be gone by the time she's around 12 months old for most low-sleep-requirement babies, and by 12 to 15 months for average-sleep-requirement babies. The following may be signs that the morning nap is no longer necessary and you need to eliminate it:

- She grizzles for a long time before she manages to fall asleep at the 8.45 a.m. bridging nap.
- She's starting to wake predictably earlier in the morning; for example, her normal waking time is 6 a.m. and she starts to wake at 5.30 a.m. each day.
- She begins to have disrupted midday sleep patterns, waking after 40 minutes and needing to be managed for 20 plus-ish minutes before she sleeps for another 40 minutes.
- It takes her longer to fall asleep at lunch time each day.

If you see this occurring for more than three days in a row and your baby is the right age with the appropriate sleep requirement to be growing out of this sleep, it's best to just drop this morning-bridge sleep immediately. Make a point of doing something extra busy at that time to help her move through the ten-minute tired period she may have for the following week. After she recovers (within ten to 20 minutes) resume your day as normal. After a week there will be no need to try and keep her busy as the old rhythm should start to diminish.

At this point your child is officially on a single, solid, midday sleep, has a solid and consistent night sleep pattern, and you can maintain her day meal plan and sleep times until she heads to kindergarten and beyond. The midday sleep will become a quiet rest time in her bed by the time she's three until she goes to school at five.

By their nature, high- and most average-sleep-requirement babies are, or should be, more flexible with their sleep times as they grow, though you'll still need to take precautions when 'doing your homework' and 'creating harmony' so they become independent with their settling and resettling skills. Anyone using these HSR routines will probably note their child isn't nearly as sensitive as her lower-sleep-requirement playmates when you manage her routine per age group.

Troubleshooting for PRM Routine 1

Q: Why is the first feed at 6.30 to 7 a.m.?

A: The first feed is at 6.30 to 7 a.m. because it affects the time your baby wakes up. A baby prepares for this first feed during her final 40-minute REM cycle before waking. If you normally feed her at 6.30 a.m. she's likely to start to stir at 5.50 a.m. the following day, and if you then feed her at 6 a.m., she's likely to stir at 5.20 a.m. the next day. So 40 minutes before her first milk feed she can start to wake the following morning. This can lead to backtracking time on feeding schedules so you have earlier waking times periodically. If you can hold out till 7 a.m. for that first feed, she's more likely to sleep up to that time the next day.

Q: How do I get her to hold out for the first feed if she wakes at 6 a.m.?

A: If she's six months old and wakes at 6 a.m. on the first few days of your schedule it may be difficult to hold out past 6.30 a.m. From 6 to 6.30 a.m. try to distract her by letting her play in the cot, changing her nappy, and taking her for a little wander while you make a cup of tea or collect the newspaper. If you can, hold out to 7 a.m. It will only take a couple of days for her to settle into the new pattern. If, after a week on your routine your six to seven month old is sleeping well till a reasonable time each morning and is hungry and not coping well with the wait in the morning, feed her at 6.30 a.m. and see if it impacts on her waking time the next morning. If it has no effect, then carry on, but if she starts to wake earlier, and that makes her tired and unhappy, you may need to work harder on distracting her in the morning.

Q: Can my baby sleep till 7 a.m.?
A: In the early stages of repairing your baby's sleep it may not be possible to get her to sleep till 7 a.m. The morning bridging nap is important for setting up a successful day so extra sleep in the early morning may affect her ability to take the morning bridge, which can then impact on her entire day. Eleven to 11½ hours of undisturbed sleep at night is excellent from six months of age. Don't feel you should let her sleep in on those first few days if you've had prolonged night wakings as that will encourage more poor night sleep. To help you cope with this waking time, make sure you go to bed early for a couple of weeks while you adjust. Eventually you'll be able to let your baby wake whenever she likes so long as it doesn't impact on the balance of her day or damage her day sleeps again.

Q: I feed on demand and I've suddenly dropped from ten to 20 plus breast-feeds a day to four on this routine. Should I do anything to prevent lactating problems?
A: Though it may be hard to wake yourself up, you should do two full expresses per night to avoid becoming engorged and getting mastitis. For the first few nights express at 10 p.m. and 2 a.m. and for the first three days massage your breasts regularly, loosening up any lumps to keep milk ducts from becoming engorged or infected. If necessary, express in the shower, after your baby's feed, or if you're feeling full. Using cool packs on your breasts can also help settle things down during the first three days. Make sure you wear a well-fitted bra for cosmetic purposes as well. As your body prepares to breastfeed, fat stores leave the breast providing room for the milk ducts to fill. Hence, when the demand and supply drops, the fat stores in your breasts start to return. If your bra isn't supportive you may experience some drooping. Wear your bra day and night for the first few weeks, and ensure you remain comfortable but firmly supported at all times.

Q: Isn't breakfast too close to the first feed of the day?

A: Given her last solid feed was at 5.20 p.m. the previous night her first milk feed will only take the edge off her hunger. If you miss the hunger window first thing in the morning, she may not be interested in eating and want to sleep to cope with her low fuel levels. Hunger and tired signs are very similar so thinking she needs a nap is misreading her body's needs. Follow through with the meal-time windows even if you can't imagine it will work, and she will settle into the program with ease.

Q: There seems to be a lot of feeds close together in the morning. Is this right?

A: There's a difference in feed quantities and frequency between the average-to-high-sleep-requirement baby's routines and the low-sleep-requirement baby's routines, particularly in the morning. This is because a LSR child's need for food increases with the reduced sleep she has in the morning. As her sleep requirement is naturally lower, you need to ensure she starts her day with appropriate windows for feeding and milk intake to be at her very best. The LSR routine has the most positive impact of any routine I've ever seen on an unsettled child.

PRM Routine 2

Babies go through typical transitional milk feed and sleep changes during the first two years and these affect their routines. The changes in sleep patterns occur whether the child has a low, average or high sleep requirement. They happen at particular age brackets and result in changing or lowering sleep and milk intake once they've been introduced to solid food in their diet. The following are the ages when changes in milk feeding times and sleep transitions occur:

- At five and a half to six and a half months solids are being established and milk feeds begin to reduce.
- At six to eight months solids will be established and milk intake will be reduced to four full feeds per day.
- At nine months full milk feeds begin to reduce to three by the tenth month.
- At 12 months LSR babies need to move to one sleep a day.
- At 14 to 15 months milk feeds should be reduced to two full feeds per day and most ASR babies need to move to one sleep a day.
- At 16 to 18 months milk feeds should be reduced to a final night feed before bed, which can be dropped at leisure. Most HSR babies need to move to one sleep a day.

Even with these natural changes, aim for your baby to have a balanced and healthy 7 p.m. settling time and 6 to 7 a.m. waking time the following morning, so adjust their routines as they transition to the next age group to achieve this.

The following routines are suggested for ASR and HSR babies who are establishing solids (at around the fifth month). Prior to that, variations between the sleep requirement groups and age transitions are vast and their needs are changing rapidly. Once your baby's night sleep is repaired to the minimum sleep suggestion for each routine, begin building up your baby's daytime sleep intake. Keep your baby well hydrated throughout the day, but don't offer water 30 minutes before solids as water will make her feel full and impede eating.

While solids are being introduced (at five and a half to six and a half months)

The following routine is the classic 'two-hours-up, two-hours-down' format, with slight variations for average- and high-sleep-requirement babies. The variation in the routine between babies still establishing solids and babies established on solids is due to lower calorie/fuel and iron intake, which creates a need for more regular sleep and more milk feeds. The dream feed is sometimes necessary when food isn't adequate due to growing hunger and a need for iron in their diet. Until these elements are provided a dream feed is appropriate for this transitioning age group.

There are two reasons you need to wake your child for a feed rather than wait for her. The first is to ensure you don't teach your baby to wake up and call out for a feed to go back to sleep which develops dependent resettling associations and will contradict your normal communication style. A child doesn't know 10 p.m. from 2 a.m. or 5 a.m., so fulfilling one request to feed to go back to sleep, but not any subsequent requests will cause tears. By waking and feeding her before she stirs and calls out you eliminate the pattern of her calling out for milk to go back to sleep.

The second reason is to try to prevent tears rather than manage them. As true hunger will typically occur between 11.30 p.m. and 1.30 a.m. and again between 2.30 and 3.30 a.m., you need to pre-empt her body's hunger and cater for that before she feels a need to cry out in hunger. That said, by the time you start this program it is better to have established solids rather than introduce or sustain a dream feed in order to avoid creating a learnt hunger pattern in your baby's circadian rhythm (which could cause her to learn to wake naturally then for a feed) or detract from your baby's daytime calorie intake as this can create a fussy feeder.

Daily routine outline for five and a half to six and a half month olds

6.00–7.00 a.m.: Natural waking

7.00: Latest waking. Milk feed

8.00: Breakfast

9.00: Mid-morning nap: ASR babies take one hour, 15 minutes; HSR babies one hour, 30 minutes

11.00: Morning tea: milk feed

12.00 p.m.: Lunch: vegetables and protein

1.00: Mid-afternoon nap: ASR babies take one hour, 30 minutes; HSR babies one hour, 45 minutes

3.00–3.30: Afternoon tea: milk feed

5.00: Dinner: vegetables with or without rice cereal

6.30: Milk feed

7.00: Bedtime for 11 to 12 hours

10.30: Dream feed

Daily routine in detail

6.00–6.30 a.m.: Natural waking. Manage any wakings before 6.00 a.m. with crying interpretation and support and aim to increase her sleep intake to encourage a later waking. Use your waking routine and allow playtime in cot for 15 to 20 minutes. Before getting her up pack away and use your wait game and cue.

7.00: Latest waking time: use your waking routine and cue and allow a brief play and pack away. Breast or bottle feed – don't allow baby to snooze. Change nappy, then allow free playtime.

7.50: Prepare baby's breakfast. Use pre-emptive language such as, 'Nearly time for breakfast', 'Nearly time to sit down and wait for Mummy, yummy food'.

8.00: Baby's breakfast. Manage her feeding and use your meal-time routine. Then dress her for the day and allow free playtime. She'll usually want to spend time with you but allow her to be free to safely explore her environment if she wishes. This is the time you might need to drop off older children to preschools or schools. If you're in the car don't let your baby fall asleep. She needs to stay awake until the morning sleep at nine o'clock. Prepare cot room for morning sleep. Use your flow of communication – 'Nearly time for stories', 'Nearly time for nigh' nigh's'.

8.45: Nappy change before beginning settling routine.

8.55: Say goodnight to anyone in the room, then complete settling routine.

9.00: Morning sleep. See sleep requirement variations. Set up play stations while she sleeps. When she wakes allow her a brief playtime in her cot, then pack away. If she wakes early encourage a longer playtime in cot. Latest waking time is 11 a.m. Change nappy.

11.00: Morning tea: breast or bottle feed. Independent playtime opportunity. Help her become comfortable with being put down to play independently, a skill she'll need for sleep – think of it as sleep-earning play. If she's not settling down to play use your flow of communication and follow through. If you leave the room, use your short-term absence cue 'I'll be back'.

12.00 p.m.: Lunch: vegetables with or without rice cereal, and protein, which should be introduced as soon as she's comfortable with vegetables. No dessert or fruit is required here. Follow your meal-time routine when feeding her and use your cues if problems arise. After lunch is complete, use the wait game and cue then get her up for a little one-on-one playtime. Give her your undivided attention for around 15 minutes. Use your pre-empting cues, 'Nearly time to pack away' towards the end of playtime.

12.40: Pack away toys completely, and prepare cot room and wrap for mid-afternoon sleep while your baby keeps you company and 'helps'. Change nappy and use pre-emptive cues for sleep – 'Nearly time for sleep, let's go find our books'.

12.45: Begin settling routine.

12.55: Final book pack away and say goodnight to everyone in the room. Complete settling routine.

1.00: Mid-afternoon sleep: check sleep requirement suggestions.

2.30–3.00: Natural waking time. Leave her in her cot as long as you can if she needs to or naturally wakes earlier. Once she's woken, use your waking routine and cues. Allow her independent play in the cot for 20 minutes or until her afternoon milk feed is due.

3.00: Afternoon tea: breast/bottle milk feed only. This milk feed will continue up to and in some cases well beyond her first birthday. Some children opt to keep this until you decide it's time to have milk in a cup with their afternoon tea.

4.15–5.00: Afternoon bridging nap for six month olds if their food is still insufficient and they appear to want the nap. This nap is strictly 20 minutes. Don't allow her to sleep more than 20 minutes. Check her every three to five minutes to see when she goes to sleep, and wake her when her allocated nap time ends, or when the sleep window ends at 5 p.m., whichever is first. Most babies have had enough of their cot by this time, and though she needs this sleep you may need to assist her to take it. As you can't assist her in her cot, this is a good sleep for her to have in the car if you're picking up older children or in her pram. If it's warm, walk her in the shade. If it's hot, raining or blowing a gale go to a shopping mall. If you can't do either, push her in the pram at home briefly until she goes to sleep, or give her another sleep in her cot. If she doesn't fall asleep early enough and doesn't nap the whole allocated time of 20 minutes, still wake her by 5 p.m.

If your baby needs this sleep at this age, indicated by her not coping when she misses it, try and make it easy for her by knowing her sleep requirement. If she's sleeping for two hours at his mid-afternoon sleep and unable to take this bridging nap but is becoming overtired by 7 p.m. after the first three days of your new routine, you will need to wake her after one hour, 15 minutes (ASR) or one hour, 30 minutes (HSR) after the mid-afternoon sleep to encourage this nap until she is seven months old and is ready to drop this bridge nap because she's starting to eat better, which will make it easier to cope with the longer afternoon.

If your six-month-old baby has difficulty going to sleep at 7 p.m. after a few consistent days on this routine, and she's taking her bridge sleep right up until 5 p.m., you'll need to taper the latest sleep time for this bridge nap back to 4.45 p.m. so she doesn't continue having difficulty falling asleep at 7 p.m. This may mean tightening her mid-afternoon sleep back a little to one hour, 15 minutes (ASR) or one hour, 30 minutes (HSR) to help her fall asleep on the bridge earlier. Her night sleep is the most important sleep to lock in first, then you can adjust her days, depending on how much sleep she has left to take. Don't steal from nights to achieve better days.

Alternatively, if she's not taking the afternoon bridge nap and is still having trouble falling asleep at 7 p.m. because she's appearing overtired, you'll need to increase her mid-afternoon sleep by limiting her mid-morning sleep slightly to one hour, 15 minutes (ASR) or one hour, 30 minutes (HSR) and not wake her at the mid-afternoon sleep, or re-assess her sleep requirement after five days of solid routine management to ensure this routine actually suits your baby's individual needs. Always allow three to five days minimum of routine management before you make any major changes as your baby needs to work through her new settling request and develop new independent associations with sleep first.

4.15–5.00: Use this time to do your final pack away for the day, and prepare for dinner, using your pre-emptive cues if she's awake.

5.00: Latest time to wake from bridging nap, using waking cues. Dinner: vegetables with or without rice cereal, then playtime in high chair as you prepare her bedroom, tidy the kitchen and organise your own evening meal for when he goes to bed at 7 p.m. It's important you eat a healthy meal at the end of your day to stave off depression and poor sleep, and it's also a good time to connect with your partner or other members of your family.

6.00: Nudie playtime, using cues for bath.

6.15: Bath time. Watch your baby the whole time. Remember your cues as you get towards 6.30 – 'Nearly time to pack away, nearly time to get out of bath.'

6.30: Take her out of the bath. The household should start to become calm. Dim lights in preparation for bed. Dry and dress baby quickly but calmly. As she'll be tired you might need to reassure her – 'It's okay, bubba, you're just tired. Nearly time for milk and nigh' nigh's.'

6.35: Breast or bottle feed, ten to 15 minutes only. Don't let her doze or even zone out during this feed as it will interrupt the settling routine.

6.45–6.50: Begin settling routine by 6.50 at the latest.

6.55: Final cue – 'Last page, then nigh' nigh's' – and pack away. Enjoy a last cuddle and complete settling routine.

7.00: Bedtime. If she cries assess the situation and interpret the cries, and be mindful of the sleep bus timetable (see page 354) before you go in and use your cues and resettling routines.

10.30: Possible dream feed. As you increase her solid intake during the day you will start to wean her off this dream feed.

Once solids have been established (at six to eight months)

By the sixth month, all the routines assume you've started solids and introduced iron into your baby's diet via a protein with her lunch-time vegetable meal. The 10.30 p.m. dream feed won't be necessary if she's eating adequate solids and getting iron in his diet. If not, it's time to reassess her solid intake before starting this routine because iron is essential for sleep between 11.30 p.m. and 3.30 a.m.

You may find it more convenient to provide your baby's independent play opportunity at 11 a.m. instead of after her mid-afternoon sleep. I've indicated both times as independent play opportunities, so choose the time that suits your day's activities. I usually suggest around 45 minutes to an hour of requested independent play followed by a solid 15 minutes of focus play.

Daily routine outline for six to eight month olds

6.00–6.30 a.m.: Natural waking

7.00: Latest waking. Milk feed

8.00: Breakfast

9.30: Mid-morning nap: ASR babies take one hour, 15 minutes; HSR babies one hour, 30 minutes

11.00: Morning tea: milk feed

12.00 p.m.: Lunch: vegetables and protein, plus dessert by eight months

1.30: Mid-afternoon nap: ASR babies take one hour, 15 minutes; HSR babies one hour, 30 minutes

3.00–3.30: Afternoon tea: milk feed

5.00: Dinner: vegetables with or without carbohydrates (rice, pasta)

6.30: Milk feed

7.00: Bedtime for 11 to 12 hours

Daily routine in detail

6.00–6.30 a.m.: Natural waking. Manage any wakings before 5.50 a.m. with crying interpretation and support. Once she's woken leave her as long as you can before entering the room using your waking routine. Playtime in cot for 15 to 20 minutes. Before getting her up pack away and use your wait game and cue.

7.00: Latest waking time – use waking routine and cue to wake her up if necessary. Allow a brief play and pack away. Breast or bottle feed – don't allow her to snooze. Change nappy, then allow free playtime.

7.50: Prepare baby's breakfast. Use pre-emptive and forewarning language – 'Nearly time for breakfast', 'Nearly time to sit down and wait for Mummy, yummy apple and oatmeal'.

8.00: Baby's breakfast. Manage her feeding and use your meal-time routine. After breakfast, dress her for the day and allow her some free playtime. She'll usually want to help you but let her venture off safely once she's mobile if she wishes. This might be the time you need to drop off older children to preschools or schools. If you're in the car don't let her fall asleep. She needs to stay awake until the morning sleep at 9.30 a.m. Before 9.15, prepare her room for morning sleep. Use your flow of communication – 'Nearly time for stories, nearly time for nigh' nigh's' in the lead-up to the settling routine.

9.15: Nappy change before beginning settling routine.

9.25: Say goodnight to everyone, then complete settling routine.

9.30: Morning sleep: allow for any sleep requirement variations. Set up play stations while she sleeps. If she wakes early, allow playtime in cot for a minimum of 20 minutes. If you're offering independent playtime when she wakes up, set up play stations while she's sleeping.

11.00: Latest waking time; allow brief playtime in cot if she wakes at 11 a.m. Pack away cot. Change nappy. Supply morning tea as soon as she gets up. Independent playtime opportunity to help her become comfortable with being put down to play independently, a skill she'll need for sleep. If she's not settling down to play use your flow of communication and follow through and position for play. If you leave the room, use your short-term absence cue, 'I'll be back'.

12.00 p.m.: Lunch: vegetables and protein every day. By eight months also offer a dessert (fruit pureed with or without rice cereal, etc.). Follow meal-time management routine while feeding her and use cues if there are problems. After lunch use your wait game and cue. Get her up for a little more independent playtime then complete her play session with some one-on-one playtime.

1.10: Pack away toys completely, prepare cot room and wrap for mid-afternoon sleep while she keeps you company and 'helps'. Change nappy and use pre-emptive cues for sleep – 'Nearly time for sleep, let's go find our books.'

1.15: Begin settling routine.

1.25: Pack away books, say goodnight to everyone and complete settling routine.

1.30: Mid-afternoon sleep. Check sleep requirements for natural waking windows and latest waking times. Leave her in her cot as long as you can if she needs to or wake her earlier. Once she's woken, use routine and cues. Allow independent play in cot until afternoon milk feed is due or for 20 minutes, whichever comes first.

3.00–3.30: Afternoon tea. This is a breast/bottle milk feed only. The milk feed will remain up to and well beyond her first birthday. Some children opt to keep this until you decide it's time for her to have milk in a cup with her afternoon tea instead. If you take up independent playtime opportunity here rather than after mid-morning sleep, your timings will look something like: 3.45 to 4.30 p.m., independent playtime, then 4.30 to 4.45 p.m., one-on-one playtime.

4.45: Time for final pack away. Say cues, 'Time to pack away, nearly time for dinner.' Put her in his high chair for quiet time, which might include her favourite DVD or books on her tray table in the kitchen while you warm her food.

5.00: Dinner time: vegetables with or without rice cereal or pasta. Then playtime in high chair as you tidy kitchen organise the family's evening meal, to be had after your baby goes to bed. It's important to eat a healthy meal at the end of your day to stave off depression and poor sleep, and connect with other members of your family. Prepare her bedroom.

6.00: Nudie playtime: use your pre-emptive cues for bath time.

6.15: Bath time. Watch your baby for her whole bath. Use your cues as you get towards 6.30 – 'Nearly time to pack away, nearly time to get out of bath'.

6.30: Take baby out of bath. The household should start to become calm. Dim lights in preparation for baby's bedtime. Dry and dress her quickly but calmly. As she'll be tired you might need to reassure her – 'It's okay, bubba, you're just tired. Nearly time for milk and nigh' nigh's.'

6.35: Breast or bottle feed for ten minutes only. Don't let her doze or even zone out at this time or it will interrupt her settling ability at 7 p.m.

6.45–6.50: Begin settling routine. This must start at 6.50 at the latest.

6.55: Final cue: 'Last page, then nigh' nigh's' and pack away. Enjoy a last cuddle and complete your settling routine.

7.00: Bedtime. If your baby cries, assess the situation and interpret the cries before you go in to resettle. Use your cues and resettling routines.

Sustaining the gap between afternoon tea and dinner

If you have a hungry baby who's not coping on just milk until 5 p.m., offer her a light snack (half a Cruskit, or some cheese, or half a piece of fruit) in addition to her 3 p.m. milk feed, and give her solids closer to 5.20 p.m. Be mindful of not filling her up so she can't eat dinner because dinner is important. Gauge her response to afternoon tea by her ability to eat dinner and decrease or increase her afternoon tea accordingly. Keep her well hydrated before you offer additional food, but don't give water 30 minutes before solids are due because this may impede her appetite.

Nine to 11 month olds

At nine months milk feeds begin to reduce and by the tenth month your baby will need only three milk feeds per day, dropping the mid-morning milk feed. If your baby is still transitioning (more common in nine month olds) and is tired despite having eaten lunch and taken her mid-morning sleep intake, you can put her down for her mid-afternoon sleep from 2 p.m. on. In this case offer her water before her sleep and give her a milk feed and snack when she wakes up to help sustain her for the longer afternoon. You can then offer dinner at 5.20 p.m. instead of 5. If this becomes his natural need for a while, ensure she has lunch closer to 12 p.m. most days. As she gets older move her second sleep to later in the afternoon, and alter her afternoon tea and dinner windows back to the suggested times in this routine.

Depending on your activities for the day, you may opt to provide her independent play opportunity after her lunch or after her mid-afternoon sleep. This is the time to help her become comfortable with being put down to play independently, a skill she needs for sleep. If she's not settling down to play use your flow of communication and follow through. If you leave the room, use your short-term absence cue, 'I'll be back'. I usually suggest around 45 minutes to an hour of requested independent play followed by a solid 15 minutes of focus play.

Daily routine outline for nine to 11 month olds

6.00–6.30 a.m.: Natural waking

7.00: Latest waking. Milk feed

7.20: Breakfast

9.30: Morning tea: fruit and water

10.00: Mid-morning nap: ASR babies take one hour, 15 minutes; HSR babies one hour, 30 minutes

11.30–12.00 p.m.: Lunch: vegetables and protein, plus dessert

2.00–2.15: Afternoon tea: milk feed and snack

2.15–2.30: Mid-afternoon nap. Option: at 2.15 p.m. ASR babies one hour, 15 minutes; at 2.30 p.m. HSR babies one hour, 30 minutes. Offer water when she wakes.

5.00: Dinner: vegetables with or without carbohydrates

6.30: Milk feed

7.00: Bedtime for 11 to 12 hours

Daily routine in detail

6.00–6.30 a.m.: Natural waking. Manage any wakings before 5.30 a.m. with crying interpretation and support to increase her sleep. If she's not awake by 6.30 a.m. on the first ten days, use your waking routine and allow playtime in cot for 15 to 20 minutes. Before getting her up pack away and use your wait game and cue.

7.00: Breast or bottle feed, but don't allow baby to snooze. Change nappy, then allow free playtime.

7.15: Prepare baby's breakfast. Use your pre-emptive and forewarning language – 'Nearly time for breakfast', 'Nearly time to sit down and wait for Mummy, yummy apple and oatmeal'.

7.20: Baby's breakfast. Manage her feed and your use meal-time routine. After breakfast, dress her for the day and then allow free playtime. She'll usually want to help you but allow her to safely venture off once mobile if she wishes. This might be the time you need to drop off older children to preschools or schools. If you're in the car try to not let her fall asleep. She needs to stay awake until the morning sleep at 10 a.m. Prepare cot room for sleep and use your flow of communication – 'nearly time for stories, nearly time for nigh' nigh's'.

9.30: Morning tea: fruit and water. During the ninth month you can offer milk *after* fruit if she's interested. By the tenth month, this milk feed is naturally dropped and she will be having only three milk feeds a day.

9.45: Nappy change, then begin settling routine.

9.55: Say goodnight to everyone, then complete settling routine.

10.00: Morning sleep begins: For ASR babies one hour, 15 minutes; for HSR babies one hour, 30 minutes. If she wakes early encourage playtime in the cot until 11.30 a.m. If you're going to offer independent playtime after lunch set up play stations while she sleeps.

11.30–12.00 p.m.: Lunch: vegetables and protein every day and offer dessert (fruit puree with or without rice cereal, yoghurt etc.). Serve as close to 11.30 as she wakes, and no later than 12 p.m. Follow your meal-time management routine when feeding her and use your cues if there are problems. After lunch is over use your wait game and cue. This is a good independent playtime opportunity.

2.00–2.15: Afternoon tea: milk feed and snack. Afternoon tea can be between 1.50 and 2.10 p.m., depending on when your baby woke and had her lunch. For example, if your ASR baby woke at 11.15 and ate lunch at 11.30 give her afternoon tea at 1.50 p.m. and put her down for her mid-afternoon nap around 2.15 p.m. The settling routine for this will begin at 2.05 p.m. If your HSR baby woke at 11.30 a.m. and ate lunch closer to 12 p.m. she can have afternoon tea at 2.05 p.m. and go down for a mid-afternoon nap around 2.30 p.m. Settling routine begins at 2.20 p.m.

2.15–2.30: Mid-afternoon sleep: for ASR babies one hour, 15 minutes; for HSR babies one hour, 30 minutes. If your baby wakes earlier than suggested, leave her in his cot as long as you can before attending to either resettle for wakings under 40 minutes or, once she's fully woken, use your waking routine and cues. Allow her independent play in her cot until the designated waking time is due or for 20 minutes, whichever occurs first. Offer her water when she wakes.

4.15: Latest sleep time allowed when building your child's daily sleep intake. Wake your baby now if she's not already awake. This is a good independent playtime opportunity if not offered after lunch.

4.45: Use this time to do your final pack away for the day, using your cues – 'Time to pack away, nearly time for dinner' – then pop her into the high chair for quiet time while you prepare her dinner. High-chair time may include her favourite Baby Einstein DVD or books on her tray table in the kitchen.

5.00: Dinner: vegetables with or without carbohydrates followed by playtime in high chair as you tidy the kitchen and organise the rest of the family's dinner and prepare their bedroom for the evening. It's important to eat a healthy meal at the end of your day to stave off depression and poor sleep and connect with other members of your family.

6.00: Nudie playtime, using cues for bath.

6.15: Bath time. You need to watch your baby the whole time. Use your cues as you get towards 6.30 – 'Nearly time to pack away, nearly time to get out of bath'.

6.30: Get baby out of bath. The household should start to calm down with the lights dimmed in preparation for her bedtime. Dry and dress her quickly but calmly. As she'll be tired you may need to reassure her – 'It's okay, bubba, you're just tired. Nearly time for milk and nigh' nigh's.'

6.35: Breast or bottle feed, ten minutes only. Don't let her doze or even zone out at this time because it will interrupt her settling ability at 7 p.m.

6.45–6.50: Begin settling routine by 6.50 at the latest.

6.55: Final cue – 'Last page, then nigh' nigh's' – and pack away. Enjoy a final cuddle and complete your settling routine.

7.00: Bedtime. If your baby cries assess the situation and interpret her cries before you go in to resettle. Use your cues and resettling routines.

12 to 13 month olds

If your baby is transitioning to this reduced sleep and feeding routine (more common in 12 month olds), and is very tired despite having her mid-morning sleep and a good lunch, you can put her down for her mid-afternoon sleep from 2.15 p.m. on. In this case either give her afternoon tea earlier or offer her water before her sleep and give her a milk feed after she wakes to sustain her for the longer afternoon. Continue to offer dinner at 5.20 p.m. As she gets older move this second sleep to later in the afternoon, and alter her afternoon tea window back to the suggested program.

Depending on your day's activities, you may opt to provide her independent play opportunity after lunch or after her mid-afternoon sleep. This is the time to help her feel comfortable with playing independently, a skill she needs for sleep. If she's not settling down to play use your flow of communication and follow through. If you leave the room, use your short-term absence cue, 'I'll be back'.

Daily routine outline for 12–13 month olds

6.00–6.30 a.m.: Natural waking

7.00: Latest waking. Milk feed

7.20: Breakfast

9.30: Morning tea: fruit and water

10.15: Mid-morning nap: for ASR babies one hour, 15 minutes; HSR babies one hour, 30 minutes. Once you've built her sleep up to this level, feed her when she wakes up.

11.30–12.00 p.m.: Lunch: vegetables and protein, plus dessert

2.00–2.30: Afternoon tea: milk feed and snack

2.30–3.00: Mid-afternoon sleep: for ASR babies one hour, 15 minutes; HSR babies one hour, 30 minutes. The latest time sleep can be built up to is 4.15 p.m.

5.20: Dinner: vegetables with or without carbohydrates

6.30: Milk feed

7.00: Bedtime for 11 to 12 hours

Daily routine in detail

6.00–6.30 a.m.: Natural waking. Manage any wakings before 5.30 a.m. with crying interpretation and support to build her sleep. If she's not awake by 6.30 on the first ten days of the routine, use your waking routine and offer playtime in cot for 15 to 20 minutes. Before getting her up pack away and use your wait game and cue.

7.00: Breast or bottle feed but don't allow your baby to snooze. Change her nappy and then offer free playtime.

7.10: Prepare her breakfast and use pre-emptive language – 'Nearly time for breakfast', 'Nearly time to sit down and wait for yummy apple and oatmeal.'

7.20: Baby's breakfast. Use your meal-time routine and manage her behaviour if she's difficult to feed. After breakfast, dress her for the day and offer free playtime. She may want to 'help' but once she's mobile allow her to be free to safely venture off. This might be the time you need to drop off older children to preschools or schools. If you're in the car don't let her fall asleep. She needs to stay awake until the morning sleep at 10.15 a.m. Prepare room for the morning sleep and use your flow of communication – 'Nearly time for stories, nearly time for nigh' nigh's'.

9.30: Morning tea: fruit and water only.

10.00: Nappy change, then begin settling routine.

10.10: Say goodnight to everyone and complete settling routine.

10.15: Morning sleep: for ASR babies one hour, 15 minutes; HSR babies one hour, 30 minutes. If she wakes early encourage playtime in her cot until 11.30. Once she's built her sleep up to the time recommended, feed him when she wakes up. If she sleeps for only 40 minutes or less when you first start the program you will need to build up his sleep. If you plan on offering independent play after lunch, set up play stations while she's asleep.

11.30–12.00 p.m.: Lunch: vegetables and protein, and also offer dessert (fruit puree with or without rice cereal, or yoghurt etc.) This should be served as close to 11.30 as she wakes. Follow your meal-time management routine and use your cues if there are problems. After lunch use your wait game and cue.

This is a good independent playtime opportunity if you aren't going to offer it after her mid-afternoon nap.

1.35: Final opportunity for a great one-on-one play with your baby.

1.50: Pack away toys, prepare cot room and wrap for mid-afternoon sleep while she keeps you company and 'helps'.

2.00: Afternoon tea: light snack and milk feed.

2.15: Begin settling routine.

2.25: Final goodnight to everyone in the room and complete settling routine.

2.30–3.00: Mid-afternoon sleep: for ASR babies one hour, 15 minutes; HSR babies one hour 30 minutes. If your baby wakes earlier than suggested, leave her in her cot as long as you can before attending to either resettle (for wakings under 40 minutes) or once she's fully woken, use your waking routine and cues. Allow her to play in her cot until the designated waking time is due or for 20 minutes, whichever is first.

Offer water when she gets up.

This is a good independent playtime opportunity if not offered after lunch.

5.00: Do the final pack away for the day, using your cues – 'Time to pack away, nearly time for dinner'. Pop her into her high chair for quiet time watching her favourite DVD or looking at books on her tray table in the kitchen while you warm her food.

5.20: Dinner: vegetables with or without carbohydrate, followed by playtime in her high chair as you tidy the kitchen, organise the family's dinner (to be eaten after your baby goes to bed) and prepare her bedroom for the evening. Always try to eat a healthy meal at the end of your day to stave off depression and poor sleep, and connect with other members of your family.

6.00: Nudie playtime, using cues for bath.

6.15: Bath time. Watch her the entire time. Use your cues as you get towards 6.30 – 'Nearly time to pack away, nearly time to get out of bath'.

6.30: Take her out of the bath. The household should be calm with the lights dimmed in preparation for her bedtime. Dry and dress her quickly but calmly. As she will be tired you might need to reassure her – 'It's okay, bubba, you're just tired. Nearly time for milk and nigh' nigh's'.

6.35: Breast or bottle feed, ten minutes only. Don't let her doze or even zone out as it will interrupt her settling ability at 7 p.m.

6.45–6.50: Begin settling routine by 6.50 at the latest.

6.55: Final cue – 'Last page, then nigh' nigh's' – and pack away. Enjoy a final cuddle and complete your settling routine.

7.00: Bedtime. If your baby cries, interpret her cries before you go in to resettle using your cues and resettling routines.

14 to 15 month olds, until they need one sleep per day

Assess your child's daily sleep intake carefully by this stage. Some ASR babies need to shift to a single-sleep-a-day routine to suit their overall daily needs (see Routine 1, variation 12 months plus). If she won't have the mid-afternoon bridging nap, she's probably ready to progress to a single sleep a day and this Routine 2 variation is not appropriate. To persist with this routine when she can't achieve a late-afternoon bridging nap will mean she's unsettled by 5 p.m. due to poor sleep and low calorie intake and you may risk causing late-afternoon tears and poor eating as well as possible multiple wakings between 7 and 10 p.m. due to overtiredness. Read my ready to move to a single sleep routine (see pages 262 and 272).

Signs and symptoms that this routine does not suit your baby's need anymore will appear in the form of:

- difficulty settling at mid-morning sleep
- inability to sleep for the rest of the day if she does have the mid-morning sleep
- wakes after 40 minutes and is unable to resettle. If she does settle well for a mid-morning sleep then take a final mid-afternoon bridging nap of 40 minutes
- not taking mid-afternoon bridging nap
- inability to settle at 7 p.m. if she does have the afternoon bridging nap
- waking after only 40 minutes if she does settle at 7 p.m., then need to be resettled for a minimum of 40 minutes.

If you see any of these signs your baby's sleep requirement has transitioned and she needs to move to a more appropriate single-sleep routine.

Depending on your activities for the day, you may opt to provide her independent playtime either after her lunch or after her mid-afternoon sleep. Help her become comfortable with being put down to play, a skill she needs for sleep. If she's not settling down to play independently use your flow of communication and follow through. If you leave the room, use your short-term absence cue, 'I'll be back'. I usually suggest around 45 minutes to an hour of requested independent play followed by a solid 15 minutes of focus play.

Daily routine outline for 14–15 month olds

6.00–6.30 a.m.: Natural waking

7.00: Latest waking. Milk feed

7.20: Breakfast

9.30: Morning tea: fruit and water

10.45: Mid-morning nap: for ASR babies one hour, 45 minutes; for HSR babies two hours, 15 minutes. Once you've built her sleep up to these recommended times, feed her when she wakes up

12.30–1.00 p.m.: Lunch: vegetables and protein, plus dessert. The lunch variation here is to cater for the two different sleep requirement groups waking at either 12.30 p.m. (ASR) or 1 p.m. (HSR)

2.30: Afternoon tea: milk feed in a cup and snack

3.30–3.45: Mid-afternoon bridging nap (20 to 40 minutes only)

4.15: Latest wake-up time: no sleeping beyond this point

5.20: Dinner: vegetables with or without carbohydrates

6.30: Milk feed

7.00: Bedtime for 11 to 12 hours

Daily routine in detail

6.00–6.30 a.m.: Natural waking. Manage any wakings before 5.30 a.m. with crying interpretation and support to build her sleep. If she's not awake by 6.30 on the first ten days of the routine, use your waking routine and offer playtime in cot for 15 to 20 minutes. Before getting her up pack away and use your wait game and cue.

7.00: Latest waking time. Breast or bottle feed but don't allow baby to snooze. Change her nappy, then offer free playtime.

7.10: Prepare her breakfast and use pre-emptive language – 'Nearly time for breakfast', 'Nearly time to sit down and wait for Mummy, yummy apple and oatmeal'.

7.20: Baby's breakfast. Use your meal-time routine and manage her behaviour if she's difficult to feed. After breakfast, dress her for the day, then offer free playtime. She may want to 'help' you but allow her to safely venture off once she's mobile. This might be the time you need to drop off older children to preschools or schools. If you're in the car don't let her fall asleep as she needs to stay awake until the morning sleep at 10.45 a.m. Prepare her room for the morning sleep and use your flow of communication – 'Nearly time for stories, nearly time for nigh' nigh's'.

9.30: Morning tea: fruit and water only.

10.30: Nappy change, then begin settling routine.

10.40: Say goodnight to everyone and complete settling routine.

10.45: Morning sleep begins: for ASR babies one hour, 45 minutes; for HSR babies two hours, 15 minutes. If she wakes early encourage playtime in the cot until 12.30. Once you've built up her sleep to the time recommended, feed her when she wakes up. If she sleeps for only 40 minutes or less when you first start your program you will need to build up her sleep. While she's asleep, set up play stations if you plan on offering her independent play after lunch.

12.30–1.00 p.m.: Lunch: vegetables and protein every day, and offer her a dessert (fruit puree with or without rice cereal, or yoghurt etc.). This should be served as close to 12.30 as she wakes. Follow your meal-time management routine and use your cues if there are problems. After lunch use your wait game and cue.

This is a good independent playtime opportunity if you aren't going to offer it after her mid-afternoon nap.

2.30: Afternoon tea: light snack and milk feed.

3.15–3.30: Begin settling routine. Depending on how long and how late she slept for her mid-morning sleep, adjust this sleep accordingly. For example: if your ASR/HSR baby slept from 10.45 a.m. to 12.30 p.m. she will be ready for a sleep again around 3.30 to 3.45 p.m. and may sleep for up to 40 minutes (if it doesn't detract from her capacity to settle at 7 p.m.). If her mid-morning sleep was longer and went later she'll need a bridging nap of only 20 minutes closer to 3.50 p.m.

Offer this bridging nap in the pram where possible.

4.15: Latest wake-up time – no sleep beyond this point.

This is a good independent playtime opportunity if you didn't offer it earlier. Don't expect her to cope with independent playtime here if she's been unable to achieve her mid-afternoon bridging nap. Reassess her sleep requirement if required and shift to Routine 1 variation 12 months.

5.00: Use this time to do your final pack away for the day, using your cues – 'Time to pack away, nearly time for dinner'. Pop her into her high chair for quiet time in the kitchen while you warm food. This may involve watching her favourite DVD or looking at books on her tray table.

5.20: Dinner: vegetables with or without carbohydrates, then playtime in high chair as you tidy kitchen, organise the family's dinner (have this after she goes to bed) and prepare her bedroom for the evening. Always try to eat a healthy meal at the end of the day to stave off depression and poor sleep, and connect with other family members.

6.00: Nudie playtime, using cues for bath.

6.15: Bath time. Watch her throughout her bathtime. Use your cues as you get towards 6.30 – 'Nearly time to pack away, nearly time to get out of bath'.

6.30: Take her out of the bath. The household should start to calm down. Dim the lights in preparation for her bedtime. Dry and dress her quickly but calmly. As she will be tired you might need to reassure her – 'It's okay, bubba, you're just tired. Nearly time for milk and nigh' nigh's'.

6.35: Breast or bottle feed, ten minutes only. Don't let her doze or even zone out at this time as it will interrupt her settling ability at 7 p.m.

6.45–6.50: Begin settling routine. This must start at 6.50 at the latest.

6.55: Final cue – 'Last page, then nigh' nigh's' – and pack away. Enjoy a last cuddle and complete your settling routine.

7.00: Bedtime. If your baby cries interpret the cries before you go in to resettle. Use your cues and resettling routines.

16 months until the day sleep is no longer needed

This is similar to Routine 1 for this age group. At this age, regardless of her sleep requirement, she's usually down to one sleep a day, with one milk feed in the evening. Most HSR babies will need to transition to this one sleep per day.

Daily routine outline

6.00–6.30 a.m.: Natural waking

7.00: Latest waking, Milk feed

7.20: Breakfast

9.30: Morning tea: fruit and water

11.20: Lunch: vegetables and protein, plus dessert

12.00 p.m.: Midday sleep

2.30: Afternoon tea: milk feed and snack

5.20: Dinner: vegetables with or without carbohydrates

6.30: Milk feed

7.00: Bedtime for 11 to 12 hours

Daily routine in detail

6.00–6.30 a.m.: Natural waking. Any wakings before 5.30 a.m. should be managed with crying interpretation and support. Waking routine and playtime in cot for 15 to 20 minutes. Throughout the day use your wait game and cues.

6.30–7.00: Breast, bottle or cup feed. Don't allow her to snooze. By around 18 months most babies are ready to start having milk in a cup after breakfast, but only if the early feed is interfering with her ability to eat breakfast.

If her breakfast isn't being affected by a first feed of the day, carry on. Her solid food diet has become her main source of nutrition and calories now so maintain her ability to eat breakfast. She'll be consuming more milk during her solid breakfast, and this will start to take the place of the morning feed. Change nappy, then free playtime.

7.15: Prepare breakfast. Use pre-emptive and forewarning language, 'Nearly time for breakfast', 'Nearly time to sit down and wait for Mummy, yummy apple and oatmeal'.

7.20: Baby's breakfast. If she's difficult to feed use meal-time routine. See meal suggestion variation on page 300 for more details.

7.50: Dress her and let her have free playtime. She'll usually want to help you but allow her to safely venture off if she wishes.

9.00–10.00: Quiet time in the high chair with favourite DVD or books.

9.30: Morning tea. Fruit and water only. See variation on page 300 for more details.

9.45: Independent playtime at play stations. This is a baby's most active, energy-burning session, so avoid the car or pram at this time if possible. This is also the time to help her feel comfortable with being put down to play independently, a skill she needs for sleep. It's also the best opportunity for you to do housework and/or cooking (try to do the whole day's cooking now to get it out of the way). The busier you are the happier she'll be to play independently. If she's not settling down to play remember your flow of communication and follow through. If you leave the room, use your short-term absence cue 'I'll be back'.

10.30: Be prepared, this is a typical ten-minute tired window for babies. It passes within ten minutes but in the early five to ten days of the new routine if your baby is getting tired and showing it, a play outside or a little cuddle time (not the kind that might make her more tired) while you play with his favourite toy for a few minutes will help. But put her down again once she calms down.

10.45: Focus one-on-one play for 15 minutes. Give her your undivided attention and don't answer the phones. Remember your cues, 'Nearly time to pack away'.

11.00: Pack away toys completely, prepare cot room for lunch sleep while she keeps you company and 'helps'. Allow ten minutes quiet time watching you do your final lunch preparations. Use your cues 'Nearly time for lunch, yummy chicken and vegetables'.

11.20: Lunch of vegetables with a protein, and offer a dessert (pureed or chopped fruit, yoghurt, custard, etc.). Follow your meal-time routine when feeding her and use your cues if there are problems.

11.40: Wait game and cue while you clean up. Change nappy if needed using cues for sleep – 'Nearly time for sleep, let's go find our books'. Begin settling routine.

11.55: Final page and pack away, using sleep cues.

12.00 p.m.: Sleep (one and a half to two and a half hours).

1.30–2.10: Natural waking time. Leave her in the cot as long as you can, allowing her to self-resettle if need be. If she wakes before 1 p.m., use your resettling routine. Once she's had a minimum of one and a half hours sleep and is fully awake, use your waking routine and cues. Latest waking should be by 2.30 p.m. until nights and days are balanced. After ten days start to build her daily sleep intake. Allow her independent play in cot up till 2.30 or for 20 minutes.

Hint: Cook up a large batch of food during sleep time once or twice a week. By 5 p.m., when children are tired and hungry, it's a dreadful time to try to cook.

2.30: Milk plus snack. See meal time suggestions pages 265–271. Snack first, milk after. This milk feed may naturally stop between the age of 12 and 15 months and she will just have the snack, but you can offer milk in a cup if she's interested.

Adventure. Time to enjoy the outdoors in a car or pram. Don't let her nap because five minutes in the car could mean a 40-minute settle window at 7 p.m.

5.00–5.10: Be at home here for the first three weeks of recovery. Use this time to do your final pack away, using cues, 'Time to pack away, nearly time for dinner'.

5.10: Allow ten minutes quiet time while you warm dinner – DVD or books in high chair or on the couch.

5.20: Dinner then playtime in high chair as you prepare her bedroom, tidy the kitchen and organise your own evening meal. Always try to eat a healthy meal to stave off depression and poor sleep, and connect with other members of your family.

6.00: Nudie playtime, using cues for bath.

6.10: Bath time. You need to watch her for the entire bath. Remember your cues as you get towards 6.30, 'Time to pack away, nearly time to get out of bath'.

6.30: Get her out of bath. Household should start to calm down and lights should be dimmed in preparation for her bedtime. Dry and dress her quickly but calmly. As she will be tired you might need to reassure her – 'It's okay, bubba, you're just tired. Nearly time for milk and nigh' nigh's.'

6.35: Breast or bottle feed for ten minutes only. Don't let her doze as it will interrupt her settling routine.

6.45–6.50: Begin settling routine at 6.50 at the latest.

6.55: Final cue – 'Last page, then nigh' nigh's', and pack away. Enjoy a final cuddle and complete settling routine.

7.00: Bed. If she cries assess the situation and interpret her cries before you go in to resettle using your cues and resettling routines.

Variations for 12 to 24 month olds

Breakfast: Rice, barley, Oat/Weet-Bix, oats, semolina, baby muesli cereal and stewed or mashed fruit, or toast fingers.

Morning tea: Fruit-and-water-only snack. No other food should be offered here.

Lunch: Vegetables, pasta, rice, couscous, meat plus dessert.

Lunch sleep: This sleep is as per ten to 12 month olds.

Afternoon tea: Between the 12th and 15th month your baby may still enjoy this breastfeed, but it's no longer a primary dietary need as solids form most of her daily calorie intake. It won't impact on her sleep or happiness if she chooses to take it or not. Offer the breast/bottle milk feed and a cuddle, but don't force it. If she doesn't have this feed she'll need to have a solid snack that's more than just fruit for afternoon tea to compensate – it's a long time between her lunch at 11.20 a.m. and her dinner at 5.20 p.m. Include yoghurt or finger foods like a Cruskit with avocado, cream cheese or ricotta, which she can eat while you're out in the afternoon, but it must be eaten in the afternoon-tea window. If the milk feed makes it hard for her to eat some solids at afternoon tea, it's vital she have solids before milk is offered. She won't be sustained by milk alone between lunch and dinner. This is about balance, so ensure she has a good snack to get her through. Don't feed her outside the meal-time windows on the recovery plan because food and sleep intake are closely linked and these plans are designed to ensure sleep is achieved as easily as possible.

Dinner: Vegetables, pasta, rice, couscous – this meal is similar to lunch though it does not include meat.

Routine 2 wisdom

- Never start before reading the philosophy behind this sleep repair program.
- Don't start your new daily routine without implementing your new settling, resettling and waking routines (see Chapter 15), and following the interpretation and assistance for crying in chapters 16 and 17.

- Regardless of her sleep lengths, when you start your new routine it can take up to a week of consistent timing for the cyclic effect to start working. Doing something for one or two days only will not achieve your results.
- When you start your new routine, don't keep changing your times based on your baby's wake-up times each sleep, or you won't achieve results. The only way to get results is to choose your sleep and meal-time windows' plan prior to starting your program, then maintain those windows regardless of earlier-than-scheduled wakings. You *can* keep her awake. Work *through* and *past* the old patterns of catnapping and tiredness, and it will pay off for everyone.

The effect of today's sleep on your baby's routine (a vital read)

The time you put a baby down for a sleep, allow her to sleep till and the length of the sleep you allow affects not only the sleep she takes today, but the amount of sleep she can take both tomorrow and during other linked sleeps.

Consider these scenarios:

- The mid-morning sleep affects the following morning's 6 and 7 a.m. waking time, and the length of time she'll be able to sleep during the afternoon sleep:
  - Too early a mid-morning sleep can cause early 6 to 7 a.m. waking times the following morning.
  - Too long a mid-morning sleep can cause a shorter mid-afternoon sleep.
- The mid-afternoon sleep affects her afternoon-bridge sleep or her 7 p.m. settle time that day, and the length of her mid-morning sleep the following day:
  - Too long a mid-afternoon sleep can lead to poor mid-morning sleep the following day because a longer sleep is often offered to compensate for a poor mid-morning sleep, thus allowing the body to sustain a shorter morning sleep in anticipation of a longer mid-afternoon sleep. By waking her after her balanced, minimum sleep-requirement suggestion, despite her early waking from her mid-morning sleep you create a demand in her body to sleep longer during the following mid-morning sleep to cope with the demand of the *shorter* mid-afternoon sleep.

  - Too long a mid-afternoon sleep can also impact on a six- to seven month olds' ability to take her afternoon bridge. The roll-on effect is an overtired baby at 7 p.m. who may settle quickly but wakes frequently between 7 and 10 p.m. Alternatively, for a baby who's not taking an afternoon bridge, a very long afternoon sleep may impact on a baby's ability to settle at 7 p.m. because she's not tired enough.
- The late afternoon bridging nap for babies six months of age has a series of side effects when used incorrectly:
  - If the late afternoon bridge is offered beyond its true need it can create significant difficulties settling her at 7 p.m. It can also create a shorter mid-afternoon sleep the following day because it is often offered to compensate for a poor mid-afternoon sleep, thus allowing the body to be able to sustain a shorter mid-afternoon sleep the following day in anticipation of a late-afternoon bridging nap. By limiting the length of sleep offered or keeping her awake until her true sleep time (7 p.m.), despite her early wakings in the mid-afternoon sleep, you create a demand in the body to sleep longer the following mid-afternoon to cope with the demand of the longer afternoon.

Increasing your baby's sleep requirement

You start with a basic amount of sleep when repairing significant sleep issues for a couple of reasons. Firstly, it's better to have a slightly tired baby who's ready to go straight to sleep and sleep for a decent amount of time at each sleep than one who may cry because of sleep caused by miscalculations. Secondly, you can't be certain if you're being fair to ask the highest amount of sleep of your baby for her sleep requirement group. So start with a reasonable and balanced amount of sleep while she starts learning how to sleep peacefully and independently. This means you're freeing her of the burden of constant disruption to her sleep from waking up crying for your help all the time. Once you've established your baby's minimum daily sleep requirement, and she's taking all three main sleep windows well, it will be time, if appropriate, to build her sleep up so she's taking more.

HSR: A high sleep requirement baby will need to sleep 7 p.m. to 6 or 7 a.m. at night and take two one–two hour day sleeps. However just because you have a high-sleep-requirement baby, it doesn't necessarily mean she'll have two × two-hour day sleeps and a 12-hour night. This

16-hour sleep requirement is tipping the highest end of the scale for this group, and while some can take it easily, others will take on a more moderate, but equally effective, version of the routine.

ASR: An average sleep requirement baby will need to sleep from 7 p.m. to 6 or 7 a.m. at night and take two one a half hour day sleeps. However, just because you have an average-sleep-requirement baby, it doesn't necessarily mean she'll have two × one hour, 30 minute day sleeps and a 12 hour night. This 15-hour sleep requirement is tipping the highest end of the scale for this group, and while some can take it easily, others will be on a more moderate, but equally effective, version of the routine.

For both groups you won't need to build their sleep up if they wake naturally on one or two of their three main sleep windows, as this would indicate you've reached their sleep need, and to offer more would only steal from other sleeps.

If your baby continues to need waking from every sleep after five days of sleep on the new routine, it's time to build up her sleep intake using a simple three-step process. Do this slowly, and wait to see if the increase (through adding more sleep at one waking window at a time) impacts on your baby anywhere else.

- Step 1. You start with the 6.30 a.m. window, offering another 15 minutes sleep to 6.45 a.m. for three days running. If you see no effect on the length of sleep she's able to take during her mid-morning sleep, that adjustment can stay and you can move on to your next window. If it does impact, don't offer the additional 15 minutes, and don't attempt to build her sleep at this window.
- Step 2. You then move to your mid-morning sleep, offering another 15 minutes to the *end* of this sleep for three days running. If it doesn't affect the length of sleep she's able to take during her mid-afternoon sleep, or on the time she starts to wake at 6.30/6.45 a.m., that adjustment can stay and you can move on to your next window. If it does have an impact, remove the additional 15 minutes offered and don't attempt to build her sleep at this window.
- Step 3. You then move to your mid-afternoon sleep, offering 15 minutes to the *end* of this sleep for three days running. If you see no effect on the length of sleep she takes during her mid-morning sleep, or on the late-afternoon bridging nap for six month olds, that adjustment can stay and you can move on to your next window. If it does have an impact, remove the additional 15 minutes offered, and don't attempt to build her sleep at this window.

Don't offer any more sleep for the later afternoon bridge for six month olds.

You have now successfully built her sleep up over a nine-day process. If your baby continues to need to be woken after every sleep on this new routine, then it's time to build her sleep up again using the same simple three-step process. Once you've reached your recommended (HSR) two × two-hourly day sleeps, and your 12-hour night or (ASR) two × one hour, 30 minute day sleeps, and your 12-hour night, hold and maintain this sleep for three weeks. Ensure she's eating enough as excessive sleep can indicate a slightly lower calorie diet. If she's eating and sleeping well, then you're welcome to repeat the same three-step growth process again until she starts to wake naturally on one or more of her three main sleeps.

How to know when your child is ready to move to one sleep a day

A HSR baby may need to transition to one sleep from the 14th to 18th month onwards. An ASR baby may need to transition to one sleep from the 12th to 15th month onwards. Clear signs of this occur after the 12th month when she's only sleeping effectively on one of her two day sleeps. This means while one sleep remains longer, the second is reduced to a catnap of 40 minutes or less. This can happen in either order through the day. It's also evidence that she's getting ready for one sleep a day when her two main day sleep times are interfering with the 6 to 7 a.m. waking time each morning and her 7 p.m. settling time each night, and are constantly needing to be reduced in order to maintain her night sleep pattern.

A final sneaky sign she may be ready to drop down to one sleep, and this can be difficult to spot without a professional's guidance, is when you start to see prolonged wakings through the night. These prolonged wakings often happen between 11.30 p.m. and 4.30 a.m. and while a baby may not need attending to, she may chat for one to two hours before she's able to go back to sleep. If she's getting iron in her diet in the form of meat about once a day as recommended, this is an indication that she's achieving too much *accumulated* daytime sleep and you either need to drop down both sleeps to her minimum sleep-requirement recommendation until the night sleep is restored, or move on to a 'single sleep a day' program.

While some parents are happy to maintain the two sleeps in this slightly unpredictable or shorter format because their baby is still happy and coping, others will see it as detracting from their baby's happy days and peaceful nights and will be motivated to transition on to the single-sleep program. This is simple. Just go to PRM Routine 1 and follow the variations for a baby 12 months old plus to be on a balanced single-sleep routine until day sleep ends.

You don't need to transition gradually, just shift her over the next morning starting at 6.30 a.m., and follow my guidelines precisely. Stay busy in the morning for the first three days with no long pram or car rides. She may be a little tired for two to three days, but on a slow progression plan she'll be tired for three weeks while you try to juggle the changes without impacting other sleeps of the day.

14

Role playing for better sleep routines

One of my most successful tools is my role-play program. Children learn as much through observing others as they do through exploring. They show more interest in participating in and mastering an observed activity than in exploring a brightly coloured toy they haven't observed someone else playing with. For this reason, your child will love your TV remote, your mobile or home phone, your handbag, your shoes, cooking pots and wooden spoons, the computer, your car keys, getting mail from the letterbox, watering the garden, opening and closing the fridge and cupboards, and squeezing the tubes of cream you use when changing his nappy.

The reason a baby finds the box his birthday present came in more interesting than the present is because you appeared to play with the box for ten minutes before you pulled the present out of it and handed it straight to him without playing with it. It's the activity of opening the box you demonstrated to your child so this is what he wants to participate in, not the object you didn't play with. Why? Because you're the one he instinctively needs to learn everything from in his first two years of life: he will literally imitate and try to master everything he sees you do.

My role-play program uses this learning tool to help babies and toddlers learn about their new settling and resettling conditions at sleep time. It also means he'll copy the way you speak to and treat others, your moods, your table manners and eating habits, your attitude to life, work, education, sharing and helping.

Role play has long been recognised by hospitals as an effective tool to help young children learn about and be prepared for painful and frightening but essential medical intervention in order to cause as little trauma to the child as possible. By incorporating role playing when teaching a baby or toddler a new routine at sleep time, I've been able to achieve the quickest and most successful transitions into independent sleep with tremendous results in the reduction of tears in all cases where the emotional foundations of the house are firmly grounded and stable.

Role-play strategies

This is essential for everyone before starting any new routine. There are two forms of role play. One is visual and this is what I mostly use with children under two. The complementary form with this age group is verbal role play, which enables you to reinforce and replay a previously conducted visual role play with a child while in the car, or while feeding him, etc. This means your baby has the chance to run through the process of events indirectly multiple times before being exposed to the experience directly. This gives him the opportunity to become familiar with the predictability of the event, start to trust your consistency within that event, and learn to cope with the emotions that may arise in this situation by looking to you for your reaction and confidence in the same situation.

Role play involves showing your child what's going to happen during a new event, such as using a teddy bear or doll to act out the entire scenario of his new settling process–word for word, action for action. You should treat the teddy bear with the same affection, love and respect you'll display to him when you start the new routine with him. Your child needs to have seen it from where you stand, and seen your intentions with this new management technique, including how you'll respond to his reaction, to accept the new routine with less confusion and stress.

This role play of your new settling routine and resettling routine (see Chapter 15) needs to be done every time someone new, such as a babysitter, is introduced to the routine, particularly when you have a child who's found sleep or any other event stressful in the past. Role playing is a key strategy in helping him quickly adjust to new conditions that would normally be stressful the first time. This is because it enables us to indirectly show our expectations of his behaviour and ensures we show ourselves to be predictable for our children, which fosters trust.

Role play also helps your child know where you're going to be once you leave his room. To him, based on the role play, it will appear you'll be waiting just outside his door should he need you. While not accurate, this is a misconception you can safely encourage because it's comforting for him. Role playing enables a child to experience the new routine while he is being held by you.

How to role play

Where possible, two adults should be present for role-play scenarios – one to hold the child and one to do the role playing with teddy. Both should remain positive, identical with actions and tones, and act as if they love teddy like they do their child, all the while giving off an air of happiness, and doing something good with teddy. This attitude should be retained, no matter how the child reacts the first few times. This is how to replace a negative association around an event with a positive association. Remember, babies learn how to react to the world around them through role play and their parents' attitude to the world around them.

However you would like your child to feel about the routine, you must first role play emotionally to him. For a settling routine you can create a positive association around his room, going to bed, you leaving the room, by simply role playing with teddy a confident and happy example as often as it takes for him to understand the game. As you do each role play, gradually pull the door towards being closed until the door is completely closed by the end of the resettle attempts with teddy, all within the same role play. By the third day of role playing, the door will be closed from the very start of the routine as your child will have had the opportunity to get used to, and become comfortable with, those conditions.

The person doing role play with teddy needs to focus on teddy, and not change the pace, tone or sequence of events, regardless of the child's reaction to the new settling routine you are demonstrating. They shouldn't keep interacting with, or focusing their attention on, the child in order to avoid confusing him about who's being put to bed. This is about the teddy going to bed, so treat the teddy as though it's your baby.

If your baby finds sleep or any other daily routine very difficult, this strategy needs to be used from six months of age. The person holding the baby needs to be aware of the role they're playing through the role play. They need to:

- hold the child in a comfortable position before entering the room and hold them reassuringly and comfortably but not too tightly

- remain entirely focused on the person doing the role play and on the teddy
- not talk to or be distracted by the baby's best tricks or verbal attention-seeking games as this might be where he's seeing what he can do to change the line of communication from being parent-directed to child-directed
- not fix it for them: if your child cries, keep holding him without squeezing, patting, rocking, shushing or talking him through it. Allow him to experience the feelings and learn he's safe and doesn't need a circus act to fix it, or you risk teaching him he'll need that when it's his turn to go to bed.

You need to provide the same conditions your child will experience at a settling routine, and for the settling routine only. This helps him get used to that unique set of conditions and experience the emotions around it while you're holding him. *He* has to find a way to calm himself down without your help, though in your arms. Allow him to witness, experience and work through events independently.

When their attention is elsewhere

If he's fighting to be put down on the floor or is moving too much in your arms while you're trying to put him in his cot, turn him to face the front and hold him firmly with his back on your tummy. If he reaches forward and tries to climb in, kick off, bite or shake the cot, step back so he can't reach the cot. If he's looking around, don't try to turn around to make him look where you want him to. Just stand still and allow him to take in the environment: walls, ceilings, curtains, darkness, door closed, you, his cot, his level of sight, everything. He'll be able to hear so that's important, and after a time the repetitious actions of the person role playing will draw his interest and attention anyway.

Stay confident, calm and interested in the role play and try not to talk at all. If he's enjoying the role play and trying to share that with you, smile and agree and point, but be careful this isn't one of his tricks to change the attention to him and his line of communication. You're equipping him with the conditions to expect at settling time which doesn't include a 'making Mummy or Daddy laugh' game because that involves a child-governed line of communication which shouldn't be used at sleep time. The idea of directing him back to the settling routine role play should be enough if you have a baby who has found going to bed challenging. If necessary, hold him firmly in the sitting position if he's challenging you.

What to expect and how to help your child through role play

It's normal to see some of the following reactions from your baby during role play:

- He laughs at your repetitious behaviour and communication: perfect, enjoy the routine with him but don't deviate from the routine and make sure you complete the role play before cuddling and kissing him.
- He tries to pat the cot: a lovely response, allow him to lean forward and pat the cot, but watch he doesn't try to climb in, or eat the bars.
- He attempts to climb in the cot with teddy: natural, but not allowed. This is where you're governing all lines of communication, and he needs to observe, not tell you what he wants to do at sleep time. Wanting to get in is a great start, but he's not ready yet and needs to know the whole process.
- He pats you while you pat the teddy: another lovely response you can allow. Don't stop him, or talk to him, just allow it to happen. Don't stop to look at him, or laugh, or change or lose focus on the flow of the settling routine. Don't ask him to do it either. If it isn't spontaneous, stay busy role playing.
- He lean towards the door with you to hear if teddy is crying: a great indication he's enjoying and participating in the role play. Carry on with the role play, looking interested in what you're doing.
- He reaches for the door handle to attend to a crying teddy: this is fine if it's not distracting. Don't go into the room if he tells you to, however, because that's a child-governed line in a settling routine that should be parent directed. Carry on, open the door when you're ready and it fits into the role play. With a toddler, perhaps remove his hand from the door before you plan to open it and say, 'Mummy do it!' (Not necessary for an under-12 month old.)
- He pretends to cry for the teddy when you ask if teddy is crying: this is fine if you plan on teddy crying and role play attending to him. However, if you've said, 'No crying from teddy', and your child still cries and reaches for the handle, insisting on you going in, don't change the line of communication to oblige his demands because it suggests to him that he governs this time and will cause tears when you try to put him to bed.
- He claps with you if teddy doesn't cry: excellent, be really excited and clap and cheer, and kiss and cuddle your baby. Praise is always encouraged. We want him to feel happy about this whole new routine.

- He shushes like you if teddy doesn't cry: lovely! Acknowledge it with something like, 'Yes, shhhhh, teddy has gone nigh' nigh's'. If you're still role playing attending to a crying teddy, don't let him tell you not to attend. Retain your parent-governed line of communication, even if he gets cross with you.
- He role plays independently without prompting: don't disturb him unless he needs help reaching teddy, or putting teddy in the cot. A good play-station idea is to set up a sleep-time-style area at home. Provide a cot (can be as simple as a box with a pillow in it) and include any environmental things you use in role play. Briefly role play his normal settling routine with teddy and allow him to role play it. It's empowering for him to govern the entire scenario himself and it's fine that you're not assuming the line of communication here.
- He sings or does the actions to 'Twinkle Twinkle Little Star' while you sing to teddy: lovely and fine to allow to occur naturally but don't respond to it during the role play. Perhaps do it together at another time of the day. Many toddlers do the actions to 'Twinkle Twinkle Little Star' as I put them down for the first time, even when they're used to hating their bed. It doesn't change the flow of my routine for settling them though.
- He tries to touch and see your face in the dark: sweet, he's trying to see how close he needs to get to see you but, alas, he begins to realise he can't see at night, no matter how big his eyes are, or how close he gets. Don't react to this, just allow him to work through it. This is the whole purpose of role playing an action as we talk it through. Your baby is learning the normal conditions of sleep while he has the security of you holding him and, since he can see you're not concerned, he can feel safe during this process.

It is normal to see the following poor reactions during role play

Poor reactions to role playing are harder for some people to handle than others, and they may be tempted to stop role playing. This isn't the right thing to do. Assess the situation and remember your motivation is to help teach your baby a better way to do something that will lead to a contented, soundly sleeping and well-fed child. There's always a transition period that feels unfamiliar to the child and this will naturally be met with temporary resistance until it becomes familiar. If you need further encouragement re-read 'Why: your movitivation for wanting balanced communication' (see pages 37–38) and work through your fears and emotions to find a better way to cope.

Following are some common poor reactions and solutions to help him:

- He doesn't want teddy to sit on your lap while you're reading a book to him: the person holding him should stop him from reaching and taking teddy off your lap. Don't try to calm him because he's learning to accept a parent-governed line of communication, and the first time he's unfamiliar with it and may try to fight it. Proceed with your routine and use enthusiastic tones to distract him. Don't confuse him by letting him cuddle teddy, or you risk teaching him to demand you let him cuddle teddy at any time during the role play, which means he'll be running the settling routine. Don't change the pace, tone or delivery of your routine role play. Quickly start to read the book to teddy in an exciting way and this should draw your baby's attention away.
- He really wants the book: don't let him have the book. Ensure he can see the book but don't try to talk him through it with remarks like 'Look Charlie, here it is' etc. as this rarely stops the demands or tears. Use enthusiastic, effective-reading skills to distract him. Carry on with your routine and allow your partner to manage the sitting or tantrum without your intervention. Don't stop at this point; it doesn't last long, and you'll get quick results.
- He may think you're putting him to bed if you're focused on him. Stick to the routine, use the cues and teddy's name and only look at teddy, asking teddy to co-operate with you. Keep going with your routine to show him you're only planning to put teddy to bed when you read and talk using teddy's name, and you only plan to put him to bed when you read and talk using his name.
- He cries as you put teddy to bed: if he's previously had difficulties settling at sleep times this is a natural way for him to express how he feels about the old conditions of sleep, which is why you're establishing new conditions. Stay confident, and work through the old emotions until you've laid the foundation for new, more positive associations with sleep.
- He wants to be taken out of the room: if you're holding him, stand, hold him, and carry on with the routine so he gets used to this parent-governed line of communication. Going to bed for you shouldn't involve him demanding to be taken out of his room. Carry on with the role play. Continue holding him firmly while watching the person with the teddy.

- He wants to attend to teddy once you leave the room on the first few role play attempts, even after you've told him teddy's stopped crying and you need to leave him to sleep: this is normal when he's experiencing a new routine through role play. But it would be confusing, stressful and compromising of trust if he didn't experience the new routine indirectly first. Carry on with your role play in a loving, reassuring and confident voice. This ensures you maintain the governing line of communication, and he gets the opportunity to learn that he needs to look to you for guidance. Once you've told him teddy isn't crying anymore and has gone to sleep, keep teddy there until you decide it's time to get teddy up. Don't ever get teddy up because he's demanding it.
- He wants to get into the cot and pat teddy: don't let him into the cot with teddy until it's his turn to go to sleep. You're teaching him that you govern sleep times, so don't let him change the routine flow, or take charge of teddy.
- He wants you to open the door: if you've assessed he needs his door shut while he's sleeping it would be dishonest to teach him he can ask to have the door opened at sleep time. He needs an opportunity to get used to this and become comfortable with the conditions of the new routine. Remember, you're learning to cater to his true needs over his short-term demands.
- He tries to open the door to leave the room: ideally he is being held but if you're on your own, he may not be, so this may arise. Simply carry on with the routine if you know he can't reach the handle. If he can reach the handle, pick him up and complete the role play while holding him. Remain confident and reassuring and complete the role play I've outlined.
- He has a tantrum: this can happen if he has very poor associations with his room, going to sleep, or if he isn't used to balanced lines of communication where you govern certain events of the day. Ensure you use your communication correctly through the day so he doesn't feel stressed by you guiding him. Carry on and complete your role play. If he's a tantrum thrower, don't feel alone because many parents are going through the same thing. Try to have help when you're role playing.
- He hits you, the cot, or the person holding him: reposition him so she can't reach the cot, the person role playing, or you. Don't speak; just stay calm and continue the role play. You don't want to teach him to

hit you if he doesn't want to go to bed, or that everything stops when he hits you.

- He wants his teddy back: be careful about the teddy or doll you use for role play. If he already has a significant bond with that teddy it's understandable if he wants to hold it when he's feeling uncertain, so choose a teddy he's not too attached to for role playing.
- He doesn't want to leave teddy to sleep in the room: this is about who is governing the situation, and how he feels about being left in his room. Remember two key things: you're governing the line of communication around all things sleep, and he needs to be reassured it's safe to leave teddy sleeping. Reassure him by responding appropriately to his reaction.
- He tries to go off to play in the room while you role play: if he's being held this isn't a problem, but if you're on your own it can be. Don't confuse him by letting him believe he can go off to play at sleep time, and don't waste any learning opportunities. It may be that he just doesn't know you'd like him to watch you so make sure he joins you, or have someone there to help you.

When role playing is running well

Both of the people involved in the role play need to stay focused, confident and interested in the role play and teddy only. If your child tries to divert your attention or change the focus back to him, your line of communication should remain the same so your child has realistic expectations of his new sleep routine and will happily look to you for guidance when you put him to bed, rather than trying to guide you.

The following reactions may occur during the role play and there is nothing wrong if they do. Your child may:

- watch teddy during story time, and try to make eye contact with teddy up close
- try to talk to teddy
- try to make teddy turn the pages of the book
- randomly kiss or cuddle teddy
- get cross at teddy
- look around the room and not always pay attention to you
- try to get your attention using his best trick, including his funniest antics, and repertoire of verbal attention seeking
- become familiar with the routine and try to lead the role play
- talk or sing endlessly through the entire role play

- go back to the door once the role play is over to see if teddy is awake or crying
- be so cute as he concentrates on listening to you that you may feel the urge to hug and kiss him.

In all these cases, just carry on and complete the role play with minimal interaction with him. Once it's done you can have one-on-one playtime with him.

Acknowledge their honesty

It's not unusual for your child to tell you how he's going to react during his direct settling event through demonstrating his response during role-playing. In a toddler, this may be demonstrated by him being happy for Mummy to settle teddy but furious if Daddy does. This essentially means he's telling you he'll settle for Mummy, but be cross if Daddy puts him to bed. You may be surprised at how clever your baby or toddler is. Try to take on board what he's telling you, and either practise role playing a bit more until he's more comfortable with it (indicating he'll be more comfortable when settled himself), or prepare yourself for a bit of a challenge at settling that day or night. After all, he's already told you he might complain about going to bed while you practised putting teddy down.

Going it alone

Even if you don't have someone who can swing by and help you, it's still very achievable to role play on your own. I often role play with toddlers and six to 12 month olds on my own, and can assure you to rest easy. You can do this!

If your baby is not yet walking, you have two choices, and the one you choose usually depends on your strength and your baby. They are:

1. Carry him throughout the whole role play. It may feel messy, but he gets the message.
2. If your child is stroppy and difficult to carry throughout, you'll need to pop him into a safe seat so he can watch you. Placing him in a baby seat, pram or high chair (if it has wheels so you can move him about as necessary), is probably the best way to manage him and your role play at the same time.

If your baby can walk you have three choices:

1. Carry him during the role play. It might feel messy, but he gets the message.

2. If he walks into the room holding your hand, then you must close the door behind you and let go of his hand and carry on with your role play. If he potters, it doesn't really matter because it's dark anyway, so he only needs to hear you. (Be careful to make the room safe from falling or other injuries if he does enjoy having a potter in the dark.) Each time you plan to leave the room and listen to teddy outside the room hold his hand and keep holding his hand, or pick him up briefly until you're back in his room with him.
3. If he's very stroppy, upset and difficult to carry, pop him into a safe seat so he can watch you. Placing him in a baby seat, pram or high chair (if it has wheels so you can move him about as necessary), is probably the best way to manage him and your role play at the same time.

Role-play routine

It generally takes between four and five role plays for your child to work past his old associations, become familiar with and start to trust the new routine, and learn he's okay and can predict this part of his day. Always make sure the room and environment is ready before you start your role play with a checklist like this:

- The cot is made.
- 'White noise' is on.
- The lights are off in the room, and in all the rooms and the hall near the room.
- The Safe T Sleep is ready if you're using one.
- Towel rolls are prepared, ready for tuck-in.
- The wrap, if you're using one, is laid out nearby.
- The book is ready on the couch (only one book required for role play).
- A clock or watch is available for timing.
- All distractions are turned off and put away.

Exclude any environmental factors not appropriate to your tailored program. For some children it's easier if you include a comfort item (like a dummy, muslin, teddy, dolly, etc.) and if it's appropriate to his needs, keep it. However, if you plan not to provide it to him during his new settling routine, remove it.

Role-play example for swaddled baby six to 12 months old

All language cues and requests I suggest here are fine for a child from around six months of age, so keep working on them. Make sure your language is predictable, clear and routine, as it's your main tool at settling time. Don't rock him to sleep, pat him to sleep, or give him things that will make him go to sleep. This is about empowering him with the tools to do this himself, so he doesn't have a stressful settling or resettling routine, and you can be at your best throughout the day as the stress of sleep time is lifted. Here you're saying to him, 'We're getting you ready to put yourself to sleep; getting the things you need to help yourself go to sleep. We love you, and if you need us, we're right outside. Goodnight.'

Remember your flow of communication. Pre-emptive language is a way of indicating what's about to happen: 'Charlie, we're going to play with our blocks, then it's time to put teddy to nigh' nigh's'. Forewarning language is the final prompt before the event begins: 'Charlie, last one, last [state event], then it's time to put teddy to nigh' nigh's'.

Initiate a parent-governed line of communication: 'Okay, Charlie, up, up.' Your partner now picks him up: 'Time to go get teddy and put her into cot for nigh' nigh's.' (Please don't say bed, as your child sleeps in a cot and doesn't know what a bed is at this stage.)

Go and get teddy together, and have a little moment of love with teddy. Pick teddy up and be really happy to see her, 'Oh, hi teddy, cuddles for Mummy, cuddles for [person carrying baby], cuddles for Charlie. Oh we love teddy, she's so soft.' From this moment on you talk only to teddy. Please always use the same teddy.

Turn teddy to face you and say, 'Okay, teddy, it's nearly time for nigh' nigh's, let's go read our book.' Take teddy into the lounge room, or another room where you plan on reading to your child (preferably not his room) and say, 'Sit down teddy, wait for Mummy.'

Show teddy the book and read to her. As you progress through the book, remember to use your language cues 'Wait for Mummy/Daddy', 'Turn the page', '*Nearly* time for nigh' nigh's', '*Nearly* last page', '*Nearly* time to pack away'. As you read to teddy, you can physically make teddy's paw turn the page, and occasionally (with children ten months plus) make teddy try to turn or pull the book down so you can correct this behaviour and set the new boundary and expectation of behaviour by using the 'Wait for Mummy' cue and action. As you reach the last half of the book, be sure to be clear to teddy that it's nearly time for sleep: 'Nearly time to pack away teddy, nearly time for nigh' nigh's'. At the last page, tell teddy, 'Last page, nearly time to pack away'.

Each time you deliver one of these new lines, make it sound more song-like by using a higher tone, and drawing out the length of the words: 'Tuuuurrrrrn the paaaaaaage'. This will help your child tune into your voice even while you're using a lot of vocabulary through the story. After the last page say 'Time to pack away' and place the book out of view. Once the story is over, stop saying 'nearly' and start saying 'time for' in your cues; for example, '*time* for nigh' nigh's'.

Turn teddy to face you and with a big smile and clear eye contact say, 'It's time for sleep, teddy. Mummy and Daddy love you, nigh' nigh's.' Have a big cuddle with teddy and give her a kiss as you repeat your cues a second time before you stand and start to walk towards the bedroom where you're going to wrap teddy.

As you walk, calmly repeat the cues every now and then until you reach where the wrap is laid out. Turn teddy in your arms so she can see the bed and repeat your cues as you give her a kiss. Point to the wrap and say 'Lie down'. Lie teddy down in the wrap in the right position to minimise any moving you may need to do. Wrap teddy casually, or practise your firm wrap. Occasionally repeat your cues.

Pick teddy up by sliding your correct arm (which will depend on which end her head lies in the cot) under teddy's neck and lift her so she remains in the lying-down position in your arms. Cover teddy's eyes with your cheek or by tucking her face into your neck as you walk from the wrapping room into the cot room. Close the door.

Walk to the side of the cot. If it's very dark, use your hand to find the position you need to be in to lie teddy into the cot in just the right position (though don't lie her down yet) and plant your feet firmly. You need to get comfortable, and slow everything down. Your voice and the rate and tone you speak with can put your baby to sleep so use it. Rock from side to side very slowly only moving your torso, or moving from the waist up, keeping your feet in the same position. Sing 'Twinkle Twinkle Little Star' in a soft, reassuring lilt and in a slow, sleep-inducing way, but loud enough to be heard. Sing the song twice, then stop swaying and singing.

Kiss teddy on the cheek or forehead (choose which one and stick to it). Say your cues in a gentle, reassuring way without even a slight hint of concern. If you smile, it will slightly lift your inflection and make you sound even more comforting as you say 'Time for sleep. Mummy and Daddy love you, nigh' nigh'. Lie down.'

Say 'Lie down' before you begin to lie teddy down. Once teddy is in the right position, pull the extra piece of free wrap material on the top left to ensure the wrap is still firm. Place teddy so she is higher up the bed, then place her lower legs under the firm sheets before you slide her down into the tucked-in bedding.

Do up the Safe T Sleep firmly. Tuck bedding in. If you're using a leg wrap only and your 12 month old has a dummy you could encourage (like a puppet) teddy to reach for her dummy and say 'Get your dummy'. Hand teddy her comfort item, saying 'Take your muslin/dolly/sooky/teddy/cuddly'. Manipulate teddy's free arm, or the preferred arm, by lifting it as though she is taking the dummy or place the comfort object parallel to her side, and drape it over her shoulder. This way is the way you would do it for your baby so he can get it himself.

Pull or attach a blocking cloth, such as a muslin wrap, to the side of the cot. Bend over behind the blocking cloth, side-on to the cot and look at your feet. Reach over the top of the cot side and into the cot and pat teddy rhythmically, saying 'Sh sh sh sh, time for sleep. Sh sh sh sh, Mummy and Daddy love you. Sh sh sh sh, time for sleep. Sh sh sh sh, Mummy and Daddy love you. Sh sh sh sh, nigh', nigh'.'

On the last word of your last cue take your hand away, stand and turn to your baby. Say 'C'mon, Charlie, let's go!' and head for the door. Once outside the room, say 'Close the door' and close it making sure it clicks (because you're learning to be honest with your child about leaving his room). Once outside, make clear eye contact with your baby who should still be in your partner's arms and say 'Is teddy crying?' Head towards the door, turn and cover your mouth and make a crying sound. Say 'Oh dear, teddy is crying. Let's go and see her.'

Walk back in the room with your partner and baby following and close the door behind you. Walk to the side of the cot and bend over behind the blocking cloth, side on to the cot and look at your feet to ensure you keep your head out of view. Reach over the top of the cot side and into the cot and pat teddy rhythmically, saying, 'Sh sh sh sh, time for sleep, sh sh sh sh, Mummy and Daddy love you. Sh sh sh sh, time for sleep. Sh sh sh sh, Mummy and Daddy love you, sh sh sh sh, nigh' nigh'.'

Again, on the last word of your last cue take your hand away, stand and turn to your baby, 'C'mon, Charlie, let's go!' and head for the door. Once outside the room, say 'Close the door', and close it, making sure it clicks. Do the 'Is teddy crying?' line. Leaning towards the door, turn and cover your mouth and make a crying sound: 'Oh dear, teddy is crying, let's go and see her'.

You will need to repeat attendances to teddy a few times but, after your final attendance, when you say 'Is teddy crying?' lean in to listen and allow a prolonged silence, even if your baby pretends to cry in the appropriate gap. Repeat the question with a little bit of a gasp and a look of surprise, 'Listen, is teddy crying?'

Allow for another pause of around ten seconds. Look happy and excited, say 'Listen, no crying', and pause again. Repeat one last time,

'No crying! Teddy's gone nigh' nigh's, yeah!' and clap and cheer. Raise your finger to your mouth and say 'Ssshhhhhh, teddy has gone nigh' nigh's. C'mon, let's go.' Carry on with your day.

For babies not swaddled, six to 12 months plus

This routine is as outlined above up until just before you read the book. Turn teddy to face you and say, 'Okay, teddy, it's nearly time for nigh' nigh's. Let's put on our sleeping bag and go read our book.' Put teddy in her sleeping bag and do up the zipper. Take teddy into the room where you plan to read to your child and say, 'Sit down teddy, wait for Mummy.' Continue on with above routine.

For toddler, 12 months plus

Place teddy in her sleeping bag prior to reading. Once teddy is in the cot and you've said, 'Lie down', pretend teddy is trying to stand up, saying, 'No, lie down, teddy.' Repeat this several times if you're expecting to have this battle with your child. When teddy is lying say, 'Good listening, teddy, good lying still.' If your child has a dummy, say 'Get your dummy' to teddy, and continue with routine as above.

Working through fear or discomfort with role play

The new sleep routine is only one of a number of skills your child will learn more quickly and less stressfully if shown through role play. Another positive application for role playing is to help a child work through a fear. This could be done to help a child instil a more positive attitude to being in an environment he's uncomfortable with or fearful of, such as a dark room. A visual role play of peek-a-boo with teddy in a dark room right from the time your child is 12 months old would be as follows:

'Mummy and Mitchell play "Where's teddy?" Mummy close the door,' and gesture closing the door.

Say, 'Mummy said, "Where's teddy?"' using a light and airy voice, as your child will be interested in a happy conversation which he might recognise. At the stage he may become still, stare off into the distance, turn to look towards the bedroom, point, or express his dislike for the feelings associated with the role play by crying. If he remains concerned throughout a verbal role play, do as much physical role playing as you can, on and off, throughout the day. Continue with the verbal role play. This is a good opportunity to expose him to the emotions of the event indirectly and to instil a new association through your happy tones and fun attitude about the peek-a-boo game you're talking through.

Continue verbally through the events of your role play by repeating the cues you used during the physical role play, including your language cues and carefree attitude about the dark, 'Oh, it's dark now, Mummy can't see teddy, where's teddy?' Find opportunities to clap or say hurray about the dark and not seeing teddy.

Complete the game with a big hurray and talk through your cuddle with teddy before moving on to another conversation.

Indirect verbal role playing

Once you've physically role played a particular sequence of events a few times it becomes so predictable to your child that you're now able to verbally role play through it. This gives you a unique chance to work through your child's anxieties without it consuming too much of your day. As you drive in the car, or go for a walk in the pram, or perhaps after dinner while he's having a little play in his high chair, talk though your role play in the same sequence as your usual visual role play. Your child will listen, look at you, or stare off into the distance as they recall the visual role-play event. Regardless of whether he gets upset at the concept, remain confident and complete the event. If he's become so relaxed about the role play and just continues to play and appears undisturbed, there's no need to repeat your verbal role play as he's indicated he's comfortable with this event. For those who struggle even with verbal role play, you'll need to persist until your baby becomes relaxed.

15

Settling, resettling and waking routines

One of the best sleep inducers you have is your ability to use your voice to soothe, comfort and reassure your child. For the purpose of putting your baby to sleep, the key to your success is understanding the effect you're having on her and how that impacts on the way she feels about going to sleep in her cot.

It's not always possible to avoid tears at bedtime. Some babies cry for 30 seconds, some for three minutes, while others have a big cry and need reassurance. Babies cry because that's what they've been taught to do. If they don't know how to self-settle and have been taught to cry to get help when they feel tired, on the first day or two of teaching them how to sleep it sometimes takes a while for them to understand and accept any change to the conditions of going to sleep. It's not easy for a child who's never been able to self-settle to *avoid* expressing herself when exposed to a new situation. It's normal and healthy for a child experiencing something new to feel uncomfortable with the unfamiliarity of the event. It's her way of saying, 'I'm not sure about this, I don't feel comfortable with it. Am I okay, Mummy/Daddy?' When you answer this question, consider the following:

- What will you tell her about the situation?
- What will your body language tell her?

- What will your facial expression tell her?
- What will your tone tell her?

Be honest and be fair

It's not fair or in the best interests of your child to let her think she's in a situation that isn't safe, perfectly healthy and normal. Think about how you move, look and sound and react when communicating with her. When you deliver visual and verbal messages what tone, facial expression and body language do you use? Do you clutch your child close, frantically soothing her like she's hurt herself or something frightening has happened? Do you tense up, yell at your partner to do something, frown or quickly take her out of the environment thereby reinforcing the fear that it's not safe? No! So please don't act this way while you teach her that sleep is a lovely thing, that she is okay, and that her cot is safe and warm and cosy.

Stay confident, and sound loving and empathetic to her tired feelings. Use a reassuring tone and make slow, soothing movements that say, 'Everything is safe, this place is good, and you're perfectly okay'. React to the new conditions or environment she may be experiencing for the first time from an adult's perspective, not in the same way she's responding, or she'll have no one to reassure her. She needs to be able to ask you if she's okay, and you need to be able to answer her truthfully about the environment she's in. You need to be her solid ground to stand on, so she can feel reassured. You're all she has to gauge if she's okay or not.

During the settling process she needs to understand *she's* okay, and she's safe and much loved. It's just her cot, it's just her room you lovingly decorated for her, and it's just her feeling the physical experience of being tired. She needs you to tell her these are all safe things, that she's okay, you can hear her, but it's definitely still sleep time, and you *can't* go to sleep for her, and she *can* do it on her own, but you will reassure her for as long as she feels the need to ask you if she's okay.

Things that can make settling confusing

Two of the most disruptive things I see in settling routines are inconsistency and mixed messages. Some settling routines advocate an approach designed to appeal to a *parent's* need to fix things, or to stay present while the child tries to work out what is being asked of her. Think about your statements and whether you're defining them correctly. If not, this is what she might be thinking:

- Why is Mummy standing there?
- Am I about to get up?
- Does she want to talk to me?
- Is this a new game?
- Should I stand like she is?
- Is she going to give me a toy?

What is your child learning from you from a particular statement or event you're governing around sleep time?

The settling routine

A settling routine is a set of predictable conditions leading up to the event of your child going into her cot and putting herself to sleep. It's important you distance the new set of sleep-time conditions from your child's old set of sleep-time conditions, because the old set will be linked to old expectations of you which could promote confusion and tears. The new set of conditions help your baby prepare for bed, relax and accept the sensation of being tired at sleep time, and gives her the chance to become accepting of your guidance ten to 15 minutes before you put her to bed. This is not what puts a child to sleep though. Only she can do that. The process of putting herself to sleep is a learnt response after she's put into her cot with these new conditions. You will have skilled her enough through homework to ensure she can start to lie there at your request and begin to accept the tired sensations, because you've defined her new settling routine and cues to always mean 'time to go to sleep' and nothing else.

If you don't provide a new set of predictable conditions around *preparing* her for sleep you perpetuate her expectation that she only needs to relax, be still and accept your guidance moments before you put her into the cot. This doesn't give her time to prepare and relax into feeling tired, and will result in her fighting you at sleep time. She'll then require intervention to help her body wind down, leading to learnt dependent sleep associations. To create a routine where she has ten to 15 minutes to settle into the feeling of being tired and preparing for sleep means if she's going to protest about going to sleep she can have her little 'Do I have to go to bed?' cry in your lap during stories or in your arms during singing time. You'll be there to reassure her she's all right and can help her move past feeling resistant to relaxing into feeling tired, so she's truly relaxed for sleep when she's put in her cot.

The normal conditions of sleep time your child will adjust to during her new settling routine, to speed up the process of her falling asleep, will be to remain still and not fight the feeling of being tired. These skills are developed and encouraged in a few important ways. Her positioning for story time helps her slow down and relax into the feeling of being tired. This is beneficial to her both now and in the future because you won't always be putting her down feeling really tired. She will often simply need to go to bed because it's bed time and healthy for her, even if she's not exhausted, so knowing what to expect and what to do when she's in her cot and starting to feel weary is empowering for her. This still time activates her body's mechanisms of slowing down and preparing for sleep. Her body temperature drops, her hormone levels drop off, she begins to breathe through her nose only, one nostril closes and the oxygen supply to her brain is lowered. This process enables her to be nicely prepared when you do put her into her cot.

To accept guidance from you is also important because going to sleep independently means you need to *ask* her to go into her cot awake and lie there until she falls asleep. The settling-routine story time allows her the opportunity to protest about you telling her the next step of the day well before you put her into the cot if she's likely to protest. This allows you to comfort her and help her relax into your governing line so all protests are over before you put her to bed. This is appropriate from six months of age.

All babies need a ten-minute wind down before bedtime to help them stay calm and learn to accept and cope with the natural body rhythms of hormone and temperature drops, and the sensation of tiredness. Read 'Sleep: Understanding the basics' and 'Solving sleep-time blues/troubleshooting' to ensure your new settling attempt won't be confusing or unexpected for your child, and will fully cater to her sleep needs. Always make sure her room and everything you need are prepared before you start your settling routine. Babies on the full recovery program require all recommended comfort items and complete stimulation reduction. For all babies, make sure:

- cot is made ready for the tuck-in technique
- white noise is on
- lights are off in her room and all the rooms and the hall near her room
- Safe T Sleep is open and ready
- towel rolls are handy ready to tuck her in with
- wrap or wraps are out on the nearest bed
- books are ready on the couch
- clock or watch is handy

- distractions are turned off and put away.

The settling routine comprises:

- reading two books together on the couch while using your pre-emptive cues and governing line of communication
- asking baby to say goodnight to others as you carry/lead her out of the room
- if wrapping your baby, doing so, ready for sleep time
- taking her into her room, close the door and carry her in a cradle position to her cot
- singing 'Twinkle Twinkle Little Star' to her
- tucking her into her cot
- using the settling cues 'Time for sleep', 'Mummy and Daddy love you' and 'Nigh' nigh''.

Use your flow of communication leading up to this settling-routine event. Once she's tucked in, say your settling cues with a soft voice, without any sounds of worry or concern, as she'll want to hear your voice even if she's cross with you. Encourage her to settle herself down by gently patting her tummy/nappy and say:

- 'Shh' four times and 'Time for sleep'.
- 'Shh' four more times and 'Mummy and Daddy love you'.
- 'Shh' four more times and 'Nigh', nigh''.

Repeat all your cues one more time then turn and leave – don't hesitate – and close the door behind you.

Outlined next is a full settling routine for a baby aged six to 15 months who is in the full swaddle. There are also variations for a leg-wrapped baby, ten to 15 months old, and an unwrapped baby 15 months plus.

Settling routine for swaddled baby, six to 15 months old

First, go into her room, turn the light on and, if required, change her nappy. Take off any bulky items of clothing down to a singlet and nappy for those being fully wrapped. For evening sleeps do the following routine after her final night feed, brush her teeth too. Then:

- Turn off the light in her room on your way out, saying 'Let's read our books'.
- Go out to the lounge chair where two or three books are ready for you.
- Sit her on your lap, facing the book in your hand, and read for about ten minutes, or until five minutes before sleep time. She may challenge

you a little when this is new; this is where you're asking her to allow you to govern this next part of her day, and defining that statement.

- As you read each book use parent-governed lines of communication and pre-emptive cues like 'Wait for Mummy', 'Turn the page', 'Grace do it' (for lifting flaps or touching texture books), 'Nearly time for nigh' nigh'', 'Last page, nearly time to pack away', and 'All finished, time to pack away'.
- Five minutes before bed put the books away and say your cue, 'It's time for sleep', and have a cuddle and a kiss with her. This story routine and final cuddle and kiss shouldn't be used as a tool to put her to sleep but as a calming pre-bed routine she'll begin to rely on to predict it's nearly time for bed.
- Have her say goodnight to everyone in the room. As you leave the room with her, others in the room should stay seated and look away to avoid confusion. Babies and toddlers can get upset if they think someone is following them, then doesn't walk behind as anticipated. On those first few days while she's adjusting to her new routine, everyone should stay put until she's out of sight.
- With five minutes to spare, keep saying 'It's time for sleep' as you walk to the room she'll be swaddled in.
- Point to the wrap (the room should be pretty dark, but light enough for you to swaddle her) and say 'Lie down', then gently lie her down and wrap her.
- Once wrapped firmly, carry her into her room in the cradle position, allowing her to snuggle her face into your cheek or neck so she's not distracted.
- Once in her room, close the door and walk to her cot, still snuggling her in a cradle position. Give her a cuddle and kiss, then sing 'Twinkle Twinkle Little Star' slowly and calmly while you gently sway with her. Sing slowly enough for her to calm down so her breathing settles into a relaxed rhythm, quietly give her a kiss and say your goodnight cues: 'Time for sleep, Mummy and Daddy love you, nigh' nigh''. Then say 'Lie down' *before* lying her down.
- Lie her in her cot regardless of her reaction.
- Avoid eye contact. Only say your cues occasionally regardless of her reaction. You're not opening up any lines of negotiation so don't add any additional language to your cues or additions to your routine or she'll think sleep is open to negotiation and unwanted tears could begin to flow.

- Do up her Safe T Sleep securely and tuck her in firmly, locking bedding in place with cloth rolls to avoid it coming loose.
- Place a muslin blocking cloth over the side of the cot and bend over so your face is behind the cloth so she has a chance to get used to her independence while she still has the reassuring and rhythmic settling cues and patting.
- Sing your cues slowly and pat her rhythmically, still avoiding eye contact until she's much better with the routine. Make sure the confident tone and reassuring warmth in your voice tells her sleep time is a beautiful thing, and she's loved and safe. Smiling can lift the inflection in your voice so you sound even more reassuring and gentle.
- Pause to go through your settling cues completely twice. Your settling cues are also your resettling cues so take the time to make them comforting for your baby in case you need to use them in the middle of the night.
- Stop patting as soon as you say your final 'Nigh' nigh''.
- Turn and leave. Don't hesitate, turn back, or change your mind. Make sure your body language is readable and consistent for your baby as she'll be taking close notice of everything you do and say.

If you hesitate or hang around a bit too long or say your cues too many times or in a concerned voice because she's unsettled she'll believe something is out of place, or misread it to mean you may pick her up and become upset when you walk out of the room. Have confidence in your actions and she too will feel confident and content very quickly because you're predictable.

Settling routine variation for a leg-wrapped baby, ten to 15 months

This strategy is identical to the settling strategy for a fully swaddled baby apart from a few minor points. Please remember movement usually equals crying, so the more firmly you make the tuck-in, the faster she'll go to sleep, the quicker she'll learn how to settle without problems, and thus the less tears she'll shed.

Don't fuss around too much with positioning but I never allow under-12 month olds to lie on their stomach for sleep time. Over that age it's fruitless to try to change a pattern of tummy sleeping if it's well established, but it is a parent's choice and sleeping on her back can still be learnt. In some cases, a 12 month old sleeping on her back has to be re-established because she's too unsettled and resistant when placed on her tummy. If you can see your child is going to fight and try extremely hard to get up when you lie her on her side or stomach, don't pursue this avenue. It's best to place her on her back and tuck her in firmly, then manage her positioning as you would for a nappy change until you leave the room.

During the settling routine, once you've leg-wrapped her, say 'Lie down' and cradle her in your arms ready to go into her room, and keep her in that position until placing her in her cot. Because her hands are free she may try to grab your top and reposition herself in an upright position. Calmly and firmly make sure you define the statement 'lie down'. This means you may need to keep one of her arms tucked under your arm. If she physically struggles to get up, calmly but continually hold and release her other hand or, if necessary, hold her hand all the time while you continue with your settling routine: entering her room, closing the door behind you, walking to the side of her cot singing 'Twinkle Twinkle Little Star'.

Give your child a chance to adjust to the idea of lying down in your arms first, rather than have her fight you if you only say 'Lie down' when you put her in the cot. This is graded exposure to sleep-time expectations and giving her the chance to adjust in your arms is a useful tool. Look at things from an adult's perspective – you've only asked her to lie down in your arms. Work up to this request with your flow of communication through the day at nappy time and getting dressed as well as through position requests and the wait game.

Once you've finished singing 'Twinkle Twinkle Little Star' to your child, kiss her gently, say your settling cues, including another 'Lie down' before you lie her in her cot. When you do this, please ensure she remains lying down and doesn't try to get up. If she does, prevent her from being able to get up by quickly tucking her in. Once tucked in, while you begin or continue singing and use your settling cues, you may still need to request her to lie down a few times and, in some cases, hold her hands to stop her trying to get up. If she's still fighting your request to lie down, use all the strategies for a nappy change until it's time to leave the room.

Settling routine variation for an unwrapped baby, 15 months plus

Once they're this age, toddlers can walk to their rooms. After reading your books, ask her to say goodnight to everyone in the room, then hold her hand while you walk out of the room and into her bedroom or carry her into her bedroom. Keep saying it's 'time for sleep' as you walk to her room. When you're in the room, ask her to close the door. If she's reluctant, take her hand and encourage her to close the door. Don't allow her to grab it and open it, this will be a confusing message to her. Stay calm during those first few attempts as she'll soon look forward to this process and start closing the door with great gusto. If, after the second day, she's still unhappy about closing the door, don't ask her to. The role of closing the door will become your responsibility, but it will be important to keep role playing this part of the routine with her, ensuring you close the door when you put teddy to bed.

Once the door is closed, walk her to her cot. Pick her up and either snuggle her in a cradle position in your arms, or gently encourage her to lie her head on your shoulder. If she won't put her head on your shoulder, lie her down in your arms before you start to sing unless she's very calm in the upright position. Often tucking her knees up onto your chest will encourage her to automatically drop her head on your shoulder so give it a go. Give her a cuddle and kiss then sing your song very slowly and calmly while you gently sway with her. Sing slow enough so she start to calm down and her breathing settles into a relaxed rhythm, then quietly give her a kiss and say your goodnight cues. Say 'Lie down' before you lie her in the cot.

Do up Safe T Sleep and tuck her in firmly, locking bedding in place with cloth rolls to avoid it coming loose, or lie her on her back, side or tummy and define your request to stay lying down if she's not tucked in. Encourage her to get any comfort items saying, 'Get your teddy/muslin', etc. If she has a dummy, use your dummy cue and game. Bend over so your face drops behind the cot bars if she's not trying to stand up, to give her a chance to get used to her independence while she still has reassuring and rhythmic settling cues and patting and your presence. This allows a final opportunity for you to step back visually from her before you leave the room so her focus shifts from you to herself before you've even left the room.

Say your cues and pat her rhythmically, avoiding eye contact, until she's better with the routine. Avoid holding her hand, because she may cry when you let go to leave. Don't allow her to tell you whether you can or can't pat her as this allows her to govern the sleep-time routine and encourages tears because you confuse her by listening to her guidance about when and if you can pat her, but not when or if you can leave the room, or will pick her up. The settling routine is a parent-governed line of communication. If you know she dislikes being patted, incorporate a 'patting the mattress' variation and role play this before you offer it in her settling routine to maintain your parent-governed line of communication.

If she's flapping, or trying to get up, or fussing with her hands, make a clear statement by holding her on her tummy and not allowing the flapping. Calmly use your settling cues until she stops fussing, at which point slowly release her to see if she's calm while continuing with your settling cues. If the fussing and flapping don't stop, hold her hands on her tummy again until she either settles completely or you've gone through your settling cues twice, then release her hands, turn and leave.

Once she's settled in and you've paused to go through your cues twice, the confident tone and reassuring warmth in your voice tells her that sleep time is a beautiful thing, and she's safe and loved. Stop patting as soon as you say your final 'nigh' nigh'' and turn and leave the room.

Resettling routine

A resettling routine is a set of familiar conditions taken from her original settling routine. It's used as a way of communicating with your baby to let her know it's still sleep time, and she needs to lie quietly until she falls asleep like you always ask her to do. The need for a resettling routine is only relevant when she's learning to sleep through the night, or if she's unwell, or if you travel into a different time zone or other changes of environment have disrupted her sleep. If you establish a resettling routine when you start your PRM you can always attend to your baby when she needs reassurance during a change in her life without her becoming stressed, and you can ensure healthy restorative sleep is maintained in your house.

To ensure your baby is comfortable with your resettling routine, invest a final minute or so in your original settling routine to lock in those basic settling cues that tell her you'd like her to put herself to sleep, and you're about to leave the room. This allows you to use the same cues when it's time to go back to sleep and she'll know what you're saying, and what she needs to do. So, during his original settling process, after you've put her into her cot, when she's lying down, just before you leave the room you establish the set of conditions via settling cues that you can use later as a resettling routine. I take the time to pause, and sing my cues and shush the baby for a soothing minute or so before I stand and leave them to go to sleep. This becomes the basis for my resettling routine. It is consistent with her settling routine, and if she knows what to do when you first put her to bed, then the use of these cues and conditions will be a clear indicator of what she needs to do to go back to sleep.

It's important to provide an immediate, distinct message when you first enter her bedroom after she's woken day or night, so she knows what's going to be asked of her. This takes a lot of stress out of resettling for her and you. The resettling-routine conditions of your walking into her room and saying nothing before you close the door behind you compared with her waking-routine conditions – you turning the light on and saying your waking cue 'Good sleeping' – will enable her to understand your request without confusion before you even reach her cot. This enables her to predict the situation, giving her a sense of control, so that within a short period, if she needs attending to, a simple attendance and your resettling routine and cue should be all you need to see her lie contently until she drifts back to sleep. Remember, you're aiming to remove the need to go in at all because she's happy to lie awake in her cot and can cope with the feeling of being tired without stress, so be careful to always assess her cries first and only attend to her if necessary.

This is an achievable result from the time your baby is six months old or even younger. Resettling routines can only be used as part of a complete PRM. Completely read and understand this chapter, as well as Chapter 2.

In brief, you walk in, say your cues and leave. The whole routine should take no more than one to two minutes during a resettle. If she cries after you leave, refer to 'Interpreting your child's cries'. As for settling above, I've provided a detailed resettling routine for a swaddled baby, six to 15 months old, and variations for a leg-wrapped baby six to 15 months and an unwrapped toddler 15 months plus.

Resettling routine for a swaddled baby, six to 15 months

When *you* decide your baby needs your assistance:

- don't turn on any lights before opening the door
- walk in and close the door fully behind you
- don't make eye contact with your baby
- with a soft, gentle voice, as your baby will want to hear from you even if she's cross with you, encourage her to settle herself down by gently patting her tummy/nappy and beginning your cues
- in the same gentle voice, without any sounds of worry or concern say 'Shh' four times and 'Time for sleep'
- say 'Shh' four more times and 'Mummy and Daddy love you'
- say 'Shh' four more times and 'Nigh', nigh''
- repeat all the cues one more time
- turn and leave without hesitating and close the door behind you.

Resettling variation for a leg-wrapped baby, ten to 15 months

All children with a leg wrap should have a Safe T Sleep to maintain consistency of environment during a 12-hour night. This strategy is identical to the resettling strategy outlined for a fully swaddled baby except for a few minor points. If your baby is trying to get up, or is overly fussing, please place her on her back, firm up her leg wrap if necessary, tuck her in securely, then manage her positioning while you calmly and reassuringly say your cues. Then turn and leave.

Resettling variation for an unwrapped baby, 15 months plus

If your toddler is standing up, ask her to lie down, or gently lie her down. Say 'Lie down' and pat her a few times on the back of her hand with one finger as a reminder you'd like her to let go and lie down. She should be used to this request from her playtime in the cot, even if she's protesting about sleep time. If she doesn't lie down for you immediately, then sit her down, then lie her on her back in a fuss-free way, ensuring she doesn't get up or roll over despite her protests. Be sure to define your request to 'lie down' with its true meaning. Once she's lying down, hold her hand and manage her position as you do for her nappy change if she's challenging you.

Regardless of her reaction, use a gentle voice, even if she's cross with you. She'll want to hear your voice and it will encourage her to settle herself down and remain calm. Gently pat the side of her nappy or tummy and in a gentle voice, without any sound of worry or concern, say your resettling cues then leave. Don't hesitate, even if she stands up straight away. Don't look back at her. She needs to learn standing up won't get your attention and the only response it will get you is leaving, which will discourage her from doing it. Close the door as you leave.

The waking routine

It's important to establish a language stream during your waking routine because if you're going to govern your child when she's going to sleep and going back to sleep, you should also govern the conditions around waking. If your child governs these areas, she'll be confused if you respond to her, 'I'm awake now come and get me' cry by sometimes asking her to go back to sleep and sometimes getting her up. When you have to wake her or you don't intend to resettle her when she's woken, observe your partial-waking pause (see page 357) and leave her as long as possible before you use this routine as a clear indicator it's okay for her to be awake and you don't expect her to go back to sleep, and her day will begin or resume again.

The waking routine is one of the two most important elements within the psychology of sleep. The kind of message you deliver at this time either confuses your child, or is in line with your settling and resettling routine. To confuse your child and damage the careful balance of sleep conditions tells her to cry to be picked up. It tells her that as soon as she's awake she should see someone enter the room very quickly or be removed from the cot immediately. It tells her the cot is not the place to be when you're awake, and if she wants to get up, she just needs to call out. This contrasts with your message at settling and resettling times, and can potentially undo all yours and your baby's work in developing trust in a predictable set of conditions around sleep time. Don't be concerned about her being awake in her cot, you want her to know it's normal and to feel comfortable to lie there and play, knowing someone will come and get her when cot time is over.

At settling and resettling times you tell your child to look to you for guidance. You tell her there's a set of conditions you always follow so there's no need for her to cry because the sleep time runs along these conditions alone (unless she's very unwell of course) and nothing else happens. You tell her it's okay to be in her cot while she's awake, and you tell her if she wakes early to lie there and relax because she may need to go back to sleep. If you were then to come in each morning when she first cries and pick her up straight away, you'll confuse her and she'll expect the same response from you at 2 a.m. and that's unrealistic. You need to develop predictable sleep conditions by always incorporating a waking routine as well as a settling and resettling routine. To not cause confusion:

- open the door and say if sleep time is over with a simple visual and verbal set of cues
- turn on the light immediately, make eye contact and smile and say 'Good sleeping, bubba.'
- teach her she needs to sit down in her cot, because standing up and asking to be picked up isn't something you want to encourage at sleep time
- teach her she always stays in her cot for a while after she first wakes up, and that time is always a happy time
- teach her that Mummy and Daddy can come and go from the room when she's in the cot, and it's normal for her to experience this, and it's okay for her to be in her cot in her room alone without you there – this will set her up and equip her with realistic expectations and skills for your resettling routine
- teach her that the process of packing away while still in the cot is what immediately precedes getting out of bed, not crying or standing and flapping

- teach her that you will always tell her when you plan on picking her up by always using your wait game and then saying a predictable 'Up, up' when she's doing the true definition of waiting.

This entire waking routine gives her all the tools she needs to cope with the task of going to sleep and going back to sleep by herself. For this reason, I often include the waking routine into a child's day while I'm incorporating my new communication, independence and meal time routines one week before I start my new daily routine, settling routines and cues, and crying interpretation and sleep repair program.

The waking routine in detail

- Walk in.
- Say 'Good sleeping', in a clear voice, not too soft, as you open the door.
- Turn light on dimly.
- Walk to cot and make eye contact with your baby, give her warm loving smiles, and say your cue again, 'Good sleeping, bubby.'
- Unwrap and undo her, and help her sit up by using one hand behind her head and upper back. Don't confuse her into thinking you're going to pick her up by putting your hands under her armpits to sit her up.
- Offer your baby her toys and establish playtime. Ensure she has plenty of time when she's playing by herself, this is her independent time, and isn't for playing or chatting with you. She'll have plenty of time for that while you're together during the rest of the day. You need to each her that eventually when she wakes up feeling happy she can chat to herself till you come in to get her.
- While you're in the room don't let your baby stand in her cot. This is a simple boundary-setting strategy to help her cope with the sleep-time expectation of lying down. Use the cue 'Sit down, wait for Mummy/ Daddy'. It's also vital to change any habits of standing as soon as she wakes up, thus lessening the chances of her accidentally waking himself up early.
- Each time you leave and return use your short-term absence cue.
- When her playtime window is drawing to a close, follow a packing-away ritual so dhe learns that it is the event, and not her crying, that determines when she can get out of her cot.
- Ask her to hand you her toys so you can pack away.
- Fold all the sheets and tidy her bed briefly; remember she must stay sitting down at all times during this.
- Play your wait game before getting her up using your cue.

Settling into your new daily routine

Within a few days, your baby will be relaxed with her settling, resettling and waking routines and your questions of her will be things of the past, but during the transition they'll be important to you. Remember, you must have role played, and role played completely, the whole routine, regardless of how insistent she is for you to stop, out of her annoyance, boredom, etc. The importance of letting her know this routine is followed through, no matter what, is vital. This means if there are going to be any major tantrums or crying while she gets used to you governing the direction of these routines, you will see them appear and be resolved mostly during the week of role play leading up to the start of implementing your new daily routines, including the settling routine. Never introduce the routines until you're prepared to define them using the crying interpretation and assistance technique.

On the first day or two of starting the new routine, your baby will quickly discover that 'these things' all mean 'it's time to go to bed'. It's normal for her to say 'Noooooo, I want to stay up and play alllll night with you guys', but it's crucial for you to say, 'You're too little and you need your sleep so, yes, it's bedtime.' Her response to going to bed does not govern the outcome. You're there to hold and reassure her, but you need to confidently put her to bed with a clear request to go to sleep, which means you follow through as calmly and as confidently as if she was lying there silently during her settling and resettling routines.

Most of the time my answer to any problems in these routines is to follow through. Be predictable. Ensure settling and resettling routines are not a negotiation, as that's probably what made her imbalanced about sleep. You need to end stress around sleep, so close off the lines of communication and say, 'From now on, this is what you can expect at sleep time, and I will always be predictable', just in your actions. Stay confident and calm, and don't hesitate at any time during your routines. Watch the currency you give certain behaviours. If you want certain behaviours to continue, stop what you're doing and start fussing around when she does them. If you'd like her to stop trying to negotiate her way out of sleep time, ignore her behaviour and follow through calmly. The message you deliver is: 'I love you, I'm always here for you, and I'll help you for as long as you need help, but it is sleep time and you need to sleep to keep yourself and the family healthy and happy, and nothing but sleep will occur from this point.' The more consistent you are, the faster she'll relax and accept this time as peaceful, predictable and lovely.

Getting it right!

A quick turnaround in results and preventing wakings is now your first priority. Once your homework is done and you've embarked on your new daily routine and sleep repair program using your new settling routines, being careful to define them using your crying interpretation and assistance techniques, it's very important to keep two thing in mind: consistency and ongoing maintenance.

Consistency

One of the fastest ways to ensure your baby or toddler can settle into her new sleep routine is to remain consistent through your management of the physiology of sleep. The importance of maintaining your child's sleep conditions in one set pattern is the only way to prevent stress to the child, avoid tears as much as possible and maintain great sleep without the need to intervene. Some of the conditions you need to consistently maintain are the environment, your communication, the carers you use and their use of your routines, and your honesty.

Environment

If she goes to sleep wrapped, she should stay wrapped. Ensure the wrap is effective enough to remain firm for the entire night or there are inconsistencies in your baby's sleep environment. If she has a dummy, make sure she has many to ensure this condition stays available to her. If the hall lights are going to be off when she wakes in the night, ensure they're off when she first goes to sleep. If she has music or white noise to fall asleep to, then have music or white noise running right through the night. If you're not going to be in the room when she wakes in the night, make sure you're honest with her and tell her when you leave when she first goes to bed.

Communication

Don't change your management halfway through a learning process. Deciding to stop working through some crying because it's been going on for a while translates to the baby as 'If I don't want to go to bed I need to cry for a long time before you'll get up'. If you're not going to be consistent during the first two to three days of teaching her a new way, don't start because it's a waste of her time and energy.

Don't change your settling or resettling cues, or open up communication by adding extra lines or asking questions, or looking to your child for guidance by obliging demands. Always retain the governing line at sleep time, even if you need to get her up to change her nappy midway through the settling routine – 'Mummy change your nappy, up up, then time for sleep' – so she knows you're governing all the events, rather than thinking that getting up has something to do with their cries.

Your voice and body language need to remain predictably reassuring and confident and soothing so your baby can trust that, although this feels new on those first few days, she's okay because you're okay.

Carers

Always use your set of predictable routines around going to sleep, going back to sleep and waking up, and ensure they're carefully aligned. Make sure your baby or toddler knows who is putting her to bed, and don't chop and change settlers at the last minute. Whenever possible, whoever puts her down should resettle, and get her up in the morning. Everyone should use the same routines for settling, resettling or waking her at home and, where possible, in other locations.

If you plan on going to the shops and leaving her with a carer while she's asleep, tell her, just in case she wakes early or if she'll be waking up with another carer. Make sure any carers are there before she goes to sleep, so she doesn't get a surprise if someone she's not expecting enters her room when she wakes up. Imagine how surprising it would be to expect your partner to walk in the front door as usual and it's your neighbour or, worse still, someone you barely knew.

Honesty

Don't be dishonest! One of the most common but trust-breaking things I see parents do is put their baby to sleep in their arms, then put them down in their cot and sneak out of the room as quietly as possible before closing the door.

Your baby has no concept of sleep, and no concept of time lapsing so she'll be surprised if she closed her eyes and relaxed in your arms or on your shoulder and opens them again to find herself in a dark room with no one in sight.

Be confident and establish your new, more honest, settling routine around going to sleep, that's in line with what she'll experience when she naturally stirs in the night. Make sure she's awake when you leave or, at the very least, hears you close the door to her room if it's impossible to keep her awake. Being dishonest creates a situation where she fights the sensation of being tired at sleep time.

Ongoing maintenance

As part of your ongoing success with this program, once you've established your sleep-time settling, resettling and waking routines, your full daily routine and recovered your sleep, maintain her sleep by ensuring you're keeping her confident in the three most basic skills she needs to keep to sleep for you: being in her cot awake, coping when you leave the room, and accepting your guidance with trust.

Independence

For anyone who scoffs at the idea of independence in a baby, I'm not suggesting you give your baby the car keys, or leave her at home while you go shopping. I'm just suggesting you empower her with a sense of security and comfort when she's in her 'own space', and help her come to terms with, and not be frightened of, certain 'normal' feelings associated with sleep.

I feel strongly about both the importance of a baby feeling comfortable with being in her cot and the importance of exposing her to the feelings associated with you being in the room, and going in and out of the room, and her *not* thinking she's in danger. Even if your child is anxious about you leaving the room, you need to let her know she is safe to have a little play in her cot. Your responses to her anxious emotions should be reassuring and confident, and certainly not indicate to her that she's in a situation she needs to be rescued from. To become as anxious as the child around these events delivers the wrong message about a safe environment by teaching her it's not safe when it's actually *perfectly* safe.

If you don't confidently work through this it means you're never exposing her to those normal emotions, thus limiting her ability to grow and become confident with coping with a normal range of feelings that come up around sleeping in her cot, or you stepping out of the room while she puts herself to sleep. Just as important as the emotionally independent sleep tools learnt around playtime in the cot, and you leaving the room for short periods, is the ability to cope with the feelings associated with sleep and you guiding them at sleep time.

To be able to deal with the feelings associated with being tired is important. You can't expect her to be content to peacefully lie in her cot as she drifts off to sleep if she's not comfortable with the feelings associated with being tired.

Coping with you leaving the room

There are two basic skills you need to empower your child with, both in the day or so leading up to implementing your new routine and in maintaining it: they are the ability to be in his cot while he's awake and the ability to cope with you leaving the room. This is where you need to implement and maintain playtime in the cot and establish short-term absence cues during both non-cot and cot playtimes.

The ability to accept your guidance

Finally, this program advocates asking your baby to go to sleep for you. This is not pot-luck sleep where you hope she's tired enough to accept your guidance. It's a clear, safe, parent-directed request to go to sleep because you think she needs a rest. This is why it's important she's able to be awake in her cot and cope with you leaving the room, and to cope with the sensation of being tired. In order to achieve and sustain good peaceful sleep in your house, you have to establish clear and consistent communication in guiding her through the days leading up to repairing her sleep respectfully, but also to maintain the ability to guide her so you can always ask her to go to sleep for you, and she's able to accept and trust your guidance.

This is probably the one part of your program that remains ongoing. Please always refer to Part 1, the communication section of this book, to maintain harmony in your house. Your flow of communication and your three lines of communication, when used as a general communication style with your child, will keep you and your family on track to *always* have 'happy days and peaceful nights'.

16

Interpreting your child's cries

Ask most grandparents and they'll generally say parenting was less complicated in their day and babies' and toddlers' sleep wasn't such a big deal for anyone. Yet reports indicate that more than half of Australian parents are struggling with persistent severe and ongoing sleep-time issues beyond their child's first birthday. Why is this generation of parents finding putting their babies to bed so much more challenging than the previous generation? Why, by six to 12 months of age, are some babies needing two or three times more night feeds than they needed when they were newborns? Do they need that level of milk intake, or are they seeking more comfort to feel safe in an environment that is already safe and nurturing? Could it simply be that we're teaching our babies to need things like breast or bottle feeding, rocking, pacing, patting as solutions to feeling tired?

Getting some perspective on crying

There are many causes of modern sleep-time challenges, ranging from changing sleep requirements as a result of healthy pregnancies and better nutrition in children and mothers, through to parents doing less labour-intensive domestic chores due to washing machines, dishwashers, etc., to fewer children per household, creating more one-on-one time between parents and their children, which occasionally tips the scales to children being fully entertained and having no quiet times to discover their own peace and happiness. I also believe one of the causes of the current sleep challenge is the fear or anxiety around a baby crying *at all* when it comes to sleep.

In 1998 some of the causes of cot death were discovered thanks to research into Sudden Infant Death Syndrome (SIDS) and parents were alerted to potentially dangerous practices that could significantly increase the risk of SIDS and saved many children's lives. However it also led to people putting their babies on their backs to sleep, reducing layers of excessive warmth and removing cot bumpers. As a result babies lost the digestive relief provided by lying on their tummies, a sense of security from the weight and warmth of extra blankets, and were exposed to more visual stimulation through the removal of the bumpers. This resulted in babies feeling less settled, more exposed and more overstimulated at bedtime.

When this became increasingly difficult for many families to deal with, some healthcare professionals started recommending a strategy commonly known as 'control crying'. Some also suggested strategies such as 'uncontrolled crying' (also called 'controlled comforting' or 'crying it out'). These methods were often implemented without any form of communication, play, independence, emotional foundation work, sleep or meal-time management strategies with their babies, and were thus doomed to fail in a large proportion of cases.

I believe most modern parenting problems involve misunderstandings about teaching babies how to go sleep. While it's important to limit the level of intervention offered to children to allow them the opportunity to try to develop independent-settling skills, the control crying method fails to prepare or empower children with the task of going to sleep by themselves and can ultimately lead to more tears and stress for babies and their parents. In addition, the control crying strategy teaches children their parents will respond to their cries in one way at night, and in a different way through the day. This is because control crying teaches babies you won't pick them up and feed them when they ask during the night, but when they wake up at a reasonable time in the morning and ask to be picked up and fed you walk straight in, pick them up, feed, cuddle and play with them.

For a baby, who doesn't know 10 p.m. from 2 a.m. from 7 a.m., it's confusing and inconsistent if one minute you say 'Don't ask to be picked up because I won't pick you up when you cry' and the next moment you say 'If you want to get up, cry out to me and I'll come and pick you up and feed and cuddle you'.

As time passed, many parents found control crying stressful and difficult, and went in the opposite direction by avoiding all crying at sleep time at any cost. This contributed to the trend of parents becoming their children's only and complete emotional solution at sleep time which, ironically, has been the cause of so many nights of crying, stress and discomfort for many children and their entire families.

In parents' efforts to avoid their baby crying in the first place, they increase the incidence of crying through the night because their child is forced to call out and recreate sleep associations to go back to sleep. While babies *don't* always cry when they learn how to settle into the feeling of being tired and going to sleep independently, some babies do, whether you hold them or not.

For babies who find falling asleep a challenge you need to be careful not to make it harder for them. Some babies become overstimulated when parents fuss, but despite their inability to cope with the conditions provided, don't know any other way to go to sleep without parents showing them. Some babies, because of discomfort from conditions like reflux, which makes lying down painful, need extra help to sleep until the conditions are resolved. But even when the problem has been resolved, these children may have learnt a sleep pattern that needs correcting to ensure they can enjoy peaceful sleeping. Initially, they may be under the impression that the cot is the cause of the pain, and perhaps insist on continuing to lie on your chest to go to sleep if that's what they've been taught, even after the reflux or other conditions have been resolved.

It's important you help your child work past his fears so he doesn't have to be fretful about things that are no longer difficult for him. And if your baby has been on a program of control crying or has failed sleep school, or you've tried a version of control crying, or had someone come in to implement control crying, and your baby has started crying more than ever, or is no better off, you're going to have to undo the learnt pattern of crying he's been taught.

Finding peace and harmony at sleep time when learning or relearning how to sleep independently by avoiding all crying is the problem, not the solution. The only two ways a child (from birth to five years of age) can go to sleep are with:

- a child-governed association to go to sleep – that is, by themselves; or
- a parent-governed association to go to sleep – you doing it for them.

A child can either be taught that he can't go to sleep without you, or taught that it's okay to lie in his cot awake after you leave the room without the need to cry for help, and therefore taught he can go to sleep peacefully on his own. This sometimes takes practice to master, and might or might not involve some tears.

It's your choice how you'd like to parent at sleep time. You can either teach your baby to rely on you, or to rely on himself. Both are effective and easy for your child and, when done correctly, both are loving and in his best long-term interests. If you like to co-sleep, and you and your family and the baby are sleeping well and happy with the arrangement, then excellent – 'Don't fix what isn't broken'. If, on the other hand, you'd like your baby to sleep in his own room after his first few months, or if he's not happy with your assistance or co-sleeping and, as a result, you're all unsettled at night, you'll need to step back and allow him the opportunity to settle himself. He either has to rely on your skills (patting, feeding, rocking, etc.) or his own skills (playing with his hair, thumb sucking, etc.).

The importance of self-settling

The reason it's so vital that a baby learns how to self-settle when put to bed is because from the age of four to six months he will naturally stir between 10 and 11 p.m., at around 2 a.m. and again between 4 and 5 a.m., and will expect and need to do the same thing he was doing when he initially fell sleep. This is because he has no concept of sleep or time lapsing. He only knows the *feeling* of being tired and what you've taught him to need when he feels that way.

I've already talked about several common things that occur when parents adopt strategies like 'avoid all crying' or 'never leave a child to fall asleep alone', particularly when a baby is learning to sleep. These include:

- a baby who once slept independently temporarily or permanently losing that ability due to a disruption like a holiday, house guest or illness
- a child being taught he should never be in his cot awake because his parents hold him in their arms to put him to sleep and/or then take him out of the cot immediately upon waking
- a child becoming fearful of his cot and crying when he realises the person who put him in his cot to sleep and was there when he closed her eyes, has disappeared – as far as the child is concerned – when he woke
- a child starting to fight sleep.

It's important not to parent from fear, so make choices based on love and what is in your child's best interests.

When you observe a child who knows how to sleep through the night, when he wakes up he will open his eyes, look around, and feel quite relaxed to be in that environment because it's familiar to him. Eventually, when he starts to drift into the next sleep cycle, his eyes just flutter closed and he goes back to sleep. If, on the other hand, you observe a baby who's been told he shouldn't be awake without intervention from an adult, he will wake and cry, look around or call out for whoever or whatever it is he's learnt she needs when he feels tired and wants to go to sleep.

Of course there is a need for comfort, nurturing, love, reassurance and responsiveness, but I rarely encounter a home where these are lacking (except in cases of profound depression, or where a mother and baby are at risk from stress and exhaustion). In fact, I often find parents who are so frightened they should never do anything but meet every demand their child makes of them at sleep time, regardless of whether it's a learnt pattern or a true need of the child. Some parents offer up to 20 feeds a night when their baby is over six months old. Some parents average no more than an hour's sleep at a time, a maximum of four hours a day, even when they and their baby are becoming ill from the level of intervention being demanded. This sometimes continues even when a relationship is about to break down due to the stress, and a parent is experiencing dangerous situations like falling asleep at the wheel or not being able to concentrate while working with heavy or dangerous machinery. To forgo sleep and focus only on meeting demands and, in doing so, allow a baby to wake repeatedly through the night, is not balanced.

I'm not saying you should or shouldn't let babies cry. I'm saying you need to look more closely at the reason babies cry in the first place, and then set about empowering them with the necessary coping skills before you ask them to try and go to sleep on their own without excessive levels of help. Crying interpretation is about listening to and understanding your child and what he's actually saying, rather than just fearing what that crying 'might mean'.

Change is challenging, but it's important to teach your child that change is not something to be frightened of. Crying is a normal, healthy way for a baby to express concern or uncertainty when placed in an unfamiliar situation. You can rarely avoid crying if you want to teach a baby, toddler or pre-schooler how to start going to sleep on his own for the first time after he's been taught something different, because children are creatures of habit. You'll literally be putting off the inevitable, or making it worse by avoiding making the transition.

Avoiding crying by fully assisting a child to sleep is one of the main causes of him waking and crying repeatedly through the night and catnapping through the day. If you believe allowing a baby to cry is unkind, your child may never learn how to breastfeed, which often involves tears and frustration, never try something new, never learn how to sit in his pram or wait in his high chair, or eat more than three mouthfuls of food or drink from a cup or eat off a spoon. He may never want to go beyond his first day at daycare or school. Eventually he will be under the impression that whenever he feels anything but happy he needs to be rescued, and that someone else should be responsible for making those feelings go away.

Everything I recommend in this book aims at helping you assist your child to be independent and equipped with the ability to cope. Learning how to sleep in the first five years of life is a healthy skill that will change his future in areas of education, personality, confidence, career prospects and more.

The Checklist

If your child has experienced difficulties with sleep in the past, before you ask him to go to sleep, ensure he's empowered with all the skills he needs to cope and is able to feel familiar and comfortable with the process of going to sleep. This means having developed communication and independence strategies and sleep-time routines to cater for his needs. Before starting sleep repair you should have:

- assessed your baby's daily sleep requirement or routine miscalculation and have adjusted these according to his age and needs
- developed predictable and soothing settling, resettling and waking routines, and have role played them so that the conditions your baby will experience in his room are so familiar he can begin to enjoy this process
- adjusted your baby's diet and fluid intake
- catered for your baby's environmental and emotional need for feelings of security and warmth with the addition of wraps, a Safe T Sleep to wear to bed, teddy bears or other comfort items, and dummy pots, etc.
- practised your wrap on a teddy so your wrapping technique is perfect before you use it the first time on your baby
- empowered your baby with feelings of security around you leaving the room for short periods, using your short-term absence cue
- helped your baby to feel comfortable to be in his cot during cot playtime

- taught your baby to understand that normal emotions are okay and that he doesn't need to be rescued from feelings like tiredness, frustration, boredom or impatience
- taught your baby how to relax and accept the feeling of being tired independently through the reading of books, rather than just by breast or bottle feeding so he can lie peacefully in his cot and be able to cope with you leaving the room when he's tired
- taught your baby to accept loving, consistent guidance from you through clear communication during the day around simple requests to sit down in the bath/car seat/pram/high chair, lie down during nappy changes, get dressed or have a milk feed without stress or resistance
- helped your baby learn he can play independently at his play stations while you do basic chores in the kitchen or around the room.

The emphasis here is on preparation and empowerment to avoid or dramatically reduce a baby crying rather than suddenly starting an action plan like control crying. This is a respectful way to do it, and the very least you can do to help a child feel in control of a brand-new situation without crying.

One thing that is crucial for me to assess and feel comfortable with before I assist parents with helping their child learn how to go to sleep independently is that the parents are prepared to give their child the time necessary to learn something new. This can involve a good three to five days working through daytime tiredness, some crying, and a few protests as the baby adjusts to the new balanced lines of communication and a new way of going to and back to sleep. I ensure that each family has made a conscious decision to invest the time and energy into following the plan 100 per cent to the letter. It is a waste of a baby's time, energy and learning ability to start something you're not willing to follow through on.

So, it's time to be sure you can use your well-developed adult coping skills, and commit to changes and remain consistent and confident when implementing them, rather than go into the same head space as your child.

Basic guidelines when introducing your new sleep routine

- Have one solid week in which you focus on repairing sleep. Take time off work if you need to, and if there's someone in your house who needs sleep, either send them to sleep elsewhere, or choose an appropriate time to work on repairing your baby's sleep. It will take a few days to help your baby to not feel the need to wake during the night, so be prepared to invest the time.

- Don't introduce your cues or new sleep times until you're ready to begin your new crying interpretation and support strategy. One of the benefits of introducing a change in sleep times through the day when correcting sleep is that it will naturally help your baby feel tired, making the settling process during those early days of sleep repair a faster and easier process for him, helping him build his confidence and adjust with less stress.
- It takes three weeks for your routine to be locked in, so plan to stay close to home during that time, not have any big changes (like going away on holidays) and be cautious of having people come to stay. It's not fair to ask your baby to look to you for guidance, then repeatedly leave him with other people while you shop or get your hair done. Try to stay close for a few weeks while he learns to settle into a guided day, and once he is more confident, start using clear language to warn him of your impending absences, even when he is six months old. Make sure carers understand your respectful, language-rich parenting style.
- Keep everything low key for half an hour before sleep time is due. It's unfair to have Grandma arrive just before his main sleep and not expect him to want to stay up and play with her. Regardless of anyone's timetable, Daddy or Mummy or anyone else needs to be there for the settling routine by 6.30 p.m., or stay out of the scene until bubby has gone to bed, particularly during the first three weeks. This doesn't mean someone arrives at 6.30 p.m., grabs a bite to eat, showers and changes and appears five minutes before he's put to bed. It means whoever is going to be there is sitting down and relaxed by 6.30 p.m. Try to get home early, and if you do get home late, stay calm and slot into the flow of the routine, focusing on what needs to be done, or there may be tears, tantrums and a very tired child.
- The settling routine can involve the entire family, or just the settling parent and the baby. If there are people not involved in the settling routine, they should say goodnight before stories start, and stay away and keep low key – no wandering around and distracting the little one.
- If you make a mistake during your settling routine, carry on. Don't tut, sigh, tense up, start again, apologise, etc. Just carry on confidently.
- Surround yourself with encouraging and positive people. You cannot be so worried about another adult not coping that you don't remain 100 per cent focused on the baby. Your baby's needs must come first. Stay confident.

- If you have a disruptive older child, have your partner read to him elsewhere on the first few days or, if you're on your own, provide distraction for him while you do your settling routine. Try to work on your communication with your older child through the day, using the language strategies highlighted in this book, so he can be involved in the process.
- No one should come into the baby's room while you're putting him to bed. If necessary, place a child safety gate further down the hall to prevent other children and pets disrupting the flow of your baby's settling routine. Even if your older child tantrums while you settle the baby, continue on with your routine. Close the door, have the white noise on, and sound unconcerned so your baby can focus on your voice, and not his sibling's tantrums. Your baby's need for sleep is a higher need than an older child's tantrum. If this is an issue for an older child, work on your short- and long-term absence cues with the older child through the day while you role play and prepare to start your new sleep program.
- Pets should not come in the room with you while you settle your baby.
- Whoever puts the baby to bed should be there to get him up.
- Once baby goes down, he should stay in his cot until he's slept as requested.
- Where possible, try to only resettle your baby during the day when you have a good chance of success. If you've taken an hour to try to get him to sleep, don't force the issue unless you're sure he'll be able to go back to sleep. Avoid 'teaching your baby to cry' by having an unsuccessful resettling attempt or the primary message you deliver is, 'If you cry for an hour I'll get you up.' I sometimes pursue sleep after a shorter sleep of 30 to 40 minutes during a day sleep session and, when I do, I always make sure I pursue the sleep to a positive outcome. Sometimes, it becomes more about defining your statement and not confusing your baby, than the amount of sleep he has. Occasionally, you may need to resettle right up until the final chance for that particular sleep window, and have him fall asleep in the last ten minutes. Still wake him in accordance with the routine.
- No matter what kind of sleep session he has, remain calm, patient, gentle and consistent.
- No matter what kind of sleep session he has, whether successful or unsuccessful, when you've reached your furthest time in that day's sleep window, use your waking routine and 'good sleeping' cues as normal and continue on as normal. Remain positive about his ability to sleep.

Always tell him he's a good sleeper even if it's through gritted teeth on those first couple of days of settling into the new routine.

- The most difficult window to resettle your baby in is between 5 and 6 a.m. after he's been asleep for ten hours. If it's close to 6 a.m., try to hold off as long as you can before attending and just start the day early, while still sticking to the routine. If he wakes at 5 a.m. and you need to resettle him, once you've asked him to go back to sleep you need to follow through until 6.30 a.m. Also, don't attend unless he's in the right cry or you risk making him very upset because you'll be asking him to go back to sleep while he's trying to insist on getting up.
- Another difficult time is if he wakes 20 to 40 minutes after going to sleep at night, or after a brief day sleep that was meant to be longer. Remain calm, work out his Sleep Bus windows based on his waking time, and settle in to help him.
- Be fair and patient. Don't expect him to learn something in one sleep session, though if it happens that way, be grateful. However, if it takes a little longer, remember he's learning something brand new. Support him patiently and consistently until he's able to understand and feel comfortable with the new way of going to sleep.
- Always make sure your baby knows you've left the room. Don't sneak off and avoid putting him to sleep. Say your cues more loudly if you suspect he's drifting off, cut the song short if needs be, shuffle out of the room so he hears you leaving and click the door shut so he hears the door close.
- Never just 'give it a try' when it comes to settling or resettling, then stop trying if he doesn't go back to sleep immediately. Be aware of the definition you're giving your settling cues and any requests to go to sleep or back to sleep. You'll need to follow through until the end of that particular (or typical) sleep window.
- Don't alter the routine backwards or forwards to suit his waking time each morning. If you want to quickly resolve his sleep, work with a set window and wait for his body to settle into the predictable pattern. If you're on a suggested routine or you've developed one of your own, lock in your windows for sleep. Once in a routine, ensure you don't overwork the hours awake between sleeps or tired signs or it can result in yoyo days and an unsettled baby who doesn't have the assistance of a locked-in settling and solid sleep window in her circadian rhythm.
- Never compensate for poor sleep at the right time with good sleep at the wrong time, or you perpetuate the cycle of poor sleep.

Before you start

Once you've ticked off your checklist above and developed a clear style of communication and established all the skills a baby or toddler needs to be confident with sleep time, any crying a child does when introduced to the settling process will be short lived and he'll soon be ready to learn to put himself to sleep without assistance. Try to see past any first few difficult days of your new sleep program, including your baby being very sleepy during the day and crying during the transition to new routines, because it's very short term compared to what might lie ahead if you don't give him a chance to find a more restful way to go to sleep and sleep through the night.

Please put a normal amount of crying/communication from your child into perspective as a natural response to new scenarios and situations. Be prepared for some tears if your baby is unfamiliar with a request, and help him through it with reassurance until he feels more comfortable about it.

If you start with a realistic expectation of your baby's response as he experiences something new, and have a realistic expectation of your role as you support him through that change, if there are no tears – which is not that uncommon with a baby under two – then it will be wonderful. If there are tears, however, be confident enough to be able to reassure him over a short period (a few days) until he learns a new peaceful, long-term solution to sleep.

So there are two things you need to bear in mind when your child starts to cry:

1. Not all crying means he's in distress, or that you need to fix it or stop it from occurring. Some cries simply mean 'Hey, I was playing with that' or 'I don't feel like doing that' or 'Pick me up please, I'm bored and want to see what you're doing' or 'I'm feeling a bit tired'. It's important to allow your child to experience this normal range of feelings because it's normal and safe to feel tired, and he shouldn't feel frightened of it.
2. Your response as a parent to your child's crying when he's feeling any of the natural array of emotions tells him whether those emotions are normal and safe and something he can cope with, or abnormal and unsafe and someone else needs to fix them for him because he's incapable of doing so.

When you over-respond to a child crying because he feels tired or hungry or frustrated, it suggests to the child that something unsafe is occurring and his response to day-to-day events can become imbalanced.

I'm not saying 'never respond to or support your child' when he feels natural and safe emotions, I'm saying 'balance' your approach to natural emotions. Overreacting to stop a child from crying does nothing to empower him with the coping skills he needs to deal with the feeling of being tired, or to learn how to go to sleep without tears. This also applies to normal and natural feelings at non-sleep times of the day, like frustration, boredom, impatience or general irritation at having to do something dull like have his nappy changed *again* when he'd rather play, or playing on his own when he'd rather you carry him all day.

However, this principle *does not* apply to emotions that clearly indicate a baby needs reassurance and comfort to feel better, like when he gets a fright, or feels pain, or is ill. A child needs help to work through these situations because it's too much for him to cope with them on his own.

Starting during the day

Helping your child feel comfortable with the array of emotions and feelings he experiences during the day will lead to him feeling secure and peaceful when he's in her own cot or bed going to sleep independently. This is achieved by remaining confident and reassuring, stopping yourself from reacting too quickly and seeing what he's actually saying or doing, and waiting to see if he can get past it without too much intervention from you if it isn't necessary.

By learning to listen to what he's trying to say throughout the day, and deciding when it's *truly* appropriate to intervene and assist him through a particular scenario, you give your child the opportunity to learn to experience, assess and become more comfortable with his natural ebbs and flows physically, emotionally and intellectually. This is crucial for managing your child's settling routines. By showing him a way to work through a situation or how to settle down from a natural feeling that doesn't require your full intervention through the day at non-sleep times, he quickly learns that there are some emotions he can trust and learn to resolve, which will no longer feel uncomfortable or unmanageable for him, particularly at sleep time.

Sometimes you can let him express frustration at a toy and then let him work through it without trying to take that feeling away by immediately fixing it. If you can teach him that lying down and waiting while you change his nappy, or waiting in the pram while you're in the check-out line, or sitting in the high chair after his meal is completed before he gets up, are normal, safe and manageable, with a little practice they'll no longer be situations that evoke protests or tears.

This is very important to understand because when you and your child have had the opportunity to feel comfortable with his natural emotional highs and lows through the day, the same principle applies to coping at sleep time, by helping and teaching a child to learn how to deal with the scenario and the feeling of being tired. When a child is tired and you know (even if he doesn't) that he's due for a sleep, tell him via your routine flow that, 'When you're tired we will always read a book, always say goodnight to everyone, I will always sing you this song, I'll always pop you in your bed' and 'I'll always leave you and you will play or lie there peacefully until you go to sleep'. Make this routine repetitious and he will love and embrace it like his favourite book, nursery rhyme or song.

Transitioning your new philosophy to sleep time

Always use an adult's perspective to assess a situation making your child cry. If he's in his room, in his cot, under a roof where he's loved, cared for and safe, asking him to have a sleep when he's tired is entirely reasonable, so you should sound confident, loving and empathetic as you work towards teaching him to go to sleep all by himself. So smile while you settle him, sound like you're singing a loving and beautiful lullaby as you settle him into his cot, even when he's feeling uncomfortable with the new conditions of a settling or resettling routine. This will reassure him, help minimise tears and lead to a quick resolution for two very good reasons: it is fair, and it treats a child in a manner according to his intelligence.

The secrets of sleeping and waking

Understanding what occurs during the process of falling asleep, sleeping and waking provides an insight into what is happening when your baby initially starts to fall asleep, or wakes and starts to cry, and what is normal and natural when teaching or observing your child during any part of his sleep-time process. There are times when your child may naturally cry during the night whether he needs your intervention or not. These times are when your child is:

- falling asleep – known as the ripple effect
- waking up prematurely – the sudden partial waking.

After discussing these, I'll introduce you to the 'Sleep Bus', to help you work out when your child will fall asleep after you first put him to bed and again during surface-sleep windows through the night. It will also give you an idea of how long it may take him to go back to sleep if he appears to be wide awake in the middle of the night. This will give you realistic expectations of your baby's sleep, reduce any confusion and help you interpret his crying during settling and resettling periods.

So let's look at what happens as your baby falls asleep.

Falling asleep: the ripple effect

A child takes around three to ten minutes from the moment he starts to drift off to sleep before he falls fully into the deeper sleep cycles. This first three to ten minutes is called a 'surface sleep'. A child may cry intermittently during this falling asleep (three- to ten-minute surface sleep) process.

When you drop a pebble in a pond, it creates ripples. This is a good analogy for falling asleep which is why falling asleep is called 'the ripple effect'. Where you drop the pebble is similar to the point of origin when falling asleep. As the ripples move away from that point of origin they are initially closer together, gradually getting further apart until they are eventually gone. These ripples are a lot like drifting consciousness as a child goes off to sleep. The peak of each ripple is where the child becomes more conscious of his environment, while the lull between the ripples is where he starts to drift into sleep and is no longer conscious of the environment around him. Babies and toddlers ripple between the two states for the first three to ten minutes before finally dropping into a deeper sleep. Remembering that a baby has no concept of sleep: whatever behaviour or crying he was engaged in at the point of origin will be repeated each time he peaks at a ripple until he begins to drift again. This is why he may cry briefly, pause for 30 seconds, then cry again briefly, then pause for a minute, cry again briefly for the last time before falling into a deeper sleep with no more ripples.

Interfering with your baby as he progresses through this pattern will prevent him from going to sleep for a further 20 to 40 minutes, so you need to be mindful of how you manage this falling-asleep process.

Understanding the Sleep Bus

This surface sleep or ripple effect also happens each time he wakes up between sleep cycles and is aligned with your baby's Sleep Bus timetable. The Sleep Bus is an easy analogy to work with. It describes your baby catching the bus, which is the ripple effect or sudden partial waking which lasts for ten minutes just like a bus stopping to pick up passengers at a bus stop. This bus is only around for three to eight minutes each time. When your child's Sleep Bus is due, two things can typically happen on the first few days of your new sleep program as your baby adjusts to falling asleep independently:

1. He resists the Sleep Bus approaching.
2. He gets on the Sleep Bus.

Resistance to the Sleep Bus as it approaches

When your baby's Sleep Bus is due, he'll start to feel the natural sensations of being tired, which include his temperature dropping, hormonal changes, irritated nose and eyes as one nostril closes to reduce oxygen supply to the brain, and light-headedness as the oxygen supply to the brain naturally lowers, helping him fall asleep.

As your baby's new sleeping environment is still to become a familiar place to him, he'll naturally become more insistent with his requests for you to provide his old sleeping conditions as the tired sensation becomes stronger for him. This is when you may hear him call out or cry quite loudly and resist the sensation of feeling tired and falling asleep for a few moments, or a minute or two, even yawning between big loud cries.

It's at this point of starting to fall asleep (the point of origin), when his body is *trying* to pull him into a sleep cycle (the ripple effect or surface sleep) you must be very conscious of not rushing in just moments before he's about to naturally fall asleep (indicated by a slightly louder call out or cry), because a poorly timed attendance won't help him. Often, going in moments before the Sleep Bus arrives will mean his behaviour and crying at the point of origin of sleep will be elevated, causing heightened crying through the ripple effect, making it possible he'll struggle to be able to settle enough to fall asleep in his three- to ten-minute surface-sleep (ripple effect) window. Any poorly timed attendance because he was crying a little louder as he resisted the sensation of feeling tired would then only serve to disrupt him to the point where he misses the Sleep Bus and has another 20 (settling) or 40 (resettling) minutes before the next bus is due and the ripple effect begins again.

Within one to three days, this new sleeping environment will be a familiar place for him, and his own self-settling skills will be his new associations, so sleep will become an easy task for him. All the weeks and months of night wakings will then be behind him because you will have empowered him with the skills to go to and go back to sleep without stress or the need to call out, and without feeling helpless without your full assistance.

Try to remember: this is an adjustment period. Just as you taught him to go to sleep with his old set of associations initially, it's no different as you teach him a new set. It's no different to a child learning to go to sleep in his daddy's arms for the first time, when he's used to being breastfed by Mummy. He just needs to find a new way and a little time and opportunity with loving predictable support.

The Sleep Bus arrives

After your child's Sleep Bus has finally arrived over the next ten minutes you'll discover if he's calm enough at the point of origin to catch the bus to sleep land, or miss it and have to wait for the next bus. Now the bus is there, with the doors open luring him to get on and relax, his cry has changed from that resistant cry to a more sleepy cry – the cry meows or slurs off at the end with what sounds like a downward inflection. Perhaps he's even in a style of cry that becomes a weary 'errr . . . errr . . . errr' though his eyes would be shut. He would do this on your shoulder or in your arms too if he was resisting sleep. This is a typical pattern in a baby who's had difficult time sleeping for weeks or months. As this subtle change appears in his cries, he may begin to have brief pauses (the ripple effect) until it becomes clear he's drifting off to sleep. You can now officially say your baby's Sleep Bus has arrived and all he needs to do is be relaxed enough to catch it.

During this process you'll hear your child starting to fall asleep. This is when he starts to drift in and out of moments of consciousness and increasing intervals of light surface sleep, indicated with pauses, for a period that lasts for no more than three to ten minutes before he becomes fully silent as he falls into a deep sleep.

After a few minutes, he stops surfacing and becoming aware, and is asleep. As a baby has no concept of sleep, or time lapsing, if he was in a settling cry before he drifted off, when he surfaces at the next ripple peak 30 seconds later, he will resume his settling cry unaware he's just been drifting. The peaks or surfaces are only brief and may involve five to ten seconds of a little sleepy cry, or whatever cry he was in when the bus arrived (the point of origin). The next ripple will then be a little further away and, despite a one-minute pause, he may briefly resume his settling cry (or whatever cry he was in when the Sleep Bus arrived) before drifting again. This will continue for a short period, and varies from baby to baby. The surface sleep ends after around three to eight minutes and he'll finally dip off into a deeper sleep cycle. Either that, or he'll climb off the bus and miss it.

Occasionally, even if he's very tired and does drift on and off while the Sleep Bus is there, if he's finding the first day or two with new sleeping conditions and/or routine challenging, or he's an unsettled baby, he may cry enough at one or more peaks to not allow him to go to sleep, and he'll get off the bus and miss it. Occasionally, if he wants you to do something, he'll remain resistant to the Sleep Bus and not even pause through the ripple effect even if he's slurring and yawning. This means you need to wait for the next Sleep Bus to arrive. Once you know he's missed the Sleep Bus, indicated by the window of opportunity ending and his cries returning to the pre-Sleep Bus elevated levels, go in and attend to him after assessing his cries, do your resettling routine, and continue to support him with consistent visits based on what he's 'saying' to you, until the next bus is due.

If he does miss the bus, don't despair. He may need some time to adjust during the first few days of learning something new. Be patient and have realistic expectations. He may just need to say, 'This is different, am I okay?' a few times until he's certain he's okay, and you're always there for him even though things have changed a bit, and he'll then fall asleep. This is particularly likely if he's been terribly unsettled, has had strategies like control crying used on him with no positive results (so he's learnt to be a resilient crier), or his or your family's health is at a crisis point. This adjustment and processing time is not uncommon but yields a calm, settled baby within two days of consistent communication and support. Stay confident that you're doing the right thing for your terribly tired baby.

Waking up prematurely: the sudden partial waking

Babies aged six to 24 months only become partially conscious when they wake up during any incomplete sleep session, and won't be fully aware of their surroundings for a full three to ten minutes. Children in this state might be standing, sitting, crying or have their eyes open, but won't yet be fully conscious. This is called a sudden partial waking and can function in a similar way to the ripple effect. At the end of this three- to eight-minute window, they will either be fully aware of their environment and awake or have gone back to sleep. This is an important part of managing their sleep and can make a big difference to your and your baby's success.

This is where the Sleep Bus analogy comes in handy again. The bus pulling up at the bus stop and opening the doors allowing time for people to get on or off the bus is similar to this transitional surface sleep.

Sudden partial waking occurs during the semi-conscious stage, surface sleep. It's the same state you might come to during the night when you adjust your pillow or change positions and go back to sleep. You can go to the bathroom quickly and if you get back into bed soon enough, and don't became too simulated, you'll fall asleep again almost immediately. This transitional window only lasts three to eight minutes, is still considered a sleep pattern, and ends as abruptly as it begins.

The key times for these brief surface-sleep transitions, based on a baby going to bed at 7 p.m., are between 10 and 11 p.m., around 2 a.m. and between 4 and 5 a.m. During the day they're in 20-minute and 40-minute cycles. There are two typical responses you can expect from your child if you go into his room during this transitional window:

1. If you go in too quickly you can quite often startle him, which can result in a very distressed cry where you can't console him which can last for up to 40 minutes.
2. If you go in quickly enough and offer a milk feed, pat on the tummy, or a dummy, you might catch him before he comes to a full waking and he will go back to sleep almost immediately.

The problem with the second response is that you're creating a learnt pattern of dependence for him in this semi-conscious state which he'll then require for all resettlings during the surface-sleep windows.

When he comes to surface sleep he needs to learn to go back to sleep without intervention using the self-settling strategies you've empowered him with through your new settling routines, crying interpretation and support. Because of the risks associated with attending during the three- to eight-minute surface sleep, ensure you create an initial pause time before going in to resettle.

Over the first five days of teaching your baby how to sleep, as he becomes more confident you'll gradually increase the pause time before attending to him and only if he's crying in a way that indicates he needs reassurance. On day one pause for a minimum of five minutes; by day five pause for a full ten minutes as a minimum based on cries. Be careful with your interpretation of his crying in those first ten minutes because attending to him could actually prevent him from going to sleep within the three- to eight-minute sudden partial waking. The result will be that he's woken up or become overstimulated enough in that first ten minutes that you'll need to wait for the next Sleep Bus to come, which won't be for another 40 minutes. This is why crying interpretation – your ability to accurately assess his cry and know when you should go in or give him some space – becomes crucial.

This is not about watching the clock, however, it's about listening to him and determining if your attendance is going to soothe or disrupt your baby.

Settling Sleep Bus timetable

Once you first put your child to bed awake, his window of opportunity to initially fall asleep lasts for three to eight minutes, and occurs only once roughly every 20 minutes from when he's put to bed, if he's on a regular routine, until he finally falls asleep again. For example, a baby who's regularly put to bed at 7 p.m. will have a Sleep Bus timetable pattern like this:

- 1st Sleep Bus arrives at 7.03 p.m. – window lasts from around 7.03 to 7.10.
- 2nd Sleep Bus arrives at 7.23 p.m. – window lasts from 7.23 to 7.30.
- 3rd Sleep Bus arrives at 7.43 p.m. – window lasts from 7.43 to 7.50.
- 4th Sleep Bus arrives at 8.03 p.m. – window lasts from 8.03 to 8.10.

This pattern of 20-minute falling-asleep windows continues in the same way until he catches the Sleep Bus. Knowing this helps when he's quiet for five minutes between buses, then makes a little noise again, because you know he's lying awake waiting for the Sleep Bus. This contrasts to the feeling of not knowing and hoping he's asleep, then hearing him again. Many parents dissolve into tears when they think their child has gone to sleep and then discover he hasn't.

This will give you realistic expectations and something more tangible to work with. Of course there is a chance you will still hear from him until the next Sleep Bus arrives if he misses the first one. Once the Sleep Bus window has passed, you can be sure of the fact that he'll be asleep, and you can expect to not hear from him. Don't be at all concerned about him being awake in her cot alone, wrapped or not. This is an important skill because it means that when the Sleep Bus does arrive, he'll be calm; meaning what he's doing at the point of origin of sleep is not crying; meaning no crying through the ripple effect; meaning your baby will be able to fall asleep. Better still, as he has no concept of sleep, there's a good chance that the next time he wakes he'll be content to lie there through his transitional surface sleep, and not wake fully. This is how your baby can successfully sleep through. This is an empowered, content and peaceful baby.

Resettling Sleep Bus timetable

A child's window of opportunity to fall *back* to sleep after waking midway through a sleep session also lasts only three to eight minutes, but this time only occurs once in about every 40 minutes for the first 80 minutes of a child's waking. If he's still awake by then, he'll return to a single opportunity once every 20 minutes. This is why night wakings are notoriously long and difficult. For example, a baby who has a sudden partial waking at 11 p.m. won't be fully conscious until after 11.10 p.m. and could fall back to sleep again quite quickly. If he doesn't fall asleep in that first three to ten minutes, he becomes fully awake and has to wait for the next Sleep Bus before he can fall asleep again. The timetable for that is as follows:

- 1st Sleep Bus arrives at 11.40 p.m. – window lasts from 11.40 to 11.48.
- 2nd Sleep Bus arrives at 12.20 a.m. – window lasts from 12.20 to 12.28.
- 3rd Sleep Bus arrives at 12.40 a.m. – window lasts from 12.40 to 12.48.
- 4th Sleep Bus arrives at 1.00 a.m. – window lasts from 1.00 to 1.08.
- 5th Sleep Bus arrives at 1.20 a.m. – window lasts from 1.20 to 1.28.

Occasionally, a baby's first bus will come at the 50-minute mark, and then follow the same format as above. This could be because he has a solid 40-minute cycle in addition to his first ten-minute surface sleep. Once you've identified if his first bus is 40 or 50 minutes, that pattern will remain his personal bus timetable. If he has a 50-minute pattern his timetable will look like the following:

- 1st Sleep Bus arrives at 11.50 p.m. – window lasts from 11.50 to 11.58.
- 2nd Sleep Bus arrives at 12.30 a.m. – window lasts from 12.30 to 12.38.
- 3rd Sleep Bus arrives at 12.50 a.m. – window lasts from 12.50 to 12.58.
- 4th Sleep Bus arrives at 1.10 a.m. – window lasts from 1.10 to 1.18.
- 5th Sleep Bus arrives at 1.30 a.m. – window lasts from 1.30 to 1.38.

If you're very lucky, after the first 40- or 50-minute pause, his buses will start to come every 20 minutes from then on. Once you identify your child's timetable, by keeping notes, his timetable will remain the same for him.

This pattern of regular falling to sleep windows continues in the same way until he falls asleep which means you have a realistic expectation of when he'll be able to fall asleep. The predictable timetable helps you not become stressed when he's quiet for five minutes then makes a little noise again, because you know he's just lying there, and there's a chance you'll still hear from him until the next Sleep Bus arrives. Once the Sleep Bus window has passed, you can be secure that he's asleep, and you can expect to not hear from him. If he's missed the bus, you can be aware of when he might be able to fall asleep next.

Locking in your settling Sleep Bus timetable

Locking in your settling Sleep Bus timetable is essential to ensuring your child is settled every time he goes to bed. This is done by developing a daily routine and following it consistently. This then programs his circadian rhythm to prepare for sleep at roughly the same time each day. By following a routine you can help him become tired at a particular time each day so he can recognise the feeling of being tired and always associate it with being put to bed and going to sleep. This means he's always ready for bed when you pop him down during the initial few weeks of his new settling routine and you lock in a settling Sleep Bus timetable.

Without a regular sleep routine, your baby won't be as predictable, but even if you're responding to his tired signs about when to put him to bed, if you pop him down when you first identify his approaching Sleep Bus within the same timeframe each day, you can anticipate the same pattern from six months on.

As discussed, there are two parts to your baby's Sleep Bus timetable:

- during settling: the predictable sleep times he has each day because of his daily routine
- during resettling: the predictable times when he'll be able to go back to sleep during his surface-sleep transitions.

The ability to predict when your baby can resettle after a full waking doesn't depend on locking in a predictable routine. You can basically assess the time he's able to go back to sleep on his waking time. But this entire holistic approach is about avoiding the wakings from happening in the first place, so you never have to deal with crying outside behaviour-based or association-based wakings. For this reason, any wakings outside the typical, transitional, surface-sleep windows of roughly 10 to 11 p.m., 2 a.m. and 4 to 5 a.m. should be investigated to ensure he's in the best position to be able to go back to sleep *before* you try any resettling attempts. If you discover the cause of his night waking you may be able to prevent it through strategic planning rather than ever having to manage crying.

This only leaves your communication ability and his associations and skills to work with at settling to sleep, and resettling back to sleep through any surface-sleep transition windows' mid-sleep cycle. This is why you've done your homework, adjusted his environment, taught him how to cope with being in his cot awake and when you leave the room as well as having developed your ability to ask him to go to sleep for you. If done correctly you can achieve instant results, or results after a 20-minute settle, or results that take a few settling and resettling attempts over a few days. Whatever time it takes, preparing for it correctly and taking every opportunity to prevent the wakings first, then ensuring he can cope with your request to go back to sleep, will be what makes this fast for your baby to learn.

The Sleep Bus gives you an opportunity to:

- be realistic about when your baby can physically fall asleep
- know when it would be destructive to attend to him during a surface sleep.

In order to understand this more clearly, let's look in depth at the settling Sleep Bus timetable of a daily routine for a low-sleep-requirement baby:

6.00 to 6.30 a.m. The Sleep Bus drops child back from dreamland.
8.46/47ish Another Sleep Bus arrives but you need to take him off that bus after his allocated bridging nap time. This means waking him at his allocated nap length. He will happily ride this Sleep Bus for a little or a lot longer time if you let the sleep run its course but then he won't be able to sleep well later the same day, and will sleep poorly that night.
12.02 to 12.05 p.m. Another bus leaves, therefore getting your baby into bed at 12.10 on the first few weeks of his new sleep program is too late and he'll become overtired by the time the next bus arrives. It would be a mistake to wait until 12.20 p.m. to put him to bed as his body will have provided hormones (adrenalin, etc.) that will make him stay awake because he's now even more overtired. If your baby misses this bus his body will send a Sleep Bus every 20 minutes until he catches one and goes to sleep. But once you put your baby into bed, he has to stay there until a Sleep Bus takes him to the land of sleep. To give up and get him up will teach him that your new settling routine and cues mean you'd like him to go to sleep but if he'd rather stay up then he should just cry. Obviously, without a concept of consequences, a baby would opt to stay up and play with Mum and Dad any day or night of the week, but it's not in his best interests to do so.

The evening bus timetable is as follows:
7.03 to 7.05 p.m. The first Sleep Bus will come, but if your baby isn't used to going to bed this early it could take a couple of nights to establish the need for a bus at that time. You may need to lie him down at 7 p.m. each night before his body recognises the need for sleep at that time, as he's already overtired. For the first couple of days, his body will try to sustain him as usual with hormones, including adrenalin, and you might

have a support session here because he's having a little trouble winding down to fall asleep. He's likely to be at his warmest at this time so make sure he doesn't get too hot, by having a fan on in his room for the first few nights, not giving him too warm a bath and not overdressing him for the settling routine. The evening bus timetable on a settling will run to the same format as the midday timetable, departing about every 20 minutes when you first put him to bed.

10.00 p.m. If he's caught the 7 p.m. Sleep Bus, his first surface sleep will be round about now. He may resettle within the first ten minutes. If not, for resettling attempts during the night, the next bus will come roughly 40 to 50 minutes after his initial waking time, then there will be either a Sleep Bus again in 40 minutes or, if you're lucky, every 20 minutes thereafter. So if he wakes at 10 p.m., the next bus will be 10.40–50, then 11.20–30, then 11.40–50, then 12.00–10, and so on. You need to check your watch and be cautious about attending to him around the time a Sleep Bus arrives.

It's vital to be totally consistent with your times in the first three weeks of any positive routine management because he'll still be learning to understand the language and its meaning. Until he's fully able to grasp that concept, work with his body's need for sleep rather than his temperament or his ability to understand that his new cues are not negotiations. After three weeks he will understand the language and be comfortable with what he needs to do, whether he's six months or 22 months old, and he'll be able to comfortably self-settle on request, which will reduce your need to work with his body's biological clock so carefully.

It's important to watch and listen for signs the Sleep Bus is near in order to give you something to target during a long assistance and warn you when it might be disruptive to attend to him. If a bus is due and you're about to attend to him, don't go in until the Sleep Bus has passed and you're sure he's missed it. It's a little difficult to establish exactly when your baby is about to go to sleep, but some things are fairly consistent with most children. Just before he's about to go to sleep and you can hear him sounding tired, he may suddenly try to fight that tired sensation. This is the time to resist the temptation to go in because this (final fight) often results in your baby going to sleep within the next three to eight minutes.

When you're trying to resettle your baby during those first few nights, you need to be prepared for the possibility that it may take you some time and patience to get him to settle himself off to sleep with your assisted self-settling strategy. Remember, there are only two ways for your baby to fall asleep, either by:

- being put to sleep by another (dependent, so will need assistance through the night); or
- putting himself to sleep (independent, so will be comfortable to put himself back to sleep).

He needs to be given the opportunity to learn how to put himself to sleep.

On the first few nights you need to be in the right head space, knowing you've worked hard to come to this new place, and that for the first night or two it will be important to communicate well with your baby so he's not confused. Embrace this time as an opportunity to teach your baby a better way to go to sleep, and go back to sleep. It's about working with all your new skills to empower your baby with the ability to understand this new process and change his sleep permanently.

Once you know your baby has fully woken and got off his Sleep Bus and you've begun the resettling process, it's best not to sleep or even lie down between attendances, even if he's quiet and only calling out occasionally, because it makes it even more tiring for you. Sit up, have a timing device, a pen and a notepad, and work out his Sleep Bus timetable so you have something to work towards. Assess any crying as outlined in the next chapter, remembering that the more you fuss the more he'll cry. Note down when she starts to yawn or sounds like he's about to settle so you can see exactly how often, to the minute, his personal Sleep Bus comes. If you can bear it, read a magazine or watch TV (don't let him hear it though).

Once he's been asleep for ten minutes, get some sleep yourself. Remember: if you do this correctly it should only last one, two or three nights and he'll have a learnt life skill forever. Compare that with your baby waking and crying every night for months or years to come.

While you're teaching him to go to sleep it's important you're considerate of his need to sleep. So:

- don't make a lot of noise right outside his room
- if you use a bathroom near his room, don't flush for a week at night or during his midday sleep
- if he stirs through the night, in the early morning, or through the main day sleeps, don't go to the toilet or make a cup of tea at those times
- don't turn on lights that create even the slightest glow around his door or he may interpret it to mean you're going to come in, and be upset if you don't.

I always say '*No one move* during the (ten-minute) surface-sleep pause time', until the sudden partial-waking phase of his sleep passes. To go in to him before this means he's only slightly aware of his environment but still essentially asleep, and you're waking him up. If you wake him up, he'll be awake for at least 40 minutes. On the first night don't go in during the first ten minutes unless it's absolutely necessary. Once the pause time has passed, you can better determine if you need to attend or not. When you know he's fully awake and you'll need to go in and manage his crying, you can go to the bathroom before attending to him.

Interpreting the cries and learning how to respond

To develop a plan that empowers your child with independent-settling skills, you need to provide assisted self-settling guidance. This is the part of most routine managements that needs extra attention and time to ensure you give him the best chance of learning to cope with the sensation of tiredness at sleep time. The key to your success is in properly assessing the type of cry you're hearing and working out what your child is saying so you can respond appropriately.

In Chapter 6, I discussed some crying you'll encounter during the daytime and playtime portion of your child's day, and typical triggers and management for those cries. However, assisting a baby while he learns how to sleep independently is an entirely different task and requires careful consideration to do correctly.

During sleep time, children's cries fall into two main groups:

- Emotion-based cries: 'I'm feeling overwhelmed. Please help me.'
- Communication-based call outs: these sound like cries because crying is a baby's main form of language.

When your baby cries, you can think 'I've heard him and he's safe, but he still needs to go to sleep and I can't do that for him.' And ask: 'Do I need to attend to him to reassure him and remind him I'm here'? or 'He's just having a grumble, squawk, or a bit of a vocal protest, but he's starting to settle himself down. Do I need to give him some more space without the need for my intervention?'

In answering these questions, be mindful not to create a pattern of attending so frequently your baby is entirely focused on calling for you to come in, meaning he'll never just lie down and to go to sleep or have a little quiet time while he's feeling tired. Before you go in ask yourself whether he's starting to settle himself. Will your attendance serve to stimulate or confuse him? If you know that when you attend to him and leave he'll be in a more elevated state than when you went in, then his cries are possibly only communication based and calling out, which you don't want to encourage so you shouldn't attend too quickly. On the other hand, if there's something wrong, or he's feeling overwhelmed, it's important he knows you'll always come in and reassure him, but your request will remain the same and though you'll help him for as long as he needs, sleep is all you'll be pursuing.

Emotion-based cries

Emotion-based cries need your intervention because they indicate your child is overwhelmed by his feelings. This is when you need to let him know that he's okay and safe, that you've heard her and you will always come if he needs you. The messages you send by the way you sound and how calm, reassuring and consistent you are with your resettling cues, will be two of the most important tools you have.

During his transition from one set of learnt sleep associations to another, you may hear any one of the following emotion-based cries:

- Distressed cry.
- Upset cry.
- Angry cry.

The distressed cry

This is where your baby becomes very upset when you attend to him or as you leave the room. This is usually only ever the extent of this cry, and you're rarely going to hear it outside those moments. It's a very prolonged cry in which he empties his lungs fully with a strong drawn-out cry then goes into a silent cry before he takes a big breath and starts again.

I virtually never hear this cry from a baby in a cot but I'm highlighting it because most people tag just about every cry as a distress cry. You need to be able to listen more carefully than that to truly hear what your child is saying. Obviously, if your child is in this cry it is difficult to listen to and you may want to go in immediately. Always attend to this cry if it does not subside within a minute and very calmly follow your resettling routine and cues.

If your baby is extremely distressed, say your cues slowly up to four times to help him calm down before leaving and giving him space to try and calm himself down. If he's under 12 months, a cry of this level may indicate you haven't catered to his need to be wrapped or tucked in firmly enough so he feels secure and held.

The upset cry

The upset cry usually happens at the end of an angry cry session and indicates your baby is tired and wants to go to sleep but doesn't know how to. This is almost always reserved for the first settling attempt and requires your intervention and reassurance. Your response to him and how confident and reassuring you sound tells him he's safe, and it won't take long before he can go to sleep all by himself. He just needs an opportunity to see that he can relax, and once he's learnt he can relax, he'll be able to self-settle. Always attend to this cry within the times stipulated in 'Supporting babies when they cry'.

The angry cry

The angry cry is very common. It's deeper and raspier than other cries and sounds more like a furious yell. During this cry a baby pauses only to take a breath between loud and furious vocal cry outs. With this cry, a baby is obviously calling out for someone to come and put him to sleep or pick him up immediately. It's deep raspy nature can quickly dry out his throat and he may cough. Unlike the distressed cry, it may not make you want to jump up immediately but it's still difficult to listen to. Your baby is feeling overwhelmed at this stage. Always attend to this cry within the times stipulated in 'Supproting babies when they cry'. Your baby is not being naughty, or having a defiant tantrum, he's feeling overwhelmed, and needs your reassurance to help him relax and understand he's okay.

Just because your child is feeling overwhelmed it doesn't mean you don't maintain your request for sleep, it just means he needs you to reassure him more often at this time, but still remind him it's still for sleep. Many parents say to me 'But he is momentarily worse once I've attended, and it makes him even more upset. Wouldn't it be easier if I don't go in?' My answer to this is always 'No, it is never easier if you don't go in.' PRM is about communication, and your baby is asking, firstly, 'I don't know about this, am I okay?' and, secondly, 'I'm tired, could you do the old things I'm used to?' while he is learning a new way to go to sleep or back to sleep. You should always address his question.

You need to be honest, and show him you'll always come for him, but that he needs to look to you for guidance and you can't go to sleep for him. If you never address this language hurdle, when you do need to attend to him to offer medication, check on him, transition him from one sleep location to another, or for other reasons, the language problem will still exist and he'll always cry, and you'll always have to walk away and leave him alone until he cries himself to sleep. That is not balanced, fair or honest and will remain a problem within your communication because you've never addressed the reason for the crying if you just ignore it.

Once you've balanced the sleep-time scales and your child learns that you govern sleep time and he needs to put himself to sleep, he'll happily sleep and you also can happily come and go from his room without tears or stress. Your baby needs to be able to accept your clear guidance or he will never stay in his room when he's transferred to a bed. By the time he's two, you'll need to have established a clear and respectful line of communication so he doesn't fuss and fight, and the transition to a 'big bed' can be a wonderful confidence-building experience for all.

Communication-based call outs and vocalisation

Communication call outs are different from emotion-based cries because your baby will stop crying out when he hears you approach his room, or turn his door knob, or sees the shadow of your feet under the door, or sees you enter the room, or when you do as he's requesting, such as pick him up, pat him, or put his dummy back in. These cry outs are often interrupted with frequent pauses to hear if you've heard and are coming as requested, or because he's momentarily distracted.

Be cautious about attending to these sorts of cries because you don't want to encourage crying or disrupt settling. These cries are far more common on this program, and the ability to understand your child's style of communication is reassuring and eye-opening for parents. With these cry outs, your child is generally saying something like 'Hey, you usually pat me to sleep, I think you forgot, can you come and do that because I don't know how to go to sleep any other way?' It's during this time when he's calling out because he wants to go to sleep, but he's not in an emotional state, that a child learns to find another way to put himself to sleep, so over-intervening will actually interfere with this very important process.

It's important to listen carefully to your child's language-based cry outs because even when he's insistent and sounds very passionate about what he's asking for, or demanding you do, a child in this state can instantly stop the crying out when the desired outcome is achieved. A good sign that he's not in a cry that is overwhelming is if he can completely stop when you come in the room, or smile at you and raise his arms up to be picked up. But remember, he's not deliberately trying to challenge you, he's just wondering how he can go to sleep without you.

This is why you need to be cautious about how frequently you attend as this can turn into a bit of a game, or he'll stay so focused on trying to get you to come into the room that he's entirely distracted from relaxing and trying to find a new way to cope with feeling tired and going to sleep. Misinterpretation and mismanagement of baby's communication are two of the main reasons a baby will cry for prolonged periods of time. They call out, you come, you go, the pattern continues and he has company while he's waiting for the Sleep Bus, and eventually he falls asleep out of exhaustion. You need to teach him that it's not time for conversations and games once sleep time begins, and if he's not upset emotionally then he needs to focus more on sleep than telling you what to do. In other words, you need to set a healthy boundary at sleep time early on. It's okay to tell your child that at sleep time he doesn't bellow if he's awake. It's okay to ask him to entertain himself until he falls asleep. You so this by not overly responding to language-based cries.

There is no need to be stressed by these cry outs. It only takes a few days for him to learn how to focus more on sleep, and learn how to go to sleep, so long as you interpret and assist his crying and communication in an appropriate manner. The main principle with crying interpretation is to help babies find a way to self-settle. One of the most important tools you can equip him with in his cot is to be okay when he's awake, and to not need entertainment or fussing. This is because when he wakes in the middle of the night, when the rest of us would roll over and drift off back to sleep if we were feeling fine, a baby who is taught to call out and expects to be fussed with simply because he's awake, will wake up and cry, and take longer to learn how to go to sleep and go back to sleep than a child whose cries are carefully interpreted and managed by pausing.

If you want him to go to sleep quickly and cry less, assess his cries. Listen to them in their natural form, not through a monitor blaring ten decibels higher and louder than your child. It's better to listen through the door, though that doesn't mean you should stand at the door. Potter over to the nearest room and listen carefully and quietly without distractions.

There are two identifiable cries in this category:

- The call out/behavioural cry.
- The settling vocal pattern or cry.

The call out/behavioural cry

As mentioned above, these long cry outs start and stop a lot and pause if a baby is distracted. There is rarely a build up in the single cry itself and the call out does not fade off towards the end of the cry. If he does trail off it's because the sensation of feeling tired is starting to take a hold and even though he's still trying to call out he's feeling weary and a bit distracted. There is a clear difference between this cry and the emotion-based cries and that becomes clear when you attend and his cry elevates to an emotion-based angry or upset cry when you leave the room without obliging his demands. If you realise you misjudged a call out and your attendance only caused him to become upset, remember this and offer a little more space before attending to this cry next time. This is not the kind of communication that should get your attention too quickly, and your child needs to take this opportunity to find a way to relax so he can go to sleep rather than rely on you to relax him in order to go to sleep. Sleep is absolutely achievable from this state, and all your child needs at this point is space and time to find his way.

If this cry is persistent and goes on for a long time you may need to think about going in to remind him it's time for sleep. However, if he's having long (a minute or more) pauses between cries, you need to give him space and time to learn how to settle herself.

It's so important that you don't interfere at this point. You want to teach him that being in his cot is normal and lovely and peaceful and nothing to be fretful of, even while he's getting used to her new conditions.

He may call out on and off for 17 minutes between long pauses before he starts to feel angry and need assistance on those first couple of days, and you need to remain focused on listening to his cries and not ignoring what he's saying and going in as soon as you can because you're watching the clock. This approach is about listening and communicating, not clock watching.

The settling vocal pattern or cry

The settling vocal pattern or cry is when a child is not calling out through the door but is vocalising to himself over a few minutes. Often babies will use the settling-down tools you've taught them, such as a rhythmic bottom pat and sh, sh, sh, sh sounds, to help them settle. You may even hear your baby make a cyclic pattern of vocalising or crying as a way of settling off to sleep. This cry will sound like 'cry hic cry, cry hic cry, cry hic cry', or other rhythmic patterns. It is often distinguished by a drop off at the end like a 'meow' or a 'mmm' or 'nnnn' sound. As soon as you hear this sound, almost like a little trailing off or settling himself, you'll know he's starting to feel the tired sensation strongly and he's close to falling asleep or trying hard to use his newfound skills to do as you've asked, fall asleep.

You need to be careful not to interfere with this natural process of falling asleep on his own. It's okay for him to feel a little uncomfortable with feeling tired the first few times you're not there to resolve it for him. This is a short-lived expression of tiredness while he gets used to the new conditions of sleep. You may also hear this cry throughout the night if he has prolonged wakings you don't need to attend to. This will be your child repeating the original settling-down patterns she was using when you first put him to bed.

During the early stages of learning how to self-settle, babies are often more vocal in their self-settling methods, using patterns such as 'uh uh uh' or groaning as they slowly start to wind down into a sleep pattern. If your baby is being vocal it doesn't mean you should intervene. Babies also have non-vocal methods of creating a rhythmic pattern such as repeated patterns with their hands, or rubbing their hair forward. As time progresses they won't need to try to consciously settle themselves (in the way adults would have previously taught them they needed to to be able to fall asleep, such as patting or loud shushing/singing or hair stroking or rapid bouncing that parents often use to teach babies). They will start to lie quietly and drift off in a more peaceful manner.

Sometimes prolonged settling cries indicate babies have come free of their wrap or it's too loose. If this happens you can generally hear movement in his cries – such as kicking in his cry in the form of a wah-ah-ah-ah-ah sound as he moves. If this occurs go in and re-wrap him if he's unable to settle without wrapping. However, try to avoid this by making sure your wrap is nice and secure in the first place or he may continue to focus his attention on getting out of his wrap. Every baby can, with a little persistence, get free of any wraps. It's when the wrap is allowing kicking or excess movement that babies don't settle, so remember the wrap is a comfort device that can prevent or greatly reduce tears if done well.

Responding appropriately to your baby's cries

The different cries are like steps on to a bus. The bottom step is his most unsettled cry (distress cry) and the furthest away from going to sleep a child can be when lying in hehisr cot. The top step is the settling vocalisation/cry, the direction your baby needs to go in to be able to fall asleep on those first few independent-settling occasions. This essentially means that your baby is accepting the sensation of feeling tired and preparing to go to sleep, essentially catching that Sleep Bus. Every time you attend to his crying, he's likely to climb down a step or two as his focus is removed from trying to calm down and go to sleep to trying to get you to pick him up or put him to sleep in the old way. If you're going to attend, you should make sure he's really needing some reassurance, not just calling out.

- Always attend to a distressed cry within a minute or two when you're sure this is the cry he's in and you can see he's feeling overwhelmed. This should rarely happen so make sure you're listening carefully.
- You might decide to repeat your resettling cues and routine three times or even four if it is necessary to help him calm down.
- Always attend to emotionally upset or angry cries within an appropriate timeframe.
- Be cautious around his language call/cry out and behavioural cries and provide more space and time for him to focus on putting himself to sleep.
- Don't disturb him if he's in a settling cry, even if he occasionally calls out.

While he learns how to settle himself off to sleep each cry needs to be consistent *without pause* for the recommended time before you offer your resettling routine. Then, as he gets better with this skill, offer a little more time each night and wean him from the process altogether.

In combination with complete PRM strategies, one in three babies will sleep through without the need for assistance on the first night, another the second night, and the last the third night. Occasionally, some children may take an extra day or so, depending on the extent of their skills before you start the program, or how significant their sleep-time disruption was prior to starting.

Once your child has had the opportunity to practice and discover he can settle himself off to sleep, he will quickly establish a peaceful pattern of going through the settling routine and having you say goodnight and leaving the room. He will feel confident and familiar enough with the new routine to not cry as he's found a new way to go to sleep. Remember that you're not putting your baby to sleep: you're supporting him as he learns how to do it himself.

If he's just calling out, he's only one small step away from trying to put himself to sleep. Attention to detail when it comes to helping him calm down by attending to the right cries at the right time is crucial in seeing him settle quickly and only cry for a short period. Even if he's making a big protest, if you hear him starting to decline in intensity or there's the odd pause, wait a minute or two, allowing him time to calm down. This is the secret to being able to achieve sleep as soon as possible: you attend when he needs reassurance as often as he needs, but as soon as he tries to calm himself down, sometimes indicated by a 'mmm' or 'nnnn' sound on the end of a cry, or the downward inflection like a meow sound, he's doing fine and settling herself well considering it is one of his first attempts.

Don't expect too much of him. Learning how to go to sleep all by yourself is a big new task, and does need a little time to adjust to, but with consistent routines and patience from loving confident parents, he will learn quickly. If you spend the whole time lost in fear and concern because he's crying, you may miss out on seeing how well he's doing. Stay optimistic, and be confident.

Finally, once your baby has shown you he can self-settle, and resettle, be careful about assisting his crying. It's no longer a question of whether he can do it or whether he can cope. You're now assessing possible causes for waking and if they're a behavioural reflection of inconsistencies in your parent-governed line during the day. For example, is he learning that a parent-governed line is negotiable, with lots of tears or tantrums? If so, he'll challenge your parent-governed line at sleep time.

17

Supporting babies when they cry

I always hesitate when parents ask me for timeframes to work with when helping their children learn how to sleep, particularly with how long to allow a child to cry. Rather than clock watching to see if a baby has settled by such-and-such a time, it's better to listen to what a baby is trying to say in order to empower her with the ability to self-settle in as brief a period as possible by accurately assessing her cries.

Having said that, in this Chapter I provide *vague* windows of opportunity to work with. These timeframes offer the *minimum* windows you should leave your child before taking further action.

When to attend after an initial settling

Always be conscious of your baby's Sleep Bus and the natural ripple effect of falling asleep on the first few days.

On day one

When initially settling your baby to sleep wait a solid five minutes after you leave the room and if she cries during that time assess her cries to determine what she's saying and if you should attend to her. If you decide not to attend to her because she's in a language-based call-out cry, you'll no longer be following any timed pause windows. Only once she begins an emotion-based cry where she appears to be finding the situation overwhelming, be it because you're not coming when she calls, or she doesn't know what do on her own when she feels tired, wait for roughly three minutes of consistent crying to be sure you've heard her correctly and to see if she can settle down before assessing her cry and choosing whether to attend to reassure her.

You may need to stop and start your timings because the cry might stop for 30 seconds to a minute, indicating she's in a language-based call-out cry rather than an emotion-based cry. It might also become a random call out between blowing raspberries after a period of time. If so there's no need to continue monitoring the cry and you don't need to attend or you risk her focusing on you rather than sleep. Reserve attending for the times when she's finding the task of sleeping a challenge.

Ensure you interpret her cries carefully after you leave the room and if her cries remain consistent for four to five minutes, with no pauses or changes and fluctuations of more settled times, go in and reassure her using your resettling routine again. Don't add to, change or lengthen the settling routine or you'll teach her to cry to achieve whatever change you've made, which turns the parent-governed line of 'I'd like you to go to sleep now!' to the child-governed line of 'I'd like you to go to sleep, but if you don't want to, just cry!' After you've finished your resettling routine, step out of the room to give her space to focus on the sensation of feeling tired. Repeat this process of assessing her cries and deciding if she's been able to settle herself down or needs to be reassured.

If your baby is feeling overwhelmed and hasn't been able to settle herself, attend to her but be careful not to deliver a message of, 'If you're awake in your cot, focus on calling out to us while you're waiting for the Sleep Bus' because this will perpetuate a cycle of crying. My methodology is about offering comfort and support when babies feel overwhelmed by a task, not if they're just awake or bored or complaining about going to bed or want you to play with them. If when you attend she's able to completely stop if you do as she says, this indicates her cry was language based and you need to set boundaries about what you'd like from her when you request she go to sleep for you.

Be honest with her and say, 'You don't just call out at sleep time, you need go to sleep. If you're having a tricky time we'll always be there for you, but if you're just fussing and being stroppy about going to bed, you need to find a new way.' This means that if her cry hasn't been consistent, or she's having pauses, or is clearly in a call-out cry or settling cry, then stop your timing as you don't need to attend to her. If she's pausing for 30 seconds or more at a time, she's not in an emotion-based cry and she's coping well enough for you to give her some more space to settle herself down. Essentially, you can stop timing her cry unless she starts a cry you interpret as an emotion-based cry, usually indicated by it being consistent, with no changes in crying style, or elevation in crying style.

If she starts crying consistently, start timing the cry again. If she cries on and off for three to five minutes and you've identified that the cry is still not an emotion-based cry, or your baby is pausing enough for you to offer her more time to try to settle herself, then no longer focus on the 'how long' and just focus on listening and interpreting her cries. But if she goes into a consistent cry for 3–5 minutes always attend to her, after timing the cry to ensure you're not disrupting and stimulating her, which will prevent her from settling herself off to sleep, particularly when a Sleep Bus is approaching. If she needs your intervention, enter the room, close the door behind you, sing your cues and leave. By pausing for three minutes once you've identified an emotional cry you ensure you're standing back long enough to hear what she's saying, and to see if she can calm down by herself. If there are no changes in the cry, however, in that next three to five minutes, she needs your reassurance and comfort and you should attend.

Once you've attended to her crying after the initial three to five minutes, try to wait for five-minute intervals before assessing her cry and attending or not attending. If you do need to go into her room, consistently use your resettling routine only, then turn and leave. One of the biggest mistakes I see people making is to focus on going in and trying to make everything better, so the baby never has an opportunity to settle down because they are overstimulated and unable to focus on sleep because they are becoming frustrated by the attendances. So make sure you're correctly interpreting her cries. If she's tired and just needs a little space to settle down, then listen carefully and determine if she's saying she's not coping, or she just needs to be left alone.

When asked to go and observe a family in distress I often feel sad to see babies pushing parents away, arching their back, kicking, screaming and biting because they are just so tired, yet they have no skills to cope on their own either. You can't always be the solution to everything, sometimes they don't want to be fussed with, and they've said 'no' to the breast five times already and no one is listening. This is where a baby needs space.

Remember, if you keep telling her that if she calls out constantly you will go in to her, she will always call out. If you teach her you will always go in when she's not coping, but when you put her to bed she doesn't need to talk through the door or walls, she will start to fill the time between you saying goodnight and her falling asleep with normal baby things such as sucking her thumb, playing with her fingers, twirling her hair or turning her head from side to side. The final result, of giving her that freedom and another way of coping when she's tired, is a more settled baby.

Maintain this management approach of attending to her around every four to five minutes of solid, uninterrupted, consistent, emotion-based style of crying, and stay confident and reassuring during your resettling attempts and cues, while continuing to step back between attendances, and patiently waiting for her to settle down enough to catch the Sleep Bus. Ensure you're assessing her cries accurately. If she's not in the right cry, then you don't need to attend. Remember: done correctly, you will teach her to sleep on the first day or two with fewer tears.

On day two

Repeat the same crying-support pattern of day one but slightly increase the time you give her to settle herself down, knowing she's learning and getting better at it. Be mindful of the ripple effect when initially putting her to bed. After you leave the room for the first time wait six to ten minutes before you assess her cries to determine if you should attend again. From that point on, wait around four to six minutes before assessing the cry and deciding whether to attend. If you have to attend to her a few times, try to wait six minutes before assessing the cry and deciding to attend or not. Again, this is about listening to what she's saying, not about watching the clock. Attend if she needs support and reassurance, but pause longer if she's just calling out or fussing about going to bed.

On day three and onwards

Repeat the same crying-support pattern of day one and day two, knowing that she's starting to know this process and getting very good at it. Move forward your *minimum* pause times by one minute. Be mindful of the ripple effect when initially putting her to bed. Wait a solid seven to ten minutes after you first leave her room before you assess her cries to determine if you should attend or not. If she starts to cry after you've decided not to attend her, then start to monitor and time that cry, waiting a minimum of five to seven minutes before you assess the cry and decide what to do. After a few initial attendances when she's consistently cried with an emotion-based cry, try to also wait seven minutes before assessing the cry again.

After day three, after you first put your baby to bed you only continue to increase the initial pause time by one minute each day until you always give her ten minutes to settle, resulting in her always settling in the first ten minutes. No time-pause changes are needed after the third day and all support from this point on will remain the same five to seven minutes.

Here is an example of what a crying-support session could look like on those first few days:

7.00 p.m.: Bubby down after settling routine completed, parent/carer leaves room.

7.02: Call-out cry begins, on and off, pausing often, no need to monitor cry or time.

7.05: Crying escalates to a more intense upset cry; begin timing, waiting three minutes before assessing crying.

7.08: Crying has not calmed, so attend and use your resettling routine calmly, then leave the room at the end of two full cycles of your singing cues.

7.09: Baby is crying an angry cry; begin monitoring and timing, but allow a three-minute pause if possible from this point on.

7.12: Crying has continued with no pauses, so calmly attend to your baby with your resettling routine before leaving and giving her some space to try again.

7.13: Baby was quiet while you were in the room doing the settling routine, but has peaked in volume since you left, with crying being assessed as upset; begin timing and wait four to five minutes if possible.

7.14: Brief pause in crying then a slight change in cry and loud call outs begin.

7.15: Longer pause in crying, one minute in total, so end timing and only start again if the emotion-based crying begins.

7.16: Call out for 20 seconds then pause. Don't begin timing.

7.17: Crying suddenly starts again and you assess it as intense upset-sounding cry, so begin timing, waiting four to five minutes, if possible, before attending.

7.21: Crying continues with no decrease in intensity and no periods of pause. Attend, do resettling routine and leave quickly. (NB: 7.21 p.m. is the latest you should leave the room if you want to give her enough time to settle down to catch the Sleep Bus.)

7.22: Baby goes into loud upset crying after you leave as she's starting to feel tired, so begin timing again, allowing four to five minutes, if possible, before attending.

7.23: Sleep Bus is due. There is a pause for 30 seconds, a call out for 20 seconds, then another pause.

7.24: Pause continues, so stop timing.

7.25: Pause continues, then a call-out cry for 30 seconds before another pause.

7.26: Call out crying for ten seconds, then a pause.

7.27: Pause continues, then a call out cry for ten seconds. Pause.

7.28: All quiet. She's caught the Sleep Bus!

Note that the Sleep Bus arrived at 7.23 p.m., according to this timetable, and the ripple effect started to slowly pull your baby down into the surface-sleep pattern before the bus doors finally closed and she caught the Sleep Bus – and hopefully it's an express! Be mindful of the typical stops the bus will make through the night when the door opens for three to ten minutes and she enters a surface sleep again.

While this is an example, your first or second crying-support session could go on for longer than this, based on the bus coming every 20 minutes or so on settling, particularly if your child is crying often through her sleep time before the program begins. Try to embrace this first day and night as an important opportunity to be consistent with your new communication, and clear about the new routine's definition and boundaries. This is when babies learn because you're actually teaching them something. Be consistent, follow through, and do your routine correctly, ensuring any crying is brief. This is a really important discussion between you and your baby which helps lift the burden of sleep time off her, helps him relax and allows you to show him a better way to sleep. Be confident about your request so she can see she's perfectly fine, despite things feeling slightly unfamiliar.

Managing sudden partial wakings

Unlike managing your baby's surface sleep from a conscious state, a sudden partial waking occurs when a child comes to a surface sleep from a deeper state of sleep consciousness.

As discussed, we cycle through four stages of consciousness during sleep. The second stage, when we are semi-conscious, is what I call 'surface sleep'. When this occurs mid sleep, it's often referred to as a 'sudden partial waking'. The first time you attend to your child during this state is an important part of sleep support, and integral to how you manage your child's sleep. In particular your use of the surface-sleep pause during this time can make a big difference to her ability to cope and resettle quickly (within ten minutes) or not (minimum of 40 minutes awake).

On the first day of supporting your baby while she learns how to self-settle, in order to avoid long periods of crying, this pause needs to be carefully considered. While you're always aiming to pause at least ten minutes, if your baby's cry sounds very elevated, and there is no pausing, then your initial pause before attending could be as short as five minutes. Please don't attend prior to this time. Seriously consider the cries your baby is having, however, and pause at least five to ten minutes. The reason for this is that once you attend she's very likely to come to a full state of consciousness and you'll need to support her for at least 40 minutes before the next bus arrives. Over the days, this initial five-minute, minimum 'wait' window will gradually build up and your surface-sleep pause times, mid sleep, will always be ten minutes. Within this first week, however, she will start to learn how to self-settle in this time without the need for intervention and you'll never need to go in as she will always resettle without coming to a full-alert state of consciousness.

Once she gets better at going to sleep independently, and the habit of calling out during a surface-sleep pattern declines, these brief sudden partial wakings will become silent. Here is a run-down of how these sudden partial waking 'wait' windows will look as your baby gets better at self-settling and self-resettling.

On day one

Before attending your baby's waking wait a minimum of five minutes, and ten if possible, then assess the cry and decide whether you need to attend or not. If your baby doesn't need attending because her cry isn't emotion-based, resume your normal crying interpretation and support pause times of three to five minutes as outlined above, after the first ten minutes have passed. If you need to attend to your baby, use your resettling routine and cues only.

On day two

Increase your initial pause time by one minute, so wait a minimum of six minutes, and ten minutes if possible, then assess the cry and decide whether you need to attend or not. If your baby doesn't need attending to because her cry is not emotion-based, resume your normal crying interpretation and support pause times of four to six minutes as outlined above, after the first ten minutes have passed. If you do need to attend to your baby, use your resettling routine and cues only.

On day three

Increase your initial pause time by one minute, so wait a minimum of seven minutes, or ten if possible, then assess the cry and decide whether you need to attend or not. If your baby does not need attending to because her cry is not emotion-based, you can resume your normal crying interpretation and support pause times of five to seven minutes as outlined above, after the first ten minutes have passed. If you do need to attend to your baby, use your resettling routine and cues only.

On day four and beyond

Wait a minimum of eight minutes initially, and ten minutes if possible, and on day five you will be pausing for ten minutes anytime she wakes mid sleep before attending. After this initial pause is observed, continue the six- to eight-minutes' pause as you monitor a consistent emotion-based cry. There will be times when you won't need to resettle your baby for a long period because her cries don't fit into the range of cries requiring your reassurance. Don't worry about these longer pauses. This support strategy is designed to promote independent resettling so if she's not getting angry or upset, she's becoming empowered and trying to resettle herself, which is why you're giving her the space to learn to achieve this skill.

Try to remember not to be frightened of her being awake in her cot. This is a life skill, that when learnt, means a healthy night's sleep, and peaceful bedtimes and night times for the whole family. This always results in you never going in before ten minutes have passed, because he will settle herself back to sleep without the need for intervention.

The following is an example of the first night-waking pause time followed by the process of interpreting the cries and pause windows you would follow. You will note that once the *initial* ten minutes of waking have passed, there's no longer a need to observe your designated surface-sleep pause window, only your *usual* pause times of three to five minutes on the first night.

11.00 p.m.: Bubby suddenly wakes after being asleep for some time. Baby is in a sleepy settling cry with the occasional call out. Don't begin timing for this cry.

11.02: Call-out cry begins solidly, pausing occasionally. Do not begin timing for this cry.

11.05: Crying has escalated to an upset cry. Begin timing the cry. As this is not the initial cry-pause window anymore, wait for your usual three to five minutes on the first night before assessing if she can settle down on her own or needs assistance and a reminder you're there, but it is sleep time. Once the initial ten minutes have passed you should be aware that she's come to a more conscious state, and is no longer at risk of creating a session of wild thrashing.

11.08: Crying has not calmed, so you attend, calmly use your resettling routine and leave within a minute.

11.09: Baby has an angry cry. Begin timing, waiting for four minutes if possible.

11.11: Crying has continued with no pauses, so calmly attend to your baby with your resettling routine and leave within a minute.

11.12: Baby was quiet while you were in the room doing the resettling routine, but has now peaked in volume with crying assessed as upset. Begin timing, waiting for four to five minutes if possible.

11.14: Brief pause and slight change in crying; loud call out begins.

11.15: Longer pause, one minute in total. End timing and begin again only if the upset crying begins again.

11.16: Call out for 20 seconds, then pause. No timing begins.

11.17: Crying suddenly starts again and you assess it as an intense upset cry. Begin timing, allowing a four- to five-minute pause, if possible.

11.21: Crying has continued with no decrease in intensity and no periods of pause. Attend to your baby and calmly use your resettling routine.

11.22: Once you've left the room, baby goes into loud frequent call outs. Begin timing, allowing four- or five-minute pause, if possible.

11.23: Crying pauses for 30 seconds, then call-out cry occurs for 20 seconds.

11.24: Pause in crying continues. End timing.

11.25: Pause continues, then call-out cry for 30 seconds, followed by another pause.

11.26: Call out cry for ten seconds, and pause again.

11.27: Pause continues, then call-out cry for ten seconds.

11.28: Angry crying begins. Start timing, allowing four- to five-minute pause, if possible.

11.32: Crying pauses for 40 seconds, followed by a single call-out cry and a pause.

11.33: All is quiet. Baby lying peacefully in bed, but possibly not asleep yet as bus is not due.

11.39: Sudden angry crying, and then pause.

11.40: Sleep bus due. There is a call out for ten seconds, then a ten-second pause.

11.41: Brief call out for five seconds, then pause.

11.43: Brief call out for five seconds, then all is quiet.

While this is an example, your crying support may or may not go on for longer than this on the first day, particularly if your child has been crying often throughout the night already.

Some common triggers of prolonged crying to avoid

These are some of the common triggers of prolonged crying and should be avoided:

- Baby not swaddled due to incorrect perception of what the wrap represents. I'm well known for quick results and one of the tools I use for immediate comfort and quick turnaround (one to three days) is the wrap because it works.
- The swaddle is not firmly enough wrapped due to poor or reluctant technique. Practise!
- Jumping, leg thumping on mattress, climbing out of cot, legs out of cot bars, kicking walls or thrashing in her cot, excessive movement. This is when an older baby needs a leg wrap or a firm tuck-in and Safe T Sleep.
- Sobbing. Some babies sob before they even cry and it's a part of their natural vocalisation in a cry. While this takes a little longer to work through, it's still important to work through their concerns about going to bed and help them learn how to sleep over a few days so they no longer feel the need to cry when placed in bed, and sobbing at sleep time will be a thing of the past.
- Vigorous eye rubbing can trigger eczema or sore eyes. Babies who do this usually need wrapping if they are under 16 months of age.
- Eczema. Needs to be treated.
- Congestion, such as production of excessive saliva or blockage in nose from crying. Some babies block up with swollen nasal passages after a minute of crying. It's unusual, except if one of the parents suffers the same problem.
- The door being open. It's unfair to expect babies to go to sleep when they can hear all their best friends (the family) still playing in the lounge room. As they need sleep, close the door so they can settle without the distraction and frustration of an open doorway that they can't walk through.

- Too many noises disrupting baby: buy a white noise CD to counteract.
- Night lights being on: turn them off.
- Being able to reach the change table so it is distracting: move the cot and change table away from each other.
- Not interpreting and timing the cries correctly: write down what you're hearing in a notepad and carefully listen to what your baby is doing. Look for change in the projection so you know if she's standing or, if she's pausing, if she sounds like she's moving, standing, lying down, kicking, if the cry is being projected for you, or if she's having a little cry to herself as she settles into the feeling of being tired. Write down any clear improvements, no matter how small, and watch out for the Sleep Bus. If you keep an ear out for the 'normal' secrets of falling asleep, it will help you understand what's going on, and to decide whether you should or should not attend.
- Attending too frequently will encourage crying, so be careful not to do so.
- Changes during their day (weekend, visitors, daycare): be prepared for how easily your child can be overstimulated. You will note a change in her sleep over the weekend with both parents home, but more commonly you will see her have a difficult time on Monday when there are less people around. Finally, if you go to a big family barbeque or get together where lots of people handle your under-two year old and take her away from you often, even when she's loving it, it can often trigger a slightly tricky settle.
- Excessive food: make sure food is balanced, and you don't overfeed your child when she sleeps poorly as it will sustain her poor sleep patterns.

When a baby wakes after a good amount of sleep

So your baby has woken at the right time, having slept what you deem a reasonable and healthy amount, and you're not sure whether to wait or go straight in. Your reaction is key to being consistent and predictable with your communication. When you put your baby to bed, you ask her to look to you for guidance and when she cries you use your settling routine and remain consistent with your reassurance but the request to go to sleep remains. If your baby wakes up and cries in the middle of the night, you ask her to look to you for guidance and your resettling routine remains consistent with your reassurance but the request to go to sleep remains the same.

If in the morning your baby wakes up, regardless of whether or not she's slept to the right time, and you immediately go in and pick her up, you're being inconsistent and not delivering the right message. In the middle of the night if she stirs you want her to look around comfortably and relax, so if her body needs her to drift back off to sleep, she's relaxed enough to do so. For this reason also, when she wakes up you need her to be happy to lie awake in her cot for a time, because the Sleep Bus has its door open for a good three to ten minutes through the transitional period or ripple effect, so you don't want to confuse her into thinking she needs you in that time, or it will keep her awake through future day and night stirrings.

If she wakes up and is happy enough, and not in any kind of cry that is concerning, then leave going in to her until the end of that natural sleep window or as close to it as possible. For example, if she usually sleeps for two and a half hours, and she wakes at the hour and a half mark and is only occasionally calling out but is happy to lie in her cot and have a rest for the remainder of the sleep window, this is best thing for her to do. If she wakes at the end of the sleep window, then still attempt to leave her for the usual surface-sleep pause of five to ten minutes to make sure she's fully awake and conscious before attending with your waking routine.

Once you've waited the initial pause, or the extended pause, whichever is more appropriate, then always enter using your waking cue and routine. Always initiate a playtime in the cot, even if it's only brief, as this is you telling her to relax and trust that you will be so predictable she can just lie back and leave all the sleep stuff to you. By the time she's six months old you have three things you generally do like clockwork for your baby at sleep time. They are:

- you ask her to go to sleep
- you ask her to go back to sleep
- you tell her it's time to get up.

This leaves your baby totally burden free and ensures there's no confusion about who is governing sleep time, thus eliminating tears.

Imagine how confusing it would be if you went to great lengths to ask her to go back to sleep when she called out during one of her wakings, yet on another you simply walked in and picked her up when she called out. This is when children become unsettled because they cannot predict your actions. And as children are creatures of habit they will start to create their own little rituals, which may not be in their best interests and can leave them overtired and overburdened with having to guide a parent through a predictable set of conditions for sleep time.

Helping a baby who vomits when she cries, day or night

It's rare for babies to vomit when they cry but it's also one of the most distressing things a parent will have to work through when sleep has gone astray. These patterns of vomiting generally result from control crying strategies that promote leaving a baby to cry in their cot as the only way of managing sleep problems, which doesn't address the real reason for the anxiety or stress the child feels in the cot. Not surprisingly, babies put through such rigorous and thoughtless strategies can become so distressed they vomit. And once a pattern of vomiting occurs, it often becomes a repeated pattern requiring patience and hard work to correct.

The first step is to address your child's settling, resettling and waking routines. You then need to look at independence issues, and encourage comfort and confidence in the cot environment through cot play at sleep time and independent floor play through the day. Assessing her level of comfort with a parent-governed line of communication is crucial. A parent with a vomiting baby at sleep time needs to have read and started to work through their communication during the day before trying to teach their child to self-settle. Once you've assessed the needs of your baby (see Dream Baby Profile pages 11–12), and empowered her with better coping skills, you'll need to embark on repairing her sleep-time difficulties. You'll only need to take some extra precautions, and use some additional gentle crying-support strategies with care and confidence to help your baby avoid vomiting.

Understanding the triggers of vomiting at sleep time

There is more than one trigger of vomiting at sleep time. Every baby is different but most fit into four main causes:

1. Stress and anxiety.
2. Physiological reasons.
3. Accidental.
4. Attention seeking.

For each trigger, there are things to consider before beginning to repair sleep. For all triggers, however, there are some environmental things that must be added to help your baby move past this situation and achieve sleep quickly.

1. Stress and anxiety around the conditions of sleep can create an elevated level of crying which can result in vomiting. This can often be identified by a baby who becomes stressed to the point of gagging or vomiting when she's taken into her room or during a role-play scenario.

This kind of vomiting is usually the result of a control crying strategy which doesn't address the child's anxieties. This vomiting pattern can also happen during the awake portion of the day if children are exposed to situations they find stressful. For example, when a parent is driving and their baby starts crying to be picked up and the parent is unable to do so for safety or other reasons, the child may become so elevated in her crying that she vomits.

2. A physiological reason for vomiting might be a certain cry – usually an angry cry – causing vibration which triggers the gag reflex or dries out the child's throat. This can often be identified by a child almost spontaneously vomiting when she cries out with a vibrating raspy cry, or starts crying or calling out at a lower level which suddenly increases in intensity resulting in a sudden vomit.

   The other physiological trigger for vomiting can be if a baby over-produces saliva or mucus in her mouth or nose, causing coughing and spluttering and, in more extreme cases, vomiting. You will know your baby has this potential if any attempt, assisted or not, to get her to go to sleep when it doesn't suit her has resulted in messy crying sessions where she coughed and spluttered on the excessive mucus. This can be stressful for her and needs to be managed carefully.

3. Accidental vomiting is more common in babies over 12 months. Some babies will automatically put three or four fingers in their mouth and rest them on their tongue or hold their bottom jaw while they cry. This pattern often happens at a younger age and would occur whether they're being held or not. It's just their way of crying. These babies are less likely to swallow their saliva as they cry and will either aspirate or inhale the pooling fluid, causing them to cough and vomit. Alternatively, the fingers in the mouth with loud crying or calling out accidentally triggers vomiting because the fingers make them gag. The child doesn't know it's her fingers triggering the vomiting so doesn't know to stop doing it when she cries.

4. Attention-seeking vomiting almost always occurs in children 18 month or older and often starts off quite innocently. Perhaps the baby has had a virus that caused vomiting and after the virus the vomiting behaviour continued. This can sometimes be identified by a child vomiting for one parent only or by it becoming a natural part of the tantrum process, or by a child being able to vomit spontaneously without crying. Often, if the parent tries to ignore the pattern, the child points out the vomit to try to achieve a response. The child is not being manipulative, but expressing herself in another way (as unpleasant and difficult as it is).

Prevention before management is my motto with vomiting. Each type of vomiting requires a slightly different approach.

1. Empower your child's emotional tool kit through the day first. Stress- or anxiety-based vomiting should be addressed through communication, solid role-play opportunities for one to two weeks, predictability in the settling, resettling and waking routines and gentle reassurance and consistent crying support. It's also vital to offer some kind of physical security, be it swaddling, a Safe T Sleep, or just the tuck-in technique if she's older. She will need to be managed carefully during the settling routine so you can stay consistent and help her find a better way to go to sleep as quickly as possible. This is vital because she shouldn't have to ever feel this way about sleep.
2. Physiology-based vomiting needs to be addressed using the strategy I outlined, plus pre-emptive crying management. Find plenty of opportunities to guide her gently through the day, for example during nappy changes, getting dressed, the car seat, high chair or quiet sitting on your lap, asking her to play on her own or not picking her up while you're washing the dishes. When you can master the language to help your child accept your guidance through the day without getting to a loud cry, she'll be more comfortable with your guidance at sleep time with less likelihood of vomiting.
3. Eliminating accident-based vomiting can be difficult to do during the day because some babies only put their fingers in their mouth at sleep time. This can be because the baby has been taught that when she feels the tired sensation she needs to have a breast or bottle in her mouth and if she doesn't have either she puts her fingers in her mouth in an attempt to soothe herself to sleep.

   If your child puts her fingers in her mouth you need to patiently discourage the habit by consistently removing her hand and saying 'Hands out of mouth' when she does it. You should make progress within a couple of days, but if not this may be her way of simply being herself and you'll have to wait until she gets used to the settling routine to stop the fingers in her mouth triggering vomiting during those. This means you'll need to manage her fingers being in her mouth, and support her until she achieves sleep. Within one to three days she'll be at ease with the request to go to sleep and the need to comfort herself with fingers in her mouth will pass.
4. Attention-seeking vomiting needs to be addressed through the day first by remaining calm, and not making a fuss about it when it occurs.

With any attention-seeking behaviour, it is the attention the behaviour receives that perpetuates the pattern. Regardless of your interpretation of the attention style you offer (being cross, for example), attention in any form is still attention. Very young children won't understand anger, so trying to be firm, cross, or any similar form of management is entirely fruitless and is likely to exacerbate the problem further.

Once you've addressed the attention-seeking vomiting through the day your baby should have less propensity to use it at sleep time. Unfortunately, if it's a part of her dialogue repertoire, it doesn't guarantee you'll eliminate it from being a part of her communication while first attempting to put her to sleep. Manage her sleep time and repair her sleep quickly to move past this.

For all triggers of vomiting at sleep time

The bulk of your work lies in preparation so your child feels familiar with her new settling routine, has had a chance to become confident with being in her cot awake, and has developed a trust in you leaving the room for short intervals. In addition to lots of predictable role play and confident parent-governed lines of communication so your baby can trust and accept your guidance, this creates a strong foundation for a quick transition into a new, relaxed sleep routine within one to three days.

Any baby or toddler who's learnt how to put *herself* to sleep when she feels tired has only achieved this with a bit of practice, and that has often entailed some crying. Don't be afraid of this crying because it's a normal way for your child to express herself, and always assist her with your regular visits and resettling routine and cues until she is comfortable to go to sleep on her own.

Most people will see a complete turnaround within three days of their child going through the program, but a baby who vomits at sleep time may need a little longer to settle down. If so, seek professional help regarding your plan before commencing. Once your plan is in place, prepare for a smooth management and transitioning from her old way of settling, into a more peaceful routine. You may have difficulty during that first settle or two but remain consistent and contained in how you manage the situation, and continue to support her while requesting sleep.

Managing the vomiting

It will take you a while to get everything organised to deal with the vomiting so plan ahead and make sure you're not rushed on the day you start:

- Put three sets of bedding on the cot mattress – a mattress protector, fitted sheet and beach towel – so if you need to strip the cot there is another layer underneath so you don't have to remake the bed and create more disruption.
- Have a plastic sheet on the floor under your baby's cot and out into the room, then place a towel over the top of that.
- Have a supply of large towels handy in case you need to change the floor towels.
- Have some small towels in the bathroom ready to assist your baby if you need to on the first night or two while you establish the new pattern.
- Have a supply of extra nappies, long-sleeved t-shirts and long, light, cotton pants in the main area of the house so you can take a change of clothes in with you rather than be scrambling around in the dark looking for them.
- Have a little wash basket outside your child's bedroom door.
- Try to have another wrap or comfort item handy just in case you need one.
- Have a beach towel or bowl in the storytelling area in case your child feels unsettled by the concept of sleep when she starts to understand the flow. This allows you to just carry on and not overreact or break the flow of storytelling if the baby vomits. Stay confident and work smoothly and calmly through the situation to help your baby calm down and rely on your comfort and reassurance, rather than be frightened by your reaction to their concerns.

In my experience, I tend to see really stressed children throw up once or twice during storytelling and in their cot once or twice. After this, which happens within the first 24 to 48 hours, the symptoms settle down and the stress is alleviated by the comfort the predictable routine provides.

As no lights can be on in her room, only dimmed lights from the hallway or a distant bedroom should be used, and while it may be a little difficult to see, you should be okay to work quickly when following the instructions.

When they are in your arms

Continue your singing or cues and don't change the tone of your voice. Lean your baby over when she throws up so it goes anywhere but on her, you or the cot, and carry on with your routine. Break your flow to say a gentle 'Oops, little vomit, Mummy wipe you' then wipe her face momentarily *as you continue* to sing and go on with the routine as calmly as normal. This means your baby can vomit if she feels a little stressed and you can reassure her that she's okay by staying calm.

If they have vomited in the cot

Walk in armed with a change of clothes, a damp cloth to wipe her and a dry cloth to wipe the cot bars. Throw these towels in the wash basket at the door while you assess the environment. If she's only thrown up on the floor then fold the towel on the floor and throw it into the basket outside her door and replace the towel. Then simply lie her back down and carry on with your resettling routine.

If she's thrown up a little on herself or the cot and you can wipe it and just remove the beach towel, then that is fine. Say, 'Oops, little vomit, Mummy/Daddy wipe it.' Even if it leaves a few little damp spots it's less disruptive than to completely change her and her bedding (when it is warmer, those small patches will dry quickly). Wipe down the cot bars quickly, then lie her down and carry on with your resettling routine. At no point should you get her out of the cot.

If she's thrown up significantly say, 'Oh dear, bubby had a vomit, Mummy fix it. Sit down, Mummy change you.' Ask her to sit, or place her at one end of the cot so she can wait while you strip the other end of the bed and strip her down. Give her a quick wipe down and wipe the bars. Move her to the dry, clean end of the bed and take the soiled bedding and clothing to the wash basket outside the door. Tell her, 'It's time to get dressed, time for sleep, Mummy and Daddy love you.' Dress her quickly in the cot, while repeating your cues. Lie her down once you've said, 'Lie down' and carry on with the resettling routine as normal.

If you'd like to offer her a sip of water, it should be within the process of the changing and reassuring and it should be predictable for her so it doesn't become too much of a child-governed line of communication during the resettling routine. Before you redress her, instigate that drink time with, 'Have a drink for Mummy please, bubba' and complete that drink time with 'Ta for Mummy' so you can retain the communication stream to ensure you're not being inconsistent or confusing.

Additional crying interpretation and support for vomiting

Some babies vomit when their voice/pitch or the vibration of their vocalisation reaches a certain point. This might be an angry yell for a toddler, or a high-tone cry. The one constant is that it's always a certain cry that triggers the vomiting. This can happen in her cot, her pram, your arms or whenever the child goes into that type of trigger cry. It's fairly common for accidental vomiters to vomit when they get upset in their car seat because they're generally saying 'Pick me up', or 'I want to be upright' and getting the same response – 'You cannot be upright at this particular time'. This is similar to what happens at sleep time when a parent is trying to nurse, rock, pat or settle a baby to sleep, so practising and becoming comfortable with positioning is vital for these particular babies.

In this situation, you need to identify the cry that always precedes your child's vomiting and enter the room quickly but calmly and follow your resettling routine. This means you should be waiting outside her door but don't let her see you or hear you during the pause. Try to wait as long as you can but as soon as you hear her trigger cry, step in and close the door behind you before resettling as usual.

Vomiting is generally a condition that goes away as babies' bodies become less responsive and sensitive to the vibrations certain cries make which stimulates their gag reflex. The purpose of this is to train the gag reflex to be less responsive to normal cries, so allow her to express herself naturally through the day and respond with your usual crying-support strategy. Only be immediately responsive to this particular cry when you know she might vomit at sleep time. Remember, though, when your baby has been asleep all night and has woken early there will probably not be as urgent a need for this pre-emptive intervention as her tummy will be empty.

Troubleshooting

Q: If my baby's been sick, can I take her out of her cot?

A: Whenever possible, after your baby vomits do everything in as smooth and uncomplicated a manner as possible to ensure you're not teaching her that she needs to vomit to be picked up. Keep her in the cot while you change her and the bedding and clean the cot.

Q: My baby did a very big vomit. Should I feed her again?

A: If your baby's done a big vomit don't feed her again. It's her overall food intake during the day that impacts on her hunger, not the last meal or milk feed of the day. If she's had a good breakfast and lunch and you've made sure she's well hydrated she'll be fine. She'll keep throwing up if you keep filling her tummy.

Q: How can I be sure it's not teething which is making my baby put her fingers in her mouth?

A: Babies don't suddenly start to teeth when you put them to bed, so if your baby hasn't been exhibiting this behaviour during the day, and she's not been teething through the day, then teething is not the cause of this behaviour. Fingers in the mouth for crying is common. If she's teething, you're more likely to hear from her between 11.30 p.m. and 1.30 a.m. or 2.30 and 3.30 a.m. If she's been teething through the day, offer pain relief or teething gel half an hour before bedtime, and keep the doses up at any required attendances through the night.

Q: Can I offer her a drink of water after she's been sick?
A: If you offer her water after she's vomited, do so using a spill-proof cup. Ensure you retain the parent-governed line of communication by saying, 'Have a drink for Mummy.' And when she's finished say, 'Ta for Mummy, Mummy take the cup.'

Q: My child is asking for things (food, drink, milk, toys, other parent, etc.) when she's sick. What should I do?
A: If your child is asking for things when she's sick, just continue your normal resettling routine. You shouldn't negotiate at sleep time while you're teaching her how to go to sleep without crying. If you allow for negotiations at sleep time, you no longer hold the governing line of communication and this will result in elevated crying when you ask her to go to sleep. As with any resettling routine, don't deviate from your clear, loving and gentle routine. If she's been sick, you can offer water as outlined above, then carry on with your resettling routine.

Q: In the morning, when my baby wakes, she goes into that trigger cry but doesn't vomit. Do I still need to pre-empt it and rush in?
A: No, if your baby wakes when she goes into her trigger cry, only respond as described in this chapter.

The three week settling window

The sudden sleep adjustment

It's not uncommon for parents to have instant success using their new routine management with an almost miraculous increase in their child's consistent sleep intake, and a dramatic increase in her overall daily sleep requirement. Suddenly their baby has gone from sleeping 30-minute catnaps and waking 12 times a night to sleeping for two and a half hours at a time during the day and 11 hours straight at night. This would be a fairy tale if it lasted but it doesn't always happen.

There may be a small price to pay if things happen really quickly. For parents who initially don't have to do much crying support there's an adjustment period in which their baby feels well slept and may wake for a period through the night. If this happens to you, don't panic or think your baby has gone back to her old ways or backwards. This is simply a balancing effect. Manage the waking with your settling or resettling routines, and maintain your routine plan, ensuring you don't suddenly offer more sleep, or longer naps, or later sleep to compensate for the waking, otherwise you'll perpetuate the prolonged wakings and encourage her to continue night after night. Whether you're on a PRM routine or following your own routine, don't compensate with excess, early or too much food or sleep.

Once the adjustment days have passed, which is usually on the third to fifth day, you'll find your baby has settled into a more average pattern of sleep.

For those who have to do some work during the first few days, this adjustment period tends not to occur as your child's need for sleep gradually increases over the one-week window rather than all at once on the first and second day.

The two- to three-week sleep adjustment

Once babies start to catch up with consistent sleep, adjustments typically occur between the second and third week. For a low-sleep-requirement child there may be a change to her midday sleep, and for a high-sleep-requirement child there may be changes to her second long sleep of the day. At some point over this time the body's need for daytime sleep drops, so she wakes early during the day sleeps and it's difficult to resettle her. It's also common to see early morning wakings for a few days also. Here are a few general rules to adhere to with your baby so it passes quickly:

- She still needs to have playtime in her cot.
- She can't have her afternoon milk feeds early.
- She doesn't go to bed earlier that night, or sleep more at another sleep window if she didn't sleep well that day.

As I've said many times already, never compensate for poor sleep at the right time with extra sleep at the wrong time. So don't let her sleep in later the next morning because she's tired after a poor night. The idea is that if she needs more sleep she has to take it when you offer it the following night or you only perpetuate more poor night sleep, making her tired and unhappy. The night-time sleep cycle should be no longer than 11 to 11½ hours initially because anything more will detract from daytime sleep patterns and encourage unsettled nights.

When the long three-week settling period is over

When you've finally reached the time in the routine management where you can almost predict your baby by your watch and everything has settled into a smooth, relaxed rhythm, it's time to gradually reintroduce normal household sounds into her sleep times. When it's time to introduce noise, don't go out and deliberately make a lot of noise because you want her to get used to it, just don't be worried about chatting near her room or as you wander around the house.

For the most part, just be considerate. Think of your baby as you would a houseguest who's really tired and needs to take a nap and if you're using a white noise CD it will take care of the rest. Gradually, over time, it will be fine to reduce the volume setting of the white noise CD so it's just audible. If, however, your baby is particularly sensitive to noise and you notice she's stirring more frequently, keep the volume up high for another three months and then try again.

This is the time you can also start to relax about when and where you take her. The rule of 'no sleep outside routine sleep times' still applies, as do routine sleep and meal times, but you can give her any of her day sleeps in the car, in the pram or at another house. If you plan on having her sleep somewhere else at night or for that dominant daytime sleep try to ensure she has familiar smells around her – worn cot sheets or perhaps one of your used pillowcases placed under her fitted cot sheets should do the trick. Be consistent with her settling routine and your cues and your support of her while she settles. This is her framework for sleep time so she'll need this to be the same in order to go to sleep and stay asleep.

The framework of the settling routine is language based and designed to be used anywhere. Predictability is what makes children comfortable. One of the biggest mistakes you can make is to change their environment *and* their settling routine. The whole world around them can change, but if you stick to the language framework of your settling routine, they have predictability and can cope.

You can go back to having dinner parties and street parties but be aware she can be disturbed by loud laughter and talking. If she wakes don't bring her out to show her off, regardless of requests to do so, unless you're really confident about retaining a parent-governed line of communication so you can pop her back to bed. It takes three weeks of consistent management to lock in a good sleep pattern and just one inconsistent resettle to confuse her and create problems again.

You'll need to settle her as usual using the crying-support technique I've shown you. If you aren't prepared to maintain this approach in front of other people because you're concerned about their reaction you'll need to rethink having guests over until your child is a bit older. For the most part she'll learn quite quickly that your expectations won't change and will settle herself off as usual.

Five out of a baby's seven main daytime sleeps should be in her cot until you're well-practised and confident at settling her. There's a seven-day theory, which says that one day in seven will be unsettled so don't over-analyse if one day isn't so good.

For the next three months make sure everyone involved in settling your child is informed of her routine management. If you haven't trained them into the settling techniques and support of crying strategies, they should not put her to bed because they may undo all the good work you've done and will be doing your baby no favours by changing things around when she's too little to understand.

After months of no sleep or stress around going to bed, and the time and effort you and your baby have put into your routine management it's always a relief to finally have your baby sleeping. I find, however, that this can make the relieved mums or dads tentative about introducing the settling routine to the other parent. If you haven't already introduced the settling routine to the other parent, do so by the three-week mark. The parent who hasn't done any settling will need to role play several times in front of bubby and have talked with you about the routine before they can confidently put the baby to bed for day sleeps first. Once they're confident with the day-sleep settling, you can start to settle your baby on alternate nights.

The general rule of keeping your baby active in the morning should always apply, as she will have good, solid night sleeps from now on. If you plan to go away and sleep somewhere new she should always have her own room. It's too difficult for babies to sleep in the same room as their parents and a lot of problems can start on holidays when a baby shares a room with her parents.

Relaxing the routine

Once you've established a consistent parent-governed line of communication around sleep you'll have earned the freedom to be more flexible. There'll soon come a time when you won't always be able to, or may not want to, put your child to bed at her designated sleep time because of an appointment or special occasion. This is often essential for families but still very much a break from 'the norm' when it comes to a sensitive sleeper. It's fine to do, and I encourage people to explore their baby's coping boundaries and relax when you put her to bed as the premise of this management strategy is to help you learn how to communicate with your baby about sleep time so she can go to sleep when you ask.

The entire program is designed to help you know how much sleep your baby is capable of taking and, therefore, help you plan day sleeps appropriately so you can avoid problems at night. It will also provide insight into knowing exactly what might happen when your child doesn't sleep her usual amount, and how best to recover the following day, so you don't have to see her unsettled and tired for days. A LSR baby can be put on a modified HSR routine (one hour, 15 minute sleeps) to accommodate special events like parties or christenings, or on a day you regularly go out, such as to church. Equally, a HSR baby can be placed on a modified LSR routine (30 to 40 minute bridge naps) to accommodate a special occasion. In both cases be sure to return to your usual routine the following day.

Coping with illness while she is learning how to sleep

It's quite common for a child who's suddenly sleeping for the first time in their entire life to get a cold, particularly a child who was sleeping very poorly before the program began. It's a similar response to when adults go on a holiday after being a little run down and not as well rested as they should be. If this occurs and your child only gets a cold, offer relief medication half an hour before sleep times, and through the night at regular intervals for the first few days of the illness, and carry on with your program as per normal. You may need to use saline drops and an aspirator to clear her nose before feeds or before she goes to bed.

If, on the other hand, your baby suddenly gets a tummy bug, a painful ear infection or a sudden raging temperature, you should stop if she's clearly not coping and needs help. It's not uncommon for a baby who's not well to just want to sleep, so you may choose to continue on your new routine flow as usual. However, if she's sleeping more or looks tired allow her to wake naturally rather than waking her. If you're unable to put her down without assistance, once you change the way you manage your baby at sleep time it's best to stop using the usual settling and resettling routines and *not use* the new language cues so you don't taint them.

The actions you take once you make a statement are what defines each word or statement, and you don't want to confuse your baby and tell her your new settling cues also mean you're going to stay and pat her, etc. To do this would cause your cues to become inconsistent streams of communication she will associate only with your help, and this will stress your baby once she recovers and you try to go back to the self-settling routine. So if she's really unwell and you can't leave her, it may be best to sleep on the couch with her so as to not confuse her about expectations in her cot. Say something like 'Bubby feels sick, Mummy help you fall asleep'. The important thing to note here is that as soon as she's 'started' to recover, you return to your program, and follow through as usual.

Coping with illness once a child has learnt to sleep so you don't lose sleep again

It's important to establish settling and resettling routines so if your child is unwell you can come and go from her room to offer medication or check her temperature without causing her distress when you leave again. It's worth investing a little bit more time into your parent-governed, language-based sleep-time conditions so you have this freedom for management of mild and common illness.

First and foremost, you need to use your instincts when it comes to your child having an illness. Obviously if she has the common cold, is teething, or is generally off colour it's important to retain her normal routine. If possible, only offer her prolonged discomfort relief in the form of approved medicines for sleep time only. Try and give it to her half an hour before you plan to put her to bed and help her settle down with regular attendances, when you can repeat your cues up to four times if she's having a little trouble when you put her to bed initially. Ensure you keep the pain relief doses up (as per the instructions on the medication) through the night if she's inclined to get upset during the night. Be mindful of typical discomfort windows and align medication relief to be at its best through those windows.

In the case of illness the most important thing to maintain during the day is hydration, and there's nothing to be concerned about if she doesn't have much of an appetite for food. This is generally the body's way of focusing on healing rather than digestion and growth, and should be accepted. If, on the other hand, you know she's finding swallowing painful because of an ear infection, blocked nose or sore throat, offering pain relief 30 minutes before a meal is important so she can eat.

Making sure she has the opportunity to drink and stay hydrated (through water and even juice if she's not eating terribly well) is important, as is making sure she's in the best possible position to eat by offering her favourite food, food that is easy, in a casual way with distractions around. When dealing with colds, tilting the bed can help, and a vaporiser is useful to reduce coughing if you keep the room slightly warmed (if it is appropriate to do so without overheating her), and then of course water and sleep are the final keys to healing.

If, however, she's running a new significant temperature and you don't know the cause, it's best to keep a vigil. If she's very hot, lying in bed with two hot bodies won't help her. You're best to stay in her room with her and help her go to sleep that way. If you have any doubt about her condition at any stage during the night always seek medical help from a qualified professional.

Tales of parents sitting up all night by their child while they're unwell are common, and this is a normal part of parenthood. It's important to remember that she would need to be quite unwell to warrant that kind of attention, so don't apply this sleep support to all forms of common illness. If she's that unwell, you would already have taken her to the doctor.

While she's unwell you may choose to put less clothing on her and allow her to sleep longer in the morning or take all the sleep she wants at whatever time during the day. If she has an ear infection, lying flat can be painful, so prop her mattress up and give her pain relief as suggested for her age on the bottle.

It's important that as soon as she starts to get better, you put her straight back on to your routine. Don't wait until she's fully recovered as bad habits can form by then and you may have a bigger job on your hands than normal. Try to keep the routine as close to normal as possible. You may have to deal with a few battles when you first go back to your normal routine. Your success will lie in how consistent and clear you are on the first day back into the routine. If you're completely consistent and clear it should only take a day, maybe two or three at the most, to get her back on track. However, if you try to introduce things gradually or in bits and pieces it's likely to go pear-shaped.

At the end of the day you will have to use your instinct and/or a doctor to determine whether you think she's recovering or not. In my experience, parents have an amazing sixth sense when it comes to their baby, so always listen to your intuition when it comes to illness.

18

Sleep resource encyclopedia

Most adults find the prospect of travel thrilling and are able to anticipate different environments with excitement. However, babies and young children are creatures of habit and like to feel in control of their surroundings by being able to predict them, so sleeping elsewhere can be challenging. This is why, to help your baby be flexible and make travel as easy as possible, you should use a language-based framework during their normal event and daily routines. Your baby then relies predominantly on your communication and a transportable series of actions around any normal daily event, like a settling routine for instance, so you can literally pick up their predictable framework and take it with you anywhere you go.

A language-based framework involves using your flow of communication around times of the day like sleeping, bathing, eating, nappy changes, dressing, going out and playtime. This ensures your child doesn't become dependent on the home environment as the only set of conditions in which he feels comfortable when given a particular request. Just because there's a cot in a new room doesn't mean the child understands you'd like him to sleep in that new room and cot. The same goes for an unfamiliar high chair, change mat, or a tent, caravan or cabin.

Classic language-based routines that are transportable and I've discussed in this book include:

- your flow of communication to keep your child well informed
- settling, resettling and waking routines for sleep time
- sit down/lie down cues for the car seat, pram, high chair, change table, bath
- role-play games and teddy-bear attachment.

In addition to the communication needs of your child being provided for, you also need to cater for the environmental needs of your baby in a new place by:

- making the sleep environment smell familiar by using his two-days' worn and unwashed cot sheets, pyjamas, wraps and comfort items, and placing one of Mum or Dad's used pillowcases under his fitted sheet to allow familiar, safe smells to permeate the cot environment
- getting him used to a travel cot at home before using it while travelling
- having environmental aids that are transportable
- creating a darker environment or darkening a room elsewhere so he's less likely to wake up and, forgetting he's somewhere new, be disorientated. The best thing to do is to limit his view of a foreign room for the first two days.

Once you're comfortable with your language-based settling routines and listening skills at home, and you've catered for his environmental needs by making sure the room smells and feels familiar to him, prepare and orientate him when you arrive at the new destination. He should see his familiar travel cot constructed, or his bed made with the usual things once she's over eight months. He needs to be told it's his cot for nigh' nigh's. By making a statement like, 'Look, Max's cot for nigh' nigh's' or 'Oh, nice cot, this is Max's time-for-sleep cot' he will quickly understand the statement because these words are a part of his usual settling cues: 'Time for sleep' and 'Mummy and Daddy love you, nigh' nigh's'. This means you're able to talk to your child, and explain that this is where he'll be sleeping well before you put him to bed, and this alone goes a long way towards being able to settle him when he goes to bed awake.

The second thing you do is role play a full settling routine with your baby. This gives your child an opportunity to become familiar with the going-to-sleep process, learn that he can not only predict you, but preempt and ultimately feel in control of the settling process because it is so familiar. Role play is the only way you can accurately explain something to a child under two years of age. It gives him an opportunity to indirectly experience the exact scenario he'll encounter at sleep time in the new environment while you're still holding him. He can see and experience going to sleep in a new room with all the familiar environmental conditions by listening to the usual songs, seeing his teddy being tucked in, and hearing his normal settling cues, then see where you'll be once you leave the room. This gives you a valuable opportunity to show you're happy and confident while you put teddy to bed in this new environment. This is one of the most important messages you can pass on to your baby or toddler. If Mummy and Daddy are okay, he can relax and trust the new situation with ease.

Role play is a predictable pattern, and like any other predictable things in early childhood, it becomes an enjoyable game and the associations linked to the settling process as a result are often feelings of warmth, fun and relaxation simply because the baby knows the scenario so well. Just as a child develops a strong sense of pleasure around a familiar book, toy or routine with a grandparent or parent, taking the time to establish and present a predictable game around teaching him the settling process can make bedtime in any environment an absolute breeze.

In this encyclopaedia I'm going to give you more practical information to help you guide your child in the following scenarios:

- Moving room/house.
- Sleeping when out:
  - Car sleep
  - Transferring to and from your car.
- Plane sleep, or sleeping in your arms.
- Sleeping in hotels/other houses.
- Adjusting to daylight savings.
- Changing time zones.
- Going back to work/others caring for your child.

Moving room/house

While some babies and toddlers may not be bothered by all the commotion and stress of moving room or house, others will find this a very challenging time. It can be particularly difficult because unpredictability makes him feel insecure. His entire universe under the age of two years generally consists of his primary carers (those living with, and taking full-time care of him) and the room he sleeps in and the house he lives in. When he starts to predict the flow of behaviour of the people in the house, he feels relaxed. When that suddenly changes, it can leave him feeling insecure, and you may find he needs to cling on to adults in order to feel more comfortable when experiencing unfamiliar events and environments.

When the whole house is being prepared and packed ready for a move, not only is the environment changing, but a parent is no longer following the usual routine. They are usually busy racing around sorting and preparing for the move. The normal flow of the day is disrupted with phone calls, packing boxes and rushed-feeling days. This results in an unsettled and clingy baby, and disrupted sleep is almost always a by-product. The following steps will help you calm your baby, keep him well informed and help you maintain his sleep through a house move:

- Keep him informed of what is going to happen using your normal flow of communication: break it down to small ten-minute increments of the day if he appears stressed.
- In the lead-up to the move, visit the new house as often as you can.
- Talk about your homes as 'Joseph's new house' and 'Joseph's old house' as you go between so he has a sense of which 'home' he's going to.
- Always sound very positive and happy about 'Joseph's new house'.
- If your child is 12 months plus, allow him to see you packing away his room to go to 'Joseph's new house'.
- If he's 18 months old or more, allow him to pack a box with his favourite things to take in the car with him to the new house.
- Try to have someone care for him on the day of the move so he doesn't need to be a part of the stress, or take him away and allow others to move you.
- Set up your child's main areas of the new house first:
  - Make his room look and feel as close to his old room as possible – you can change it around later if you like, but for the initial few days, it's nice for him to have predictability.
  - Make the cot with used sheets, and dress him in used sleepwear, wraps and comfort items so he has familiar smells on the first night.
  - Prepare the bedroom so it will be darker than the old room for the first week or so to help prevent him becoming confused when he first wakes up and forgets he's in a new house.
  - Set up the lounge room and play areas next.
  - Get the kitchen and his eating environment organised for feeding times.
- Introduce him to the new set-up before you expect him to sleep, play or eat in that new environment, and sound really enthusiastic.

- Role play your sleep settling routine with teddy several times before you put him to bed in his new room the first time.
- Stay with him to play during morning play sessions for the first few days if he's a little unsure, and really enjoy exploring his new environment together.
- Keep him close until he's ready to move away from you rather than just expecting him to be fine.
- Stay confident and relaxed, because your response to the environment will tell him if his feeling of concern is shared by you. You are the one who lets him know that everything is okay by showing that you're okay.
- Be patient and attend to him as often as he needs, but remain consistent. His settling routine and your usual pattern of behaviour are the two predictable things left during a big change. Some parents think they should be different as it's a new place, but this unsettles a child even more.

Sleeping when out

Car sleep

Asking a child to sleep in the car is achievable from six months of age if you continue to work with his normal settling routine, regular sleep times and your predictable communication. Most people just hope their baby will conk out once they start driving, but it is also possible to ask your baby to go to sleep, and help him understand he needs to do what he usually does to fall asleep but, this time, in the car. This is possible because you've taught him a clear set of language cues, and attached strong associations to those cues at home through the use of a predictable settling routine. This means he understands you and knows what to do.

Encouraging sleep time in the car is useful for many reasons. It is more pleasant for him on long trips to utilise his sleep time so the trip appears faster for him. It enables you to go on school runs with older siblings and means you can communicate your desire for him to go to sleep, and he will try to go to sleep for you. The following tips will help you encourage sleep in the car:

- If you're planning a two- to three-hour car trip, leave it until his longest daytime sleep session.
- Tell him 'It's nearly time for nigh' nigh's', 'nearly time to sleep in car'.
- Do your normal settling routine at home before you leave, reminding him during stories it's 'Nearly time for nigh' nigh's in Mummy's/ Daddy's car'.

- Once you pop him in the car, buckle him in and offer him comfort items (teddy, dummy, dolly, etc.) – use a dummy chain and clip if he has a dummy, and encourage him to get his dummy by using the language cue 'get your dummy'.
- He obviously can't be wrapped for a car trip so, once he's buckled in, snuggle the muslin around his legs and over him like a sheet – the familiar smell, texture and contact of it as you use your settling-routine language will trigger all the usual sleepy feelings.
- After saying your settling-routine cues, close off all lines of communication, hop in the car and begin your trip, stay quiet until he drifts off to sleep.
- On a long trip, play his usual CD or one of his white noise CDs as these might trigger the old sleepy feelings.
- If you've left earlier than his due sleep time and it is a family outing, get someone to sit in the back seat with him and keep him awake by playing and having some fun games until it's time to stop for lunch – if he is due for morning tea, it can be had on the move (unless it is a breastfeed, naturally) but always try to stop for a leg stretch and little run around at lunch time, maybe in a café or park, before heading back to the car for his settling routine – after which both parents can be in the front seat again and can sit quietly, not talking to him but quietly to each other, until he goes off to sleep.
- If your child becomes upset, respond to his cries and communication as you normally would when assisting him to self-settle. If you do need to offer some support and remind him it's sleep time you should only do it by singing your cues without turning around so you can maintain management if you're driving alone, without becoming distracted from watching the road.
- Continue with appropriate crying pauses, offering support when necessary, but remembering to listen to what he is saying and assessing the request from an adult's perspective; stay confident, loving and calm until he settles down.
- If he chats happily to himself, don't worry, just relax and enjoy your trip knowing he will eventually drift off to sleep.
- When he wakes up, wait your initial surface-sleep pause to ensure he is fully awake and not about to drift off back to sleep then use your usual waking cues and have a chat with him so he knows your sleep-time request is over.
- If you plan on transferring him to a cot, if he wakes when you stop the car, say, 'Time for sleep' and carry on as usual with your settling

routine. Make sure you've set up his room and wraps before you left, knowing you may come home and transition him into his cot. This is far more achievable at night than during the day but can be achieved in the day on a longer sleep window if he hasn't been asleep for too long (longer than one hour, 15 minutes).

- Don't leave him unattended in the car – if you want him to continue sleeping, either take a scenic route until the sleep time is complete or stay in the vehicle with your child with the air conditioning running in a safe, well-shaded place until he wakes up at the appropriate time.
- Make sure your baby is wearing sunscreen for long car trips, and provide a shade cloth on the window nearest him for sun protection and any glare.
- Bridging naps are great sleeps for the car when you have older children who need to be taken to school, even if you need to take a little detour to make your trip home a few minutes longer. It's a great opportunity to drop children off, let your baby have his bridge nap until you arrive at the shops to get any grocery items you may need, then head home in time for morning tea.

Transferring your sleeping baby to and from your car

Transferring a baby or todder without waking him is a fairly difficult task during the day. Some transfer well, others don't. Night transferring is easier because it is dark and during a baby's longest sleep sessions. Below are the strategies that will make the movement of your baby more calm, but I suggest you master the transfer method at night first, always make sure your baby is able to go to sleep for you ordinarily with the settling routine and not cry if he is awake for a short period, and ensure he can play happily in his cot before you attempt to transfer him during day sleeps. If he does wake up during the transfer for day sleeps, what you're aiming for is him lying in his cot quite contentedly until the end of his usual, natural sleep session.

Okay, so you're at your parents' house and your baby was bathed and put down at his usual 7 p.m. sleep time before all the adults ate together. The evening has come to an end, and it's now time to go home. You need to make sure your baby is disrupted as little as possible when getting him from a bed to the car. To do this, say your goodnights to everyone, get yourself organised and pack your car before you go in and get your baby. When it's time to make the move, make sure just Mummy and Daddy are involved. Granny and Grandpa are way too exciting to ensure your baby sustains sleep so he should have already said goodbye before he first went to bed. If you know he is sensitive, ask his adoring grandparents to peep at him from a distance as you leave so your child can't see them.

As you pick up your baby quietly say, 'Time for sleep' and hide his face in your neck while you cradle him to guard his eyes from light or other stimulation. If he is older, encourage him to lie his head on your shoulder by tucking his knees up on your chest and quietly whisper your cues to him. Don't worry if he wakes up, just repeat your cues and buckle him into his car seat telling him, 'You're going home for nigh' nigh' in your cot'. This ensures he knows your intention is to put him in his cot.

You will need to unwrap a swaddled baby first to pop him in his car seat, but just try to keep all stimulation, including eye contact, to a minimum. Respond to any cries he has as you would if he were in his cot, and only use your language cues in the usual way of repeating them twice before staying quiet again and giving him an opportunity to settle down. The cues are meant to reassure him and remind him it's time for sleep, not to make him go to sleep. Only he can do that.

Remember, the more you fuss, the more he'll fuss; so be calm and consistent. If he wakes up fully and is happily looking around all the way home, don't worry; it's okay for him to have a little awake window, but if you become stressed about it he will pick up on your mood and may become difficult to resettle. Remember: you've taught him through his settling routine that it's normal to go into her bed awake, so there is nothing to be anxious about if he wakes up during transfer.

Before you left for your evening out you should have prepared his sleep environment, including putting wraps out on the bed, switching lights off, etc., so everything is ready for your settling routine when you walk back into your house. If he's awake when you get home, tell him, 'It's time for sleep'. When you unbuckle him, either cradle him, shielding his eyes, or carry him, encouraging him to put his head on to your shoulder, and only say your cues to him as you would after stories, and nothing else, while you walk to his room. Respond to any crying in the same way you would during an ordinary settling routine. Once you've practised and mastered this for a good week or two at his usual bedtime, your baby will be familiar with the routine, so there really shouldn't be any tears if you stay confident and remain consistent.

If he's asleep when you take him from the car, stay quiet and take him to his wrap environment to swaddle before going to his room, or take him directly to his room if not swaddling. Close the door and follow your normal settling routine. If he remains sleepy, then skip the song, and just follow your normal settling routine from the tuck-in or lying in the cot portion onwards. Only say your cues once before you leave. Manage any subsequent crying consistently with your usual resettling routine until he settles. Try to remember his Sleep Bus, and his surface-sleep window. Be realistic, if he does stir and become partially aware of his environment you have ten minutes only to get him into bed and to leave him to get himself to sleep. If he doesn't resettle within the surface-sleep window, refer to the resettling Sleep Bus timetable for an idea of how long he could stay awake for.

Pram sleep

Just like car sleep, most people think it's pot luck if your baby or toddler falls asleep in the pram. But once you've established settling, resettling and waking routines, and your child understands the cues, you can step out and *ask* your baby or toddler to go to sleep for you on request, and he will be able to fall asleep with relative ease. Almost every baby I've worked with, who has never slept in their pram before, is able to do so the first day I attempt pram sleep with their settling conditions if I remain calm and consistent with my routine, environment and support.

If you have a child under 12 months of age who still needs a super-snuggly wrap for sleep time at home, then he will need the consistency of being wrapped in the pram too. Once he no longer needs the wrap in his cot, he'll no longer need the wrap in his pram. Make the task of going to sleep easier by both reclining the pram and reducing visual stimulation completely. For under-two year olds have a pram that can be covered so they can go to sleep with as little disruption as possible. Use two muslins in the initial training stage, one that is white and a second that is navy blue, to darken the pram. A mesh sun cover has the added advantage of providing your child a clear signal that it's time for a little snooze. Once he is asleep, you can lift the mesh cover and allow him to sleep under the muslin. When babies or toddlers are tired they become extremely sensitive to stimulation, which is why they become so unsettled. Often, time in the pram is the most stimulating part of the day because there is so much to look at, so if you can reduce that distraction, a tired baby will be able to calm and settle himself quickly.

Babies who know how to go to sleep at home will happily chat to themselves or lie peacefully in the pram until they drop off to sleep. The golden rule of sleep in any new environment is to ensure you've prepared your child well. For pram sleep make the environment clear to him, and ensure he understands your intentions and what you'd like him to do. Any new sleep environment needs to feel familiar to him, and he must be able to cope with the skills required for sleeping or being in any environment. So before you ask your baby to sleep in the pram, help him be comfortable with just sitting in the pram on request, and being still. Obviously sleeping in a pram is harder than sleeping in a cot, so he must be well versed with going to sleep in his cot with your settling routine at home before he experiences the request to put himself to sleep in the pram for the first time. The exception to the rule is the afternoon bridge on PRM 1 where he must sleep from day one.

For babies on a PRM routine, you will need to role play the settling routine with teddy in the pram at home in much the same way you would for the settling routine in the cot, but cover the pram as opposed to closing the door during cot sleep-time role play. When you first try to help him sleep in the pram I usually suggest you stay close to home, and do it during a cooler time of the day. If you're outside, walk in the shade so there isn't too much direct light on the pram, and the pram stays cool. If it's too hot, perhaps head to a local mall that is air conditioned.

There's no need to use the full settling routine for the pram when you're out, but the use of your flow of communication and his normal settling cues and comfort items will help him predict events. Saying, 'Nearly time for sleep, bubba, nearly time for nigh' nigh's' five minutes before you begin your settling routine in the pram will be enough to help him be relaxed when you say, 'It's time for sleep' at the beginning of his sleep time. Once you complete the pram-settling routine (wrap, sing, cues, cover over), if he continues to have a difficult time, use your resettling routine and cues and support of crying technique to help him settle down.

If, however, you're planning to take a walk around your local neighbourhood, you can do the full settling routine at home the first few times you attempt a pram sleep before following through with settling him in the pram, then saying your cues and covering him over. Be ready with your shoes on, bags packed, house keys and mobile phone in your hand, so you can head straight out the door and he is in the best possible position to go to sleep when you use the full settling routine to help him relax. Use this kind of settling routine for pram sleep before attempting to settle him in a more foreign environment without the benefit of calming him down with books.

If your only intention of settling him in the pram is to teach him how to sleep in places other than his cot, before going on a holiday for instance, once he's asleep you can park him quietly under a cool tree where you can see him, or stop at a coffee shop and let him snooze or even come home again. Always apply the pram brake when the pram is stationary, and never let him out of your sight if he is not in a house with you. When you head home, wheel his pram into his room so he can finish his sleep session in the pram. Because the pram is covered, the environment won't have changed. Because he's learnt to sleep in his cot at other times of the day, these sleep associations will not be foreign.

Try to always settle your baby in the pram to sleep for his normal sleep-time duration but be realistic. Babies don't sleep *as* well in their prams or any other environment as they do in their cots or usual sleep locations. Expect him to sleep about half the normal amount of sleep he'd ordinarily take. Don't worry about the shorter sleeps, just stick to your normal daily routine and he'll be perfectly okay.

Pram sleep for an evening meal at a restaurant

If you're going out to dinner and you need to drive to the location of the restaurant, allow a little extra time so your baby or toddler can be walked off to sleep in the pram before you take him into the restaurant. Don't let him go to sleep in the car on the way to the restaurant as this could be problematic for a baby who has had difficulty with settling. Once the pram is set up with his usual comfort items, including his sleeping bag, take him out of the car to wrap him, if doing so. If you have a car with a hatch back or door-opening rear, you can wrap him on a soft blanket in the back of the car, otherwise wrap him in the pram. Ensure you use your usual pre-wrapping and wrapping language cues so he isn't fazed by the unfamiliar wrapping environment. Once wrapped, cradle him in your arms, say your settling cues and sing your settling song before asking him to 'lie down' and putting him in the pram.

Make sure you have all your bags ready and have locked the car before you say your goodnight cues so you can start walking as soon as you cover the pram. Once he's asleep (which won't take long – about five to ten minutes for a baby in a good routine) go in to the restaurant and tuck his pram neatly beside you. Choose an outside table in summer as it's a little quieter, or a corner table so he can be shielded from the bulk of the restaurant chatter by being placed near the wall.

If your baby wakes, try to leave him for the first five to ten minutes in the pram to resettle *if possible*, and then offer a gentle rock of the pram. If he starts crying immediately, give him a gentle rock as soon as you deem necessary to get him to sleep. If you need to use your cues, then just pop your hand in under the cover and pat him and quietly shush him and repeat your cues before continuing the pram rock. If he appears very awake and the chances of resettling him are remote, you can either get him up using your waking cue and allow him to sit and play in his pram or, if you know he really needs to sleep, someone could take him for a bit of a stroll until he drifts off again. It's best to have practised pram sleep outdoors before you brave a restaurant with a troubled sleeper.

Once you've enjoyed your meal out, and hopefully your baby has slept peacefully, remember not to fuss. If he is sleeping, leave him be and don't keep peeping in or disrupting him. When you transfer her back into the car, follow the instructions for car sleep to transition from one sleep environment to the next. The biggest obstacle when it comes to helping your baby become flexible with his sleeping environment is your own fear of it not working. If you adopt an attitude of 'I'll give it a go, it can't hurt', then you can't really go wrong. You will then discover your child's limitations and can plan around those. Some children are just better off sleeping in their cot peacefully with a babysitter than going to a restaurant with you, but if you go on holiday, pram sleep is a valuable skill to have taught him, and very achievable with a bit of persistence and practice even with a previously poor sleeper.

Plane sleep, or sleeping in your arms

Most people find the idea of getting babies to sleep on a plane daunting, but there are only two positions in which they can go to sleep: in someone's arms or in a bassinet. If you face a particularly long flight, it's worth checking in online as soon as the flight opens or getting to the airport as early as possible to secure a bassinet seat, but if this is not possible it is easy to have your baby fall asleep in your arms.

To help you and your baby have an enjoyable flight, make sure you've prepared him for the conditions he will encounter on the plane. If you know he's likely to resist you on the plane, there are a few positioning things you can practise at home to minimise problems. He'll need to know how to sit calmly on your lap and accept your guidance so you can entertain him, or he can entertain himself, on the plane. He will need to remain buckled at least for take-off and landing, and whenever seated for safety reasons, so being able to sit calmly will help reduce the chance of tears or stress for him.

In readiness for plane sleep your baby also needs to be able to lie in your arms as you sing the settling song to him. Practise sitting on a chair in his bedroom for his song for a week prior to the flight so he is familiar with this request. Don't let him get up during the song, or insist on getting into his bed before the song is complete. Ensure you sing the song through twice fully before you place him in his cot. Be very consistent with your request to 'lie down' in your arms at home and be sure to define that statement when it is just the two of you at home. This means any challenge to sit up will have been worked through and he will happily accept your request to lie down for the song on the plane as a result.

If you haven't been allocated a bassinet, once on the plane go to the bathroom and make sure you're comfortable so that once you're back at your seat you can bear the full weight of your baby sleeping in your arms. Ask for a couple of pillows or blankets and get yourself warm and cosy before beginning the settling routine. Use your pre-emptive language, 'Nearly time for sleep', as you read him stories. Complete your stories and pack away as usual, then get him to say goodnight to you and your partner before putting on his sleeping bag or wrapping him on your lap if you're able to – it's a good idea to practise this at home so he is used to you wrapping her this way – then say 'Lie down' as you cradle him in your arms for the usual settling-routine song.

For safety reasons, always ensure his seat belt is fitted to yours and placed around him after he is zipped into his sleeping bag or wrap. That way you won't have to disturb him by putting it on mid sleep if the captain requests it. Draw the window blinds and drape a muslin over your shoulder and your baby so he's only able to see your face and the wall of the plane or the back of your seat if you're not near a window, then begin your settling song. As you sing ensure he stays lying in your arms, even if he resists for a little until he falls asleep.

You will need to be consistent and not worry about others and what they may think if your baby has a temporary protest, even if it is a passionate and loud one. Carry on and know that he will settle down when he can see that this is one of those times when Mummy and Daddy are governing the situation calmly and consistently. Ensure you haven't created a situation where he can negotiate about who is putting him to bed at home or he will try to chop and change settling parents, and sleep is less likely to come peacefully. Once he is asleep and settled, you can either place him calmly into his bassinet, if you have one, or get him comfy on the pillows on your lap and free your arms so you can eat, read or stretch.

Sleeping in hotels/other houses

Establishing a parent-governed, consistent settling routine at home is vital before transferring your request for your baby go to sleep in a new location. You also need to be conscious of making his sleep environment as familiar and safe as possible by catering for his environmental needs, and through role playing. Do this by:

- using unwashed (but not dirty) cot sheets, one of your used pillowcases under the fitted sheet, and used wraps, pyjamas or sleeping bags for familiar smells
- getting your baby used to sleeping in the travel cot at home first
- ensuring he has his own room or space in the new environment by giving him the room you were all offered at, say, a friend's house and you sleeping in the lounge room, or by placing a visual curtain up to separate your child's sleep zone from your own; or at a hotel put up some temporary hooks on the wall and drape a dark sheet over some fishing wire to provide a visual block
- taking any comfort items, white noise or CDs you use at home.

In addition to catering to environmental needs, make sure going to sleep is as easy as possible for him. Be considerate and don't expect him to go to sleep in an unfamiliar environment with a television on, lights blazing and adults chatting within eyeshot. A simple, full visual block like a dark sheet and quietness will simulate an independent sleep environment and make settling much easier for her.

Before you put him to bed for the first time in a foreign environment, role play (for children six to eight months and older) with his normal teddy and usual settling routine. This means he will know where you'll be (on the other side of the sheet), he'll understand your request to go to sleep, and he'll be aware that if he cries you will come. If you're in a hotel, follow your settling routine through in the same way as at home, with two books etc.

If you're staying at a friend's or relative's house, allowing grandparents, cousins or friends to run around while he's settling may make going to bed a challenge. It's best to allow your baby a fun bath time with his grandparents, friends or cousins around but, whether he is six months or two years old, he should say goodnight to others before his final milk feed and settling routine. Once his settling routine begins, he should not see any of the other house guests. Give him around 15 minutes to settle down and get used to a less stimulating environment, before placing him in his cot awake and saying goodnight.

If your baby is upset, be consistent. When things around him change, you shouldn't take away the only predictable thing he has left, which is you and your normal behaviour and communication style. Many people make the mistake of changing the way they support their child in a completely different environment, but to change what he expects actually stresses the child even more. Remember to assess the environment and request from an adult's perspective, and decide if he is or isn't safe. If he's safe, it's in his best interests for you to convey that by remaining calm, confident, reassuring and consistent to help him settle quickly. This means you now do in this new sleep environment just what you would do at home.

Use the same resettling routine and crying-support plan, and the same waking routine and 'playtime in the cot' routine before you pack away and get him up for the rest of his day as at home. This ensures he can rely on you for guidance, can see that everything is predictable, and is able to see that you don't consider this changed environment as anything to be rescued from, thus enabling him to feel more confident about the changes. Maintain your confident parent-governed line of communication and keep him well informed and be the one consistent thing in an inconsistent environment.

Adjusting to daylight saving

On a Sunday morning in spring most Australians and New Zealanders turn their clocks forward an hour, from 2 a.m. to 3 a.m. On a Sunday morning in autumn we turn our clocks back an hour, from 3 a.m. to 2 a.m. It's only an hour, but for a baby it can pose a few problems.

When daylight saving begins – spring forward

The warmer months when we have daylight saving are a lovely time of the year. Because of the movement of the clock, it doesn't feel as hard to wake up or as though there is no day left to yourself when your children go to bed at the end of a long day. The sunrise is at a more social hour of the day (6 a.m. instead of 5 a.m., or sometimes earlier), and your baby's natural alarm clocks (the birds, sun and traffic) peep and zoom happily when the sun comes up, which, conveniently, is the time when your body wants to wake up, and not before.

Before daylight saving begins in the wee small hours of the Sunday morning, let your normal day routine run as usual the day before you change your clocks and, just before you go to bed on the Saturday night, turn your clocks forward an hour. Try and go to bed earlier on that Saturday night because you will, in effect, be losing an hour's sleep because that Sunday will only be 23 hours long.

For those of you on a PRM or time-managed routine with your baby, the transition is simple. Pre-daylight saving, your baby was probably rising a little too early by the clock because the sun was rising earlier, so he will now wake at a more reasonable hour for you by the clock because the sun will be rising later. So set your alarm for your child's designated wake-up time according to the new adjusted time. Hence if your baby has been waking too early, like 5.30 a.m. (normal standard time) because of the light or birds, then the daylight-saving's change will see him now waking at 6.30 a.m. If he doesn't wake naturally by 6.30 a.m. daylight-saving's time, you'll need to wake him, if this is his latest waking time according to his routine.

Without wanting to complicate things, your baby is waking according to his normal routine, or old waking time, but everything on his routine during the day will be shifted forward an hour. When you feed him at 7 a.m. after daylight saving starts, it will be 8 a.m. old time. Once you've woken your child at her routine waking time, follow through with your routine according to the new clock time. Everything will be an hour later than his natural body clock tells him, so don't worry if he takes a little while to fall asleep initially and is a little off his food and yawning at odd times through the day. His body's natural rhythm will settle into the new pattern within one to three days. It takes around three weeks to lock in a new circadian rhythm so stick to your usual routine times for the next three weeks to ensure the best results.

End of daylight saving – fall back

The end of daylight saving is more challenging than the beginning and is more likely to result in early wakings and tired babies for a few days. Stay strong, be patient, and know it's only temporary. You're turning the clock back one hour so 6 a.m. (daylight-saving's time) will become 5 a.m. (standard time) again. In effect, there are 25 hours in this one day.

Based on the standard time, adjust his first day sleep window by pushing it out 30 minutes (see example below). Based on the new time, the adjustment on his second sleep window will be another 30 minutes. An example of this for babies on LSR morning bridge follows.

Daylight-saving time (old time)	Standard time (new time)	Strategy
6 a.m.	5 a.m.	Ideal situation: baby wakes at 6 to 6.30 a.m. and you maintain your routine without changes. Run your day according to the routine, based on the new clock. Worst-case scenario: your baby wakes at 5 a.m. thinking it's 6 a.m. Push the start of the next sleep-window back by 30 minutes (see below). Any further changes below are designed to get him through the day if he's started it an hour early.

Daylight-saving time (old time)	Standard time (new time)	Strategy
8.45	7.45	For LSR morning bridge, begin sleep window half an hour earlier at 8.15 am, standard time.
1 p.m.	12 p.m.	For babies who go to sleep at 12 p.m., keep them up now and they will go down at 12 p.m. standard time. Expect babies to be tired as their morning will be one hour longer than normal if they wake at 5 a.m. and you have to push their sleep windows out.
2	1	Worst-case scenario: babies wake before 1 p.m. They'll need to be resettled until 2.30 p.m. standard time. Any early waking at lunch can only be corrected by putting them down at the right time for the next sleep, according to the new adjusted clock. Either 4.15 p.m. (if bridging) or 7 p.m. (if not bridging).
5.15	4.15	This window is now adjusted. Put your baby down at 4.15 p.m. standard time. Maintain your routine according to your personalised chart. Evening bedtime should be at standard time as per your positive routine management.

The full adjustment is made by the end of the first day. This is just an example, so adjust the times according to your baby's personalised routine management.

If your baby wakes at 5 a.m. new time thinking it's 6 a.m., don't fret. Just expect he'll be a little tired on the first day or two while you make the push into the new clock after a few days of early wakings. His circadian rhythm will still flow in its old pattern for a few days more so don't be alarmed if he still shows tired signs (those waking early for a few days) or alert signs (those waking at the normal time but have to adjust their circadian hunger and tired rhythm to new clock times) according to old daylight-saving's times. You will need to work your way through this patiently; make playtime after dinner longer to pep him up, take a walk in the garden to find the 'birdies' until the sleep waves pass (they should only be ten minutes' long), then carry on as normal.

Don't be tempted to put him down early on the first night back on standard time. His body won't shift into this new time and you'll have the same battle the next morning. This will promote a cycle of early wakings resulting in a tired baby through the day. Babies can make the shift very quickly and be back on track by the next morning if you stick to your plan. This is a new rhythm and, as with all other changes to the body's rhythm, you need to be consistent with your new times until the pattern is established (usually one to three weeks).

When you don't have daylight saving

For those of you who don't have daylight saving but are suffering from the early morning starts of summer, here are some tips to help you get a sleep in past 5 a.m.:

- Reduce the light in your child's room with blackout curtaining. Start with the room being extra dark and then, gradually, as he starts to sleep in longer, begin to introduce more light if he can tolerate it.
- If your child is woken by birds chirping happily in the wee early hours of the day, desensitise him to the noise by using a white noise machine – simply adjust the device to eliminate the sound of the birds chatting without creating a sleep association.
- Don't compensate for a poor sleep at the right time with a good sleep at the wrong time. The best plan with a baby over six months is to find a standard routine that suits and stick to it, regardless of when he wakes. This will take a couple of days and requires patience on your part, but will prevent your baby from waking at 5 a.m. and going back to bed by 7 a.m. to take the remainder of his sleep that should have happened *between* 5 and 7 a.m.

Changing time zones

When you have to make significant time-zone changes, or you're transitioning through multiple time zones in a short period, some juggling may be necessary to help your baby settle into his new surroundings and help you all recover from jet-lag effects quickly. Some babies and parents are very relaxed and don't plan ahead, while others find it crucial. If you don't mind when your baby wakes or falls asleep on your holiday, and he's flexible with sleep, these planning measures aren't likely to be necessary and you'll all fall into a natural pattern.

If, on the other hand, you've had a difficult time with sleep in the past, or are particularly anxious about your child's sleep on holidays from past experience or for other reasons, then these kinds of plans are helpful and comforting and, in some cases, essential in ensuring your holiday isn't a disaster. The strategies in this book are about finding a balance based on yours and your child's needs.

Two common scenarios often occur with domestic and international travel:

- Multiple time-zone changes.
- Single time-zone transitions.

Multiple time-zone changes

In multi-stopover trips it's best to shift your baby's routine into the time zone of the place you'll be staying the longest, rather than change it too often. If, for example, you're travelling from Perth via Melbourne for one day, Sydney for two days then Brisbane for a two-week holiday, you'd work on Brisbane time during the three days in Melbourne and Sydney so your baby is adjusted and settled by the time you arrive in Brisbane.

To do this, the morning your holiday begins, wake your baby so he starts the day on your destination time, then run your routine for the rest of the day based on the times at your destination, even when you're in the stopover places. This may mean that your baby goes to bed for the entire night in the first stopover at 6 p.m., which may be 4 p.m. at home but 7 p.m. in your final destination. This is your ultimate goal, and the reason for waking him early on the morning of your intended travel day: to shift your baby's body clock quickly rather than have him waking at odd times for up to seven days before his body adjusts to the new times.

Some parents like their children to sleep in longer on holidays, and go to bed later at night for convenience's sake, but it doesn't always work. What may happen is your baby ends up waking with the sun occasionally, and sleeping in on other days, which throws his body clock completely, and makes him tired. The ability to transition children quickly into the new time zone is the key to a happy holiday.

Whether it's a trip from London to Turkey, or Perth to Sydney, slight changes in time zones are best dealt with by shifting over into the new time zone on the morning you plan on leaving for your holiday. Bear in mind, you're aiming to achieve a full night's sleep from 7 p.m. (new time zone) to 6 or 7 a.m. (new time zone). Once you have a base to work with (the night settling time on 7 p.m. new time zone, for instance), you can arrange his day sleeps in the right pattern to encourage him at his normal, daily nap intervals.

If the transition is in the reverse order and you have a time shift that requires your baby to sleep in until 9 a.m. in order to fall into a new time zone of 7 a.m., it's not always an easy task. I tend to adjust the routine from the afternoon/evening before and try for a later settling time to push a child into the new pattern. With a six- to 12-month-old baby this can be helped by offering a late nap, between 6 and 7 p.m., of around 20 minutes (low-sleep-requirement babies) or 40 minutes (high-sleep-requirement babies) to help her achieve a later settling time the night before. If he is 12 months plus, you can offer him a bridge nap at 5 or 6 p.m. for 20 minutes to encourage the later settling time.

The later afternoon bridge will ensure your baby stays awake until 9 p.m. to encourage a later sleep in, and a faster transition into the new time zone. If your baby still wakes at his usual 6 to 7 a.m. time on the morning of your trip, you can feed him and resettle him to encourage a wake-up time closer to the time you're wanting to achieve. You will need to adjust his meal plan as well as his sleeping plan. The two run parallel to each other when it comes to adjusting his circadian rhythm. This may mean your baby is up a little at night when you make a stopover, and sleeps more during the day, but this will give you the flexibility to explore new places as he sleeps in his pram, and enjoy some late evening meals and walks.

The most important thing to remember with multi-stopover travel when the transition is the reverse order (9 a.m. = 7 a.m.) is to adjust his night-time sleeping pattern to align with your destination's time zone the evening before you plan on arriving, even if this means his final night cycle happens on the airplane. Be sure to plan your arrival time carefully. Arriving in the middle of the night or at 4 a.m. is never a good thing when you want to adjust body clock quickly. Precious days could be wasted with an exhausted baby and exhausted parents before you all settle into a good rhythm. Book a flight that will have you landing first thing in the morning, preferably, or, at the very least, some time during the day so you can always work your previous, evening sleep cycle around that.

If you land in the morning, it will work in your favour as you can check into your hotel, get his sleep environment organised, and head out for the day, encouraging day sleeps at appropriate times in the pram, and not fall prey to the ever-inviting jet-lag day sleeps that ruin yours and your child's chances of quickly adjusting to the new time zone by discouraging a good first full-night's sleep.

For example, if you're on a 24-hour flight that lands in Italy at 7 a.m. Italian time, ensure you keep your baby going with naps, healthy snacks and well-spaced meal times during the first part of the flight. Then settle him down for a full night's sleep for the final ten to 12 hours of the flight. Alternatively, if your flight lands at 5 p.m. Italian time, ensure he's been up for the day and progressed through the normal breakfast, lunch and dinner times and all his usual sleep times for ten hours prior to landing. This way, he'll be ready to go to bed at 7 to 7.30 p.m. Italian time after you've checked in, set up his cot and role played through the settling routine.

The final leg of your flight should align with your destination time zone so that by the time you land, your child and you will have already started to adjust, and there'll be less chance of him being awake all night and wanting to sleep all day. Obviously, in order to adjust his body clock, you'll need to wake him after appropriate lengths of time, and feed him and provide naps rather than allowing long, full-night sleep patterns through the day, to transition into the new time zone.

Single time-zone transitions

If the amount of time you're going to spend in the first time zone exceeds three days, you should transition your baby into the first stopover's time zone in much the same way you would for domestic or international travel with a single time-zone change. This can be done in two ways depending on whether the time zone you're moving into is earlier or later than your city's time zone. They are:

1. Provide an extra nap later in the day to help him stay awake longer for a late settle time.
2. Wake him earlier on the morning of your travel so he can go to bed earlier in the afternoon for his usual full-night cycle in the new time zone.

This is done in the same way as described in the international zone transition. Plan the previous day to align his night sleep cycle to be in the destination's time zone and ensure his meal times through the day run in correlation with those sleep times. For example, your child's routine at home may look something like this:

6 a.m.: wake
7.00: feed
7.30: breakfast
9.00: nap
9.30: feed
11.30: lunch
12 p.m.: sleep

2.30: feed
4.15: nap
5.30: dinner
6.30: feed
7.00: sleep

If your destination is three hours behind these times, to adjust his and your body clock quickly, adjust him into the new time the morning you plan on flying out. This may appear daunting, but you will have to make the transition anyway, so you're best to adjust on the day of your travel, than waste a day of your holiday adjusting his body clock, or worse still, have a baby or toddler who becomes overtired or is overwhelmed by inconsistent sleep on a number of days.

To do this, you adjust your leaving day's routine to:

4 a.m.: wake
5.00: feed
5.30: breakfast
7.00: nap
7.30: feed
8.30: lunch
9.00: sleep
11.30: feed
1.15 p.m.: nap
2.30: dinner
3.30: feed
4.00: sleep

But your destination's routine clock will read:

6 a.m.: wake
7.00: feed
7.30: breakfast
9.00: nap
9.30: feed
11.30: lunch
12 p.m.: sleep
2.30: feed
4.15: nap
5.30: dinner
6.30: feed
7.00: sleep

This means your child's body clock will be adjusting, and you can adjust him to the new environment with ease and as little stress to him and you as possible.

Going back to work/others caring for your child

Returning to work and leaving their child with a carer is often a great concern for parents planning on maintaining their career. Regardless of a mother's or father's preconceived ideas of what returning to work will be like, the realities of doing so can be extremely daunting and emotionally difficult. The primary concern of most mothers is how her baby, who has virtually been with her from the moment he was conceived, will cope without her present to cater to his emotional needs.

There are many choices of care and environment for your child. You can have him cared for at home, at a family member's house, at a friend's house, in family daycare or in a childcare centre. You can have your child cared for by a nanny, a grandparent, a friend, or a trained childcare worker or teacher in a centre. You can have your child in care full time, part time, or cared for as little as half a day a week.

When returning to work, be conscious of the following things to make the transition as easy as possible for your child:

- Continuity.
- Predictability.
- Frequency.

One of the more difficult scenarios you can place your child in when he's adjusting to you going back to work is allowing a lot of inconsistencies in his week. Having to adjust to three or more carers and multiple environments can leave a child feeling unable to establish himself in any one environment and unsettled as a result. Sleep generally suffers when a child feels nothing is predictable in his day.

As far as possible, try to limit his carers to you and his other parent, plus one other carer, and try to limit his care environment to home plus one other location. When placing a child into care, consecutive days are almost always easier for him to adjust to and recover from each week, than staggered days.

When placing a child into a childcare situation with other children, a minimum of two days is recommended rather than a single day. After working in childcare centres and preschools for many years, the slowest and most difficult adjustments I witnessed occurred when children were only attending the centre one day a week. On the single attendance days, they took longer to become familiar with the carers, the other children and the routine flow of the day.

When placing a child into care in any environment other than home, take the time to have an orientation and slow introduction to that environment. Spend time exploring and enjoying the environment together and start to develop predictable but brief arrival and departure routines. An example of an arrival routine could be something as simple as:

- greet his carer enthusiastically
- unpack his milk cup/bottles/food into the fridge together
- unpack his sleep comforters, whether they're dummies, a wrap or sleeping bag, or his dolly/teddy and place it in or near his cot
- put his bag away and play two activities together before saying goodbye. You could do something fun like put a lipstick kiss on his hand, or a little stamp if he is 12 months or older, then sing a funny little song as the last thing you do before saying a cheery bye bye (long-term absence cues) and heading off to work.

Once you leave, don't return so you can give him a chance to be comforted by his temporary primary caregiver. If you teach your baby that when he cries you will return he's more likely to naturally want you to stay, so he may be more inclined to cry expecting this style of communication to yield the same results of you returning each time. This makes it harder for him to accept comfort from his carer and usually promotes crying and clinginess while you're in that environment. This becomes confusing for him and for you, so make sure you give your child and his new carer a good opportunity to find a way together. Most children settle down very quickly when distracted and will quickly bond with an attentive carer.

Always remember to assess the environment and situation from an adult's perspective. If he is safe but feeling a little unsure of the changes, your response should be empathetic but reassuring and you should remain confident and happy even when he's expressing some concern. Your confidence will be the most reassuring and comforting thing you can provide him in this situation. If his mummy and daddy are okay, he'll generally be able to trust and accept the situation far more quickly than if a parent appears as concerned or unsure as him.

Before you leave him for the first time, be sure he's familiar and confident with the new environment and his carer. He needs to be able to cope with you slowly pulling back your involvement during his play, and learn to eventually cope with short absences while he plays, before you leave for gradually longer intervals.

Initial absences could be as brief as a trip to the toilet using the short-term absence cue you've established and practised at home. Gradually you can step out to make and enjoy a cup of tea, remembering to use your short-term absence cues for an absence of under 15 minutes. Eventually you will build this time and leave him for a few hours in the morning before returning to take him home for a sleep, or attempting a sleep in that environment (depending on where he's being cared for).

If his care environment is a place you often visit as a family as well as have him cared for there (such as a grandparent's or friend's house) establish a clear language cue for the two different scenarios he'll encounter at that house. One cue for your work days, that you use as a part of your flow of communication so he can have forewarning you're planning on leaving him there, and another that will enable him to predict the occasions you will stay with him.

These cues should be a simple language cue like, 'It's Mummy's working day today, Noah's turn to play', or a little routine like a song to the tune of 'This Is the Way We Clap Our Hands' on the way like:

This is the day Mum goes to work, goes to work, goes to work,
This is the day Mum goes to work
And Noah has a play day.

For the occasions you don't plan on leaving your baby, have a very different language cue so your child can predict your movements and not become clingy for the entire visit to the house in anticipation of you leaving him.

When looking for an appropriate centre, look for the more obvious signs of a settled and well-flowing environment as well as for good accreditation. Often people are really impressed with the programming and planning done by long daycare staff and can become easily sold on these points. We're blessed to have high standards of care which are continuously assessed to ensure our children are catered for in the best possible way.

Some of the things to look for when visiting a new centre are:

- staff communication dynamics, including staff–parent, staff–director, director–parent, staff–children and children–staff relationships
- environment: art displayed well with names and dates, which looks as if it's changed regularly; toys put away, and the environment tidy and organised. (If staff don't have time to pack away correctly, or clean up

after meal times in a reasonable timeframe, then they may be under tremendous pressure and not have enough time to really invest in the care of the children and their other duties. This can be problematic because it can mean staff are not happy and, if your child is overly stressed or distracted, this can impact on the children indirectly. This is generally a management or communication problem.)

- a good staff-retention rate
- well-established and practised system of communication between staff and with the parents including daily events, routines and weekly programs
- happy children busily exploring their environment
- flexibility to accept transferable communication; that is, predictable routines that can be transferred from you (the parent) to the new primary caregiver, which is a lovely way of helping your child feel comfortable and able to predict his day even when you aren't there for a little while.

First and foremost, establish a sleep-time settling, resettling and waking routine. Ensure a predictable environment for him to sleep in, and make sure that you, where possible, role play through his usual settling routine in the new cot environment. In addition to developing a language-based settling, resettling and waking routine and teaching it to his carers, ensure you've worked on a long- and short-term absence cue, and some basic forewarning and guiding cues around sitting or lying down for typical events like nappy change, meal times, pram play and getting into the car.

Other carers and your child's sleep

Your child's sleep is an important consideration when deciding who will care for him. If sleep time was challenging for you to repair, maintaining good sleep and your child's trust in his sleep routine and environment will be a priority. The importance of role play and consistency cannot be underestimated in children from eight months onwards, but is still a valuable tool from six months in a child who has found sleep particularly stressful in the past. Once your new carer (in any environment other than a childcare centre) is familiar with his settling routine, your child should be given the opportunity to witness her settling teddy so he can see this is a normal set of conditions to expect from this person, and so avoid tears when he experiences it for the first time with his new minder while you're at work. You've established a predictable set of cues and events that empowers your baby, and it is much easier for your carer to adjust to change and settle your baby a new way, than it is for your baby to adjust to change and settle the way your carer wants to do things. Stick to your sleep routines, and train anyone settling your baby into them. If she is experienced, this should be a simple task for her.

If you have a carer who wants to let your baby guide sleep time, you can run into serious problems. Once you've corrected your sleep-time difficulties by re-establishing a confident guiding style of parenting, it can be confusing for a child to have to deal with a sudden reversal of roles again at sleep time, particularly in those first few months after his sleep disruption has been repaired.

When a child is cared for by grandparents, I think it's important to maintain the child's full sleep-time program and management in order to help him stay calm and relaxed. This also ensures he doesn't become upset when he comes home and has changed sleep association, even if his grandparents are caring for him.

This is often easier said than done, however, and there are certain cultures I've come to understand very well where the concept of asking the grandparent to put the child down for sleep time would be laughable. This means that unless your carers (grandparents or otherwise) are willing to maintain your child's new peaceful sleep program, it's probably easier on the child in the long and short term that you find someone who'll be able to provide the predictability your child needs.

The end result of someone physically teaching a child to rely heavily on others to settle again during the day, particularly after he's learnt the skills of independent settling and been able to go to sleep and stay asleep peacefully, is that the child will suddenly become unsettled again day and night, and will cry when you put him to bed. Try to make sure the person caring for your child understands the difficulty your little one may have had in the past and is respectful of not taking him back to the old ways that made sleep time so difficult for him.

If your child is in a daycare centre environment, time is far more precious to the carers and while all good centres are happy to accommodate your daily sleep routines and incorporate certain aspects of your settling routine, no centre can afford to allocate one entire staff member to a ten-minute settling routine. Stories are not necessary but it's reasonable to expect a staff member to use your pre-emptive language such as, 'It's nearly time for sleep/nigh' nigh's' and your child's normal sleep-time song and settling cues when they are putting your baby/toddler to bed.

If, while in daycare, your baby or toddler is on a little mattress out in the main room with the 'big babies' there's a chance the staff may assist him to go off to sleep with a pat or hair stroke. If your child has just recovered from unsettled sleep patterns and is now able to self-settle, you can request the staff use your usual cues and requests to lie down, etc., but not assist him to sleep through patting or stroking to avoid creating old patterns of expectation which will make sleep at home challenging again.

If your child is upset you can suggest a carer sit next to him, perhaps have a hand gently resting on his back for reassurance, or even sing the sleep-time song to help him settle down, but try to stop all those aids and just sit quietly next to him once he's calmed and is starting to fall asleep.

What to expect when you collect your baby after care

While all our children are so unique, there are some very predictable patterns of behaviour when a parent collects their child from care, whether the child has been there for two hours or a full day. Most people write the behaviour off as tiredness, and in some cases that's true; it can take a good one to two full days to get your child to settle back down and stop being so reactive or grouchy after daycare.

When a child who has been very unsettled but has finally relaxed through balanced communication and confident guidance at home through the PRM program, transitions to being much more self-directed in child-care or care in general, reverting to accepting balanced guidance can be a little challenging for hin at the end of the day. Often, the emotions of seeing one of his parents can be a bit overwhelming, and his desire to have a big cuddle may be quickly followed by him pushing you away. All of this can be a bit unnerving for even the most confident of parents but he's likely to be emotional at seeing you and unsure what to do with himself when he feels this way. Stay confident, smile and take the pressure and focus off him by taking the time to sit and have a little play with his toys until he settles down and comes to you for a cuddle or to join in.

Now is the time to put your flow of communication in place so you can resume guiding and empowering him (right from six to eight months of age) with what is coming next so he too can feel in control. Maintain your usual arrival and departure routine and keep him well informed and well involved in the process through your flow of communication.

If he resists, which children often do, remain consistent, confident and follow your flow plan of defining your statements clearly and following through. If you re-assume your usual, confident, guiding-parenting role, he'll quickly settle back into sharing the control of his day, and you won't have the 24- to 48-hour transition of grouchy and teary or challenging behaviour until he settles back down.

What is positive routine management?

The primary goal of parents with children under the age of two is to *be understood*. Once children are six months old they can understand you. If you create a pattern of routine communication ('language cues') during an everyday routine event (such as nappy changing time, going to bed and meal times) you develop predictable associations around those cues. Your baby will be able to learn any new process or language in less than 12 hours. By the time he is six months old, you will have a well-balanced and well-defined style of communication with your baby.

Meeting a child's every demand doesn't always mean meeting a child's every need

Using predictable and consistent ways of communicating with your baby throughout the day is the only way to reduce or eliminate tears significantly when teaching him a new routine around sleeping, eating, or playing independently.

Make sure you allow the time to set your child up and equip him for coping in the world so he can confidently and happily engage with his peers and his carers.

It is in the first two years of a child's life that the emphasis on his responses to you and the environment around him is aimed squarely at his ability to understand, predict and therefore trust his mummy and daddy.

By adopting a balanced, healthy parenting philosophy, in which you convey your wishes and intentions clearly to your baby or toddler, you can open simple, easy-to-understand, trustworthy lines of communication.

When someone asks me, 'When is my baby going to learn how to sleep?', my only answer is, 'When you teach him!'

The six steps of the flow of communication

For a baby to become comfortable with you providing a predictable style of language, you should start when your baby is six months old.

The following six steps of communication are important for children ranging from eight to ten months of age and absolutely vital for 12 to 15 month olds plus. Use this flow of communication in all aspects of his day, not just areas he's having difficulty with so your child develops good associations with this style of language and feels confident that understanding is achievable.

1. Pre-empting

State what you're doing now and what you will be doing next. For example: 'Now we are ____A____, but soon it will be time to ____B____.'

2. Forewarning

Provide a final warning to your baby that transition is about to take place: 'Last one bubby, nearly time to ____B____.'

3. Stating event and expectation

For example, you can say 'Time to change your nappy, time to lie down and wait for Mummy.'

4. Defining your statement

Define each statement with its true definition; for example, 'Lie down and wait' does not mean 'Roll over and get on your knees'; it means, 'Lie down and wait'.

5. Following through

Regardless of your baby's reaction to the request or statement you've made, continue enthusiastically until the task is completed.

6. Completion

Wrap up the event with a clear statement indicating it's all finished now and he can guide you again.

These six steps are important and you should refer back to them. A good idea would be to flag this page with a Post-it Note so you can find it easily.

Hot tip: Use your flow of communication prior to predictable trouble times, such as meals, nappy changing, bedtime or going to daycare. You'll reassure your baby and get him ready to smoothly transition from one event to another.

Your primary intention when communicating with children under the age of two years should be to fully focus on being understood. This means being 100 per cent accountable for what you say and the clarity of each statement.

The way you respectfully use a parent-governed line of communication with your child is very important to the way he perceives your guidance.

Defusing meal-time tears

Imagine you have a ten month old who is getting a little grumpy about eating dinner. He's tired, has had a big day and isn't feeling inclined to be patient. He's frowning, lowering his chin into his chest and pouting. He looks to be on the brink of losing it and, finally, he gives a kick and squirms in his chair as he grizzles a complaint at you. You're on the threshold of meal-time hell. Do you become tense?

Parents in this situation often try to distract their baby by overwhelming the baby with choice. While distraction is sometimes a helpful tool, it can also escalate a situation, and frustrated crying and tantrums can follow. My suggestion for dealing with a toddler when you can see he's getting a little edgy is to try to defuse things with humour. But how?

When he does his little kick and grizzle at you, respond with a little surprise jump in your seat (and a blink and shake of the head) and offer a high tone, '*Oh!*', and stop and smile at him. He now has your attention and he can see you're waiting for him to respond. This will change the flow of what is starting to occur, which you can lock in by being repetitive. Your baby will likely repeat the behaviour because you were responsive, so repeat your response. If he is reacting well, get a little more dramatic with your surprise. Raise your hands, jump a little higher, anything to make him interested in your little interaction. This should start a meal-time laugh session. Then it's official, you've defused the situation and this will allow you the opportunity to start the meal with one of those gooey laughs (all food and gums).

Defusing an embarrassing situation

Imagine your 22 month old bumps his head on the table and plops down on his bottom. There are three people sitting nearby watching, and all react with a little 'Oo-ohhh' when he does it. The bump wasn't so hard, but the emotions that have come up around that event are potentially overwhelming when all eyes are suddenly on him. Most people pre-empt what will follow and rush forward when they can see their child is about to cry. Others in the room offer a hand as well and it all becomes too much for the toddler. This sudden overload of input tips him over the edge, and tears and shying away from the crowd begin. These episodes can take a while to recover from. Toddlers tend to want to hide their face, and sit still with their parents for a while, and can be a little clingy afterwards. Rather than risk this scenario, try to defuse the situation on a one-on-one level if you can. How?

If you can see it is going to take more than an, 'Oops, up you get' and a 'Hurray' clap and cheer, then keep him close, make eye contact and act as though you got the bump like him. Pull a funny face, lift your tone, look a little surprised and say, 'Oh bump' as you touch your head. Repeat it a few times and gauge his response. At this point he might laugh, in which case the people around him join in, and he thinks he is quite funny. On the other hand he may just cry or shy away anyway. This is normal with an older age group, and at least you can rest assured that you gave it a try. If he does react poorly to the situation, all focus should be removed, and a quiet cuddle with Mummy while you chat to the guests should take the pressure off him. Once he's calm, offer a distraction but don't be surprised if he doesn't want this, preferring to sit snuggled in your lap. Many mistake this for being tired but it's a normal response from a toddler to others seeing him hurt himself.

What tone is that?

Say the statement 'Lie down and wait for Mummy' using different tones. First, say it as though you're talking to your child. Now repeat the statement like you're concerned he's going to cry and resist your guidance when you ask him. Did your inflection lift, was your voice low and soft, did you skim over the words, did you pull a funny face where your eyebrows went up in the centre and down at the ends? Imagine this from your baby's perspective. You look like something bad is about to happen, and you feel bad about it. This means every time he's asked to do something, he assumes the asker is doing something awful and feels bad.

Now try it with a bossy tone. Did you sound angry? Did you frown and open your eyes? Did you finish the statement with a pout and retain your frown and stare? Imagine this from your baby's perspective. Your simple request looks like you're angry at him. This means every time he's asked to do something, he assumes the asker is angry.

Now try and say the statement politely. Did you smile? Did you make clear eye contact? Did you sound happy with a higher tone right through the sentence? Did you raise your eyebrows and open your eyes? This last way is how I'd like you to deliver every parent-governed line within your PRM. This ensures respect through guidance, and establishes a positive and healthy association and attitude for your baby towards education. It will also benefit your child in the long term by encouraging healthy expectations from friendships and relationships in the future.

The case of baby Corbin

One of the most upsetting things I come across with young mums and dads is the misinformation, or misunderstanding of information, that occurs when parents are told about body language and the importance of and appropriate use of eye contact. I had a first-time young mum come to listen to a lecture I gave, after which she approached me to tell me about her five-month-old son, who was only able to sleep for 15 minutes at a time, 24 hours a day. He was sitting quietly in his pram, and when I got down to his level to greet him, he made no eye contact, deliberately avoiding my gaze. I sat next to his mother to talk with her about the situation and observed her communicating with her son. Neither looked at each other, and when he became upset he looked away as she patted his tummy looking at the floor.

I asked her to communicate with Corbin more directly, so she said his name, touched his hands, reassured him, but continued to avoid eye contact. If she did look at his face, she was averting her gaze, and vice versa. When I enquired about the avoidance of eye contact she told me she'd been told by a healthcare professional to avoid eye contact and he would settle down. The only result of avoiding eye contact altogether, however, was an emotionally unsettled little baby.

I immediately put strategies in place to encourage an intimate connection with baby massage, swimming lessons and lots of songs, nursery rhymes and one-on-one focus playtime . . . with lots of eye contact. That day, she went home, had a bath with her baby, and talked while he lay on her chest for over an hour. They connected and Corbin got the giggles. For four days straight Corbin giggled every time his mother looked at him.

Corbin's first sleep after that intimate and close interaction was established, as well as a few other basic routine adjustments, was for three hours straight and then right through that first night. I had only encountered this once previously, and the same level of unsettled behaviour accompanied this pattern of body language.

Sebastian wants a biscuit

I stayed in a house with a family in Melbourne who had 19-month-old twins, Lucy and Sebastian. The mother was concerned about how many tantrums Sebastian was having, and how difficult she was finding it to manage his behaviour. Sebastian was a poor eater, had a low iron-absorption rate and low iron stores and was struggling to cope during the day and unsettled at night. His biggest problem was snacking, so we were trying to establish a balanced eating plan for him to encourage better overall nutrition to improve his general demeanour.

We were taking a two-pronged approach: we needed to be clear with our communication to ensure we weren't triggering the tantrums; and we also needed to correct his eating habits to restore a balance to his system so he wasn't so depleted nutritionally, and that his threshold for coping with normal emotions wasn't so low.

On the first day Sebastian approached his mother at the kitchen bench while she was serving dinner and asked for a biscuit. He stood with his feet firmly together, one hand in the air pointing to the biscuit tin, his eyes clearly fixed on his mother. 'Biscuit,' he said. His mother said, 'Look Sebastian, Mummy has made some yummy dinner, chicken, your favourite.' Sebastian looked at the food, which smelled lovely and was making him feel hungry, but continued to point to the tin. 'Biscuit!' he repeated. This time his mother sighed and said, 'Here you are, can you take your spoon to the table for Mummy?' Sebastian took the spoon, dropped it on the floor, then bounced on his knees as his frustration clearly started to grow.

'Biscuit,' he insisted, just about to cry. His mother took his hand and said, 'Come on, let's go and wash our hands for our yummy dinner,' and tried to lead him out the door. At this point Sebastian continued to point at the biscuit tin and tried to look back at it as he was guided out of the room, crying. He then dropped his weight and went into a full tantrum before they reached the hallway.

The problem for Sebastian was that he was trying to tell his mother something, but she didn't acknowledge that she'd heard or understood his request, and never answered his question. This avoidance strategy only frustrated him, and made him ask more and more passionately. This common communication error often happens when a parent is nervous and not sure how to say 'no'.

Olivia learns a new way

Little Olivia was ten months old when I worked with her mother and father to help her sleep. Olivia and her mother were having a terrible time when it came to going to sleep, and an equally difficult time throughout the night with resettling. Olivia had been guiding her mother through a settling routine that was clearly not working as her mother needed to breastfeed her for up to three hours to get her to sleep. This was making both mother and baby exhausted, and wasting precious energy on an event that did not need to be so difficult.

We set about developing a new routine for sleep time. From the day we were to start the new routine Olivia could predict the following events:

- Breastfeed on couch.
- Cooing and cuddles with Mum and Dad.
- Kiss Dad goodnight (he would learn to settle her in a week).
- Walk up to parents' room to be wrapped (one arm out to suck her thumb).
- Be taken into her room.
- Have a cuddle and a song.
- Get a kiss on the cheek.
- Be put into her cot to be tucked in.

- Cues.
- Mummy leaving room so Olivia can put herself to sleep.

We role played for a couple of days leading up to the first day, and had been working very hard on our communication. Olivia was ready to try it all by herself.

Olivia's mum called me in tears on the second day of their new routine. Concerned, I asked her if Olivia was okay and she told me the reason she was crying was because Olivia was not only comfortable with the routine, but had taken control of it. After her mother gave her a cuddle and sang 'Twinkle Twinkle Little Star', Olivia stretched up and kissed her mother's cheek, then reached out to her cot to be laid down. Her mother was thrilled that by creating a predictable routine she'd empowered Olivia with a lovely way to go to sleep that suited both her and Olivia.

New basic cues

Here are some simple language cues to use in some of your event routines:

Pre-empting

'Now we're doing ______, but soon we will ______.'

'Nearly time to ______.'

'Sit/lie down, and wait for Mummy.'

Forewarning

'Last one, nearly time to ______.'

'Time to pack away.'

'Time to sit/lie down, wait for Daddy.'

Saying 'no' when you have other plans

'Say bye bye, ______.'

Boundary setting

'No touch. Hot/break/hurt/sore.'

Request to keep shoes and socks on as you drive in the car

'Socks on. Shoes on.' But remember to define this!

Distraction or redirection

'Where's your ______ (sound effects are sometimes good here: buck buck beguck, for chicken)?'

Self-help skills for feeding

'Scoop it up, in your mouth.'

Retaining a governing line when your baby is challenging you
'Daddy do it.'

Meal-time management
'Hands down.'
'Fingers out of mouth.'
'Bite.'
'Mummy/Daddy do it.'

Asking to give you something or put it somewhere
'Ta for Mummy/Daddy/toy box.'

Offering something
'Ta for (baby's name).'

'Woke up on the wrong side of the bed' babies

Alex was the beautiful 18-month-old baby boy of two very loving, working parents. He'd recently experienced a significant trauma when introduced to a childcare centre without the usual orientation and gradual introduction to his new carers and the environment. After four days he was so unsettled he cried for two days straight. Despite a lengthy stay in the local hospital and every test the emergency department had to offer, Alex was sent home with a clean bill of physical health. But he was far from emotionally healthy. He was screaming, and continued to do so for another 48 hours straight. No breaks, no sleep, no food or water, just inconsolable crying from a baby who'd crossed the emotional line from distress into the realm of trauma.

Alex's absolutely distraught parents rang me sounding utterly consumed about what could have happened while he was in the centre's care to cause this reaction. As a childcare worker myself who'd helped thousands of children adjust to daycare, I'd rarely seen such a strong reaction from a child. As I got to know Alex over the next week, what had happened at his childcare centre became clear.

Alex was a child who needed time to warm up to his environment, and the extra people in it, even at home. He was still young and he interacted predominantly with one carer at a time prior to childcare. As his parents shared his primary care equally, he was comfortable with both parents nurturing him. When Alex shifted from one location to the next, from sleeping to coming out to be with his family for instance, he would become very distressed. People would try to talk with him, offer him toys, everyone would look and fuss, try to make him feel better and, when all that failed, they'd assume he must feel sick. In fact, he just needed to sit, get comfortable in that space without too many people focusing on him, and be gently encouraged to start playing by the person who brought him into that situation.

Alex wasn't ready to interact with others until he'd had some adjustment time, even at home. Imagine how he felt being taken to childcare for the first time, with no warm-up days when his parents were with him, no time to get to know his carers, no orientation to get to know the environment, no time to watch the other children play and see how much fun they had, and without his favourite teddy. He was just taken there, and at the centre staff's encouragement, was simply left there. Clearly this was a traumatic event for him, and could be stressful for any child under two.

The centre claimed they 'forgot' his orientation process and apologised for their error. Alex regained his trust within five days of starting this program and now attends a new daycare centre after careful preparation. He loves it. Our strategy to help him through this 'stage' of his life at home was simple. Before being introduced to a new scenario he needed lots of forewarning. We would tell him in happy tones who he would see, and what toys there were to play with, and let him know he could have a cuddle with Daddy/Mummy until he was ready to play. As we entered the room, we would play a peek-a-boo game, asking the other adults in the room not to respond to our entry. Unless he indicated he was ready to say hello to other people, we kept things low key and didn't push things for a few minutes.

His initial response was always the same. One finger in his mouth, head tilted looking shy and firmly attached to whoever brought him into the room. Once he was sitting, we encouraged the adults to start natural communication with one another and just leave him be. He would sit, listen quietly, and eventually start to look around the room. When we saw this we would slowly point out his toys with a little bit of humour. We didn't offer the toys to him though. He would stay on our lap, and we would have a little play with the toy but leave it on the floor.

Within moments he would be giggling at our crazy play, and then suddenly pop down, still holding one of our legs and reach for his toy. If he couldn't reach, we would hold his hand and with gentle encouragement he'd slowly step away from us, and then come back with his toy. He would generally start to play at our feet, and the other carers could talk about the toy from that point on. As soon as he was ready, he would respond to the other carers and suddenly feel completely relaxed and move on as though nothing extraordinary was happening.

This was Alex's warm-up time. It took about two or three minutes for him to adjust to a new environment each time he initially entered it. Within three weeks, the need to warm up had disappeared because he always knew he had the time he needed to adjust without the pressure of everyone overwhelming him. He had regained his trust. While Alex's case was extreme because of the childcare centre incident, it is actually a common phenomenon in early childhood.

Max and the great 'carry me' debate

Young 19-month-old Max had taken quite a liking to being carried. Not just carried here or there, but everywhere. He would not go in the pram, he refused to walk, and he would not let his mum put him down to play unless she sat down while he clung desperately on to her, then sat on her as soon as she sat. He was glued to his mother's hip unless he decided otherwise, which was rare. His mother was six months' pregnant and not sure what she was going to do over the coming weeks if this behaviour continued. As he grew and his weight increased, so too did the stress on his mum's shoulders and she ended up with severe shoulder strain, resulting in significant pain. She was instructed by her doctor not to carry her son at all.

This was clearly going to be a challenge for Max's mum and me. Max would throw a tantrum if his mother didn't carry him in exactly the position he preferred. This was putting her back and her unborn baby at risk, so we needed to help him learn how to accept the boundary of not being carried everywhere. This was all about balance, so we said we would sit down for cuddles, but Mummy couldn't carry him. We set up a new management plan by pre-empting the situation. We explained that Mummy had a sore back and a sore shoulder and couldn't lift him, and soon he would be able to have a lovely play with his toys while Mummy did some cooking. We set up play activities for him near his mother, showed him how much fun they were by playing for a few minutes, and then popped him down to have a play. Mum stayed for a few minutes then informed him that soon she would stand up to do some cooking. Finally, as promised, she praised his lovely playing and told him she was going to cook and she wanted him to play with his toys.

Max stood up at the same time and asked to be picked up. His mother reminded him she couldn't pick him up but that she would sit down for a cuddle on the couch. This was not what Max was demanding and a tantrum ensued in which he pulled at her arms, tried to push her to stand, tried to push her off the chair and refused her gentle offers of a cuddle.

This is a good example of when you need to adopt a no-nonsense approach. Once you've made your decision, offered a sensible solution and patiently given the child a minute to accept it, there is nothing more to be done. To stay would only drag out this process, and to pick the baby up wouldn't resolve the situation. The only thing left to do is go back to your chores and ignore the behaviour, and give him three to five minutes to calm down.

These were the new boundaries I asked Max's mother to set:

- If he pulled at her, and hung off her hands, she was to lie him down on the floor and release his hand from hers and say 'Okay, Max is too cross, Mummy is going to do her jobs.' Then she was to stand up and go back to her chores.

- When she was to lay Max down, she had to provide a soft area with pillows, soft toys and books.
- He was not allowed to grab her hands, drag her, move her, push her or make her do anything. She had to keep busy with her chores, and occasionally remind him, 'No, Max, Mummy can't pick you up now, when you feel better Mummy will come and have a cuddle on the couch', then offer a line of redirection like, 'Where's your books?'
- When the three to five minutes were up, she was to try again by saying, 'Okay, Max, let's have a cuddle on the couch?' before going and sitting on the couch with an offer of arms.

If the tantrum repeated itself, she was to repeat the above sequence. Once the tantrum subsided, Max would either accept the cuddle or not. If he accepted the cuddle, she used the flow of communication so he knew that after the cuddle it was time to go back to his toys and play again, because there was more cooking to be done by Mummy. She persisted with this strategy for two days until there were no more battles. Max was able to predict the times he would be playing, and knew that if he needed a cuddle he could ask for one.

This is the kind of response – ignoring a tantrum or just letting it take its natural course without actively intervening or trying to fix it – that will help the situation come to an end much quicker than it would if you were intervening. If a child is just upset with what you've said, and it was a reasonable boundary, ignoring the tantrum for brief intervals will allow it to subside. When a child is being very stroppy because he's impatient or is demanding to be picked up, or rejects offers of toys on the high chair, etc., it's best to pretend you didn't see the tantrum behaviour begin. If he's very cross, sit quietly near him doing something else until he calms down. You can say, 'Too loud for Mummy's ears. When Sam feels better, Mummy get you up.'

Playing to find emotional solutions

You're equipping your baby with emotional coping tools when you foster role-playing strategies. I call this a child's 'emotional tool kit'. This means that when he feels an emotion he can go to his emotional tool kit to find a solution to resolve the way he feels. If he opens the tool kit up and the only tool he can use is Mum or a cuddle, this leaves him very disempowered, especially if the parent isn't with him 24 hours a day. What may seem a reasonably simple solution – giving a child a breastfeed when he's angry that he needs to stay in his cot to play – isn't going to be much use when he goes to daycare or starts kindergarten, spends the day with Daddy, goes to Granny's, or if his mother has to go away or gets ill. His mother won't always be there to give him a breastfeed then.

Think about what other tools/skills you've empowered your child with to cope in these situations. Mummy, Daddy and a good old cuddle and feed offers the most basic and important solution, but because you're looking to provide balance, you want to ensure you're empowering your child with more than one solution to a problem. Your child's emotional tool kit needs to hold a variety of coping skills/tools you've helped him to learn in order to empower him. These skills/tools will be used by him on a daily basis, and are a combination of learnt and instinctive coping and resolution strategies around certain types of feelings and emotions.

Naturally, there will be times when he will have some emotional response to his surroundings and he will have an instinctive need to be close to a primary nurturer. These are typically around illness and basic dependency needs, such as hunger, warmth, love, comfort, fear and so on. When you respond to these emotions with physical intervention, you tell your baby he needs your help and this is something he can't resolve on his own, *yet*. This enhances the foundation to all bonding, growth and development. When you lump every single emotional response he has into that emotional dependency basket, however, you're not truly listening to your child, and you're limiting his ability to start to understand a normal range of human responses, leaving him disempowered and vulnerable.

It's normal to have to wait, and the feeling of impatience is not an indication that a child is emotionally at risk and, therefore, not an emotion he needs to be rescued from all the time. It is better to equip him with appropriate coping strategies instead. In this case, learning to challenge the environment around him and start to play is an appropriate response. To always rescue him from these normal feelings (like impatience) is to tell him that those feelings are not safe, and should not happen, and Mummy/Daddy is the only one to make him feel better. This is not the case, and you're teaching him that he can't cope with a simple non-threatening feeling. It is important to truly watch and listen to your child and ensure that your responses are appropriate and on a graded scale of intervention.

When I was teaching in the daycare and kindergarten settings, I would often see two- to three-year-old children come into centres and find it extremely hard to cope on their own. Even their most basic feelings had always been resolved for them by being picked up and having their immediate demands met. This created an unrealistic transition into a normal social environment. I often observed these same children make a request to their friends (all developmentally egocentric at this age) and when their friends didn't oblige, they became upset and began to tantrum. This scenario is also common in other settings.

Little children are often surprised then frustrated when their new friends lack the willingness to meet their demands as their parents have done for most of their lives, but it's when they reach into their emotional tool kits to find the tool they should have been empowered with, and discover it missing, that things can become stressful for them. Some children are taught to cry, or tantrum, if they really want their parents to do as they've asked. Often the parents' reasoning is that it's just too hard to do it any other way. Sadly, these little children then try to use these tools at kindergarten and have a tantrum with their friends, who may look on briefly with interest, then walk away and continue playing. These children find it difficult to integrate and socialise initially, and often need lots of assistance from carers to learn the basics of social interaction and balanced expectations around communication.

However, to not provide multiple tools for coping with the multitudes of emotions or typical situations children experience is not only unfair, but also neglects our duty as carers to impart our wisdom to our children, and prepare them to cope and integrate into a social world where they are independent of their mum and dad.

Set their sights on play

Your baby needs you to create a clear, simple, clean environment for him before he'll feel comfortable enough to step away from you and explore that space. Overly colourful and busy play mats may be disruptive to play. Primary colours are often used in the design of children's toys to make them eye-catching and attractive. However these same primary colours are also used in the design of baby play mats. All too often I see parents, with the best of intentions and the desire to create an inviting environment, place a brightly coloured mat, pattern side facing up, with multi-coloured toys on the top and then wonder why their baby either cries immediately when placed in that environment or will only play with his fingers, barely touching the toys. Unfortunately, his beautiful and eye-catching toys are now camouflaged on their overly busy play mat, and it is all a bit too much.

Less is more when it comes to children's play stations. Use a play mat with a single colour so your child can see the colourful toys on top of it. Only provide a small number of toys in each play area to ensure that when you offer toys, they are easy to see, and inviting to play with.

The simple idea of setting up several play stations in a room in well-spaced positions creates a flowing, inviting, continually refreshing environment for your child, and helps him to learn how to transition from one activity to another.

Toy/activity inspiration list

Here are some ideas for toys or activities at various play stations. Catalogue your toys to get you thinking about specific areas of development and plan the stations.

For cognitive/problem solving

- Simple three- to ten-piece puzzles with large handles (gradually make more challenging as baby's skills increase)
- Posting boxes and shape sorters
- Nesting cups
- Stacking rings
- Earlyears inside out cube
- Fisher-Price pop and slide animal pop-up board
- Bead puzzles
- Fisher-Price Peek-a-Blocks 2-in-1 activity wagon

Social/role play

- Fisher-Price Little People yellow school bus
- Toy mobile phone
- Fisher-Price Chatter Telephone
- Mega Bloks Musical Farm
- Amazing Animals Sing & Go Choo-Choo

Physical development

- Laugh & Learn Stride-to-Ride Learning Walker
- Homemade pillow pit (made with your couch cushions)
- Cars
- Balls
- Pull-along toys
- Activities that encourage throwing, rolling, stacking or transferring
- Different handbags (your old ones or from an op shop) with different clasps – zipper, magnetic stud, draw-string, twist clasp – containing coloured scarves in one, blocks in another, spoons in another, small soft toys in another

Construction/Destruction

- Large Duplo
- Large foam blocks

- Simple, light, wooden stackable blocks
- Fisher-Price Peek-a-Blocks
- Any activity that can be pulled apart/put together
- Plasticant Mobilo building and construction toy (for 18 months and over)
- Four 1.25-litre bottles filled with coloured water with added sparkles or other interesting additions with lids Super Glued shut – show him how to roll the bottles down a simple homemade ramp

Language
- Puzzles
- Books (hard-backed)
- Small tent filled with pillows and hard backed books
- Magnetic storyboards (Maisy) for the fridge or white board
- Soft toys
- Puppets

The case of James

Seven-month-old James was a very tired, overstimulated and anxious little boy when I arrived to help him and his family find a little peace. His mother had carefully filmed James's play prior to my arrival, and as I sat on the floor getting to know James, she showed me what it was like on a normal day to try and put him down on the floor for even the most simple of playtimes. At this stage his mother was suffering from a strained shoulder and was finding it very difficult to hold him all day, every day, but James wouldn't let her put him down on the floor.

I watched the video, which showed James sitting happily on his mother's lap, feeling safe and secure, watching his very theatrical three-year-old sister dance and sing and rolly polly over everything. His mother then lifted him out of her lap and lay him down right next to her. He burst into tears immediately and became frantic, kicking and flapping wildly. His sister leant over to try and help him stop crying and tried to tickle his tummy, which only upset him more. His mother got frustrated with big sister and used a firm tone to ask her to 'just leave him be'. His mother then lay down next to him and offered him toys and shook his rattles in front of him to try and distract him. He tried to hit them away kicking and crying, all the while watching his sister dancing. He then started to rub his eyes and cry in long deep howls. Within two minutes of being put down to play, his mum commented that he was obviously tired and that was why he couldn't play, and proceeded to pick him up. Once she picked him up, his crying stopped immediately and he'd smile as she perched him on her hip.

James was often put to bed because his reaction was being misunderstood and this had created serious sleep-time problems as well. It's not uncommon for a child's dislike of environmental conditions to be misinterpreted as tiredness.

What I could see from this simple video was a whole series of other things causing James stress and frustration. Firstly, he wasn't given any warning he was going to be laid down on the floor. So the first new rule of communication was a consistent pre-emptive cue to indicate he was about to be put down before it was done. The second very clear problem was his concerns about his very gorgeous but overexcited sister playing Mummy. She would cramp his space all of a sudden, tickle his tummy and make a lot of noise. Some clear boundaries needed to be set around him when he was playing by himself on the floor. Then we looked at positioning. When his sister was around, sitting him up was more appropriate than lying him down because it left him feeling less vulnerable. The problem he had with sitting was that with very little practice he was not very good at staying upright, which resulted in him falling, which then created a poor association for him.

It took us one morning with the new boundaries and positioning rules in place to regain his trust and establish positive independent play. The results for him and his family were wonderful. This highlights the need to look at all aspects of the problem to help resolve a baby's daytime blues.

The case of James and Oliver

James was a sweet little eight-month-old baby who had a lovely older brother called Oliver. Oliver loved the company of his mother Sarah and his baby brother James. But James was finding it extremely difficult to be put down at any time during the day. While it was difficult for Sarah, she reasoned it wasn't too bad because sleep time was not an issue. But within a month of showing a dislike of his mother putting him down during the day, James started experiencing the same concerns at sleep time. My investigation revealed this pattern of behaviour began during playtime.

I sat on the floor and got acquainted with Sarah, James and Oliver. As Sarah and I sat and chatted, little Oliver sat playing quietly on his mum's legs showing me all his favourite toys. I asked Sarah to show me what she normally did when it was time to put James down. She rolled her eyes and said, 'Okay, cover your ears', then briefly turned James to face her, gave him a little kiss and said, 'C'mon little man, time to lie down and have a play'. I was pleased to see she was using clear pre-emptive language with him.

James was placed carefully on the floor but he lay there stiffly, straining to look down towards his toes. There were no tears, but he was clearly watching for something and his tummy muscles were straining. He had absolutely no interest in the toys his mother was offering him but I could see James watching his brother. Oliver, having seen his brother being put down, immediately set about gathering up toys in the room and then placing them on his baby brother's tummy.

This had become a ritual, his mother claimed. She hadn't wanted to damage the strong bond developing between her sons so she initially fostered this behaviour by rewarding Oliver. She was so pleased to see him being so kind and generous towards his sibling. Within a few short months though, this pattern of behaviour got completely out of hand and was now causing James and Sarah considerable stress.

Oliver had now gathered up a fair few toys for his brother, and Sarah said, 'No more toys, Oliver,' as she watched him continue to gather even more. Thirty seconds later James was becoming excited with the amount of toys, but was still not crying. 'Oliver, Mummy said no more, now listen to me,' Sarah said in a firm voice, but Oliver continued to offer more toys, just one at a time now. James started to try to roll towards his mother and moan. Sarah raised her voice sharply, 'Oliver, that's enough. Now Mummy's cross!' By now James started to cry. As Sarah picked him up she said, 'I'm sorry, Oliver keeps spoiling your play.'

As I watched, the same pattern repeated itself. James wasn't concerned about his brother bringing him toys; in fact he was quite used to it and watched with great interest. What bothered him was the fact that his mother yelled every time she put him down. Because Oliver always got James's toys, and his mother had accidentally defined the statement 'No more toys' to mean 'Get more toys until I yell and pick him up' by not following through, Sarah yelled every single time she put James down. This meant James, being a baby and not understanding her behaviour, was getting a fright each time he was out of her arms. As this didn't happen when he was in her arms, he'd decided to stay in her arms so he didn't get yelled at.

Together we worked on the flow of communication, at rebuilding James' trust in play when put down. Within 24 hours, James was sleeping and playing without a hitch. This highlights the importance of setting boundaries politely and consistently with an older sibling around the baby without raising your voice.

The case of Andrew and Olivia

Andrew and Olivia were beautiful six-month-old twins who kept their adoring parents on their toes every night with two-hourly bottle feeds. Every time Mum fed one twin, she would feed the other just so she didn't have to get up in ten minutes' time, but the twins often then stayed awake for hours during the night, needing snuggles and reassurance. During the day, the babies were tired but happy. They spent a lot of time awake each day and were classic catnappers.

Olivia was content to play and enjoyed the company of her brother but didn't have difficulty playing on her own. Andrew, on the other hand, was a very adoring big brother. He would snuggle and smooch his twin sister endlessly, and would be at his happiest when he was right on top of her sucking her cheek. Olivia loved him very much but found this arrangement unsatisfactory because she clearly had toys to explore, and a slobbering brother was cramping her style. Eventually she would get upset by her brother's antics, and her frustrated cries would send Andrew into a complete emotional meltdown. This ultimately meant that play sessions were over within 15 minutes and both babies needed to be held until the next feed or nap time.

The general strategy I work with when dealing with unsettled twins is to offer graded exposure to a less dependent form of play at least once a day. We decided they needed time together towards the end of an hour-long play session, as this was when they were both less able to cope on their own and were ready to be together. So their first play station was designed to encourage a visually close environment where they could coo and smile at one another but from a slight distance. This resulted in Olivia chatting away happily with an occasional smile for her brother, and Andrew gazing starry-eyed at her, while still playing happily with his toys.

Gradually, we'd bring them closer and closer together in 15-minute intervals. The second play station offered them feet-to-feet playtime, which was delightful to watch. With bare feet they would lock toes immediately, and both of them would play and chat happily without visual contact, content knowing the other was near. Next we progressed them to head-to-toe play where they would lie next to each other but at opposite ends. Eventually, they would play alongside one another and Olivia, having had her busy free play, was more content to play and smooch her brother in return. Play became more settled and enjoyable for both babies and Andrew learnt he could be as content looking at his sister as sucking her cheek.

One of the most empowering aspects of this form of play for Andrew was to be seen at sleep time. Andrew found it very stressful if he was unable to see his sister when he woke up and would often cry until she woke up and cried too. When he was able to hear her crying, he would settle down immediately and go back to sleep. Unfortunately, this now meant his little sister was wide awake and cross about it. Once these play strategies were incorporated into his day, and we made some careful adjustments to their sleeping arrangements, Andrew was content to sleep without the need for tears or disrupting his sister.

Body language

Initially, it's common for babies to have expectations their parents will pick them up, so ensure you don't confuse them with your body language.

- Don't lean over the cot with two hands, like an invitation for him to ask you to pick him up.
- Only ever stand side on to the cot to talk to him and only use one arm in the cot at a time until he's used to playing after sleep rather than being picked up immediately when you enter the room.
- Don't try and offer a semi-hug over the bars or by placing your hands under his armpits as your child may think you're going to pick him up and will be disappointed when it doesn't happen.

If your child can't start to play in his cot, or starts to kick excitedly, misreading your intentions, sit down or stand side on to the cot and chat to him through the bars and keep your hands busy by perhaps folding a towel.

Good high chair play hints

- Use your flow of communication at all times of high chair play, particularly if you're going to duck out of his line of sight. Always be conscious of letting him know 'I'll be back' if you plan on going for a short period of time.
- Moving the high chair to a window or to a new section of the room may create a new feel to the play and keep him interested for a little longer.
- When you start to play and he is about to cry, try to distract him quickly. Call out to your dog or cat, asking him, 'Where has Jessy dog gone? Jeeesssy?' This should buy you some time and help her forget what he was going to cry about so you can introduce a new toy and move him into the kitchen with you.
- If your partner comes home, it's natural to want to chat to them but be sure to stay emotionally available to your baby so you're conscious of what he's doing and saying to you or he'll want to come and be with you rather than staying in his high chair.
- I often notice that when fathers come in, they kiss their wife and, with the intention of getting changed for a fun play with their child, race off to their room without greeting bubba effectively. It's better for fathers to take a moment to go and see their baby, get down on his level, greet him and have a quick chat about his toys then tell him what you're about to do: 'Daddy is going to get changed, I'll be back,

nearly playtime!' This means your baby can start to anticipate one last little play before you always come back for a great fun nudie playtime. Or you could sneak in and get changed without your baby noticing before you enter the room to say hello and get him straight up.

Food as a distraction

Whether to use food as a distraction when a baby is in the pram is a question that comes up all the time when I am visiting families. Here a battle occurs between encouraging effective coping skills in children when it comes to entertaining themselves, and what has become quite the norm: giving children food so they don't complain when they start to get bored when you're not entertaining them. My main concern with this distraction strategy is that parents are essentially teaching their children to eat if they are bored or frustrated.

I am very conscious not to avoid an easily resolved situation or a normal healthy interaction for the sake of short-term peace. I prefer to work through demanding behaviour and answer it appropriately and teach children a healthy coping skill than provide a short-term relief strategy like feeding that potentially teaches them poor emotional coping strategies for patience or boredom in the future. It is better that a baby learns life is not always about being entertained because the true reality of it is they have to learn that a lot of time is actually spent 'waiting'. Doctors run late, dentists can take forever, the queue at the checkout is usually long enough to send most new mums into a state of panic. We stand in endless lines to pay for products, and even a walk down the road involves your baby sitting and waiting at several sets of traffic lights. It's important to teach babies that sometimes they'll need to entertain themselves in ways that don't involve food, to help them develop the essential life skills of patience and waiting.

Obviously, those parents on the full recovery program will have very specific meal plans so this will not be an option for you anyway. For everyone else, if you provide food to stop your baby from being bored it will not help him get back on track with healthy and more effective eating. Snacking in the pram would also be potentially very disruptive to his next meal time. Therefore, no food in the pram unless it is in a designated snack time is the rule for all.

Hot Tip

One of the biggest mistakes I see many people make, even though it is a lovely, sweet and almost instinctive pattern, is to over-rock or jiggle a baby in a pram when they stop it. Even when the baby is content to sit and wait happily, parents continue to rock the pram energetically. This can, for some babies, set them up to need constant rocking or movement to stay calm. In turn it creates difficult expectations around play and, worse still, develops a dependency on rocking that could turn into a sleep solution that needs to be done over and over again all night, every night. This means that as children get older, they'll have been taught that sitting still is not normal and this makes play and sleep a more difficult task.

Simple solution: don't jiggle or rock the pram when you stop. When you're walking the pram moves. If you stop, let the pram be still.

Tips for trolley times

The same principles apply to high chair play before you attempt a restaurant visit as they do to a shopping trolley expedition.

- Don't forget how amazing the world is to your baby. There are thousands of things he's never seen before. Make your trips interesting and exciting.
- Always stay calm, happy and consistent even if he is becoming demanding or making a baby racket.
- The ability to stay emotionally available to your child, even while you're busy doing the weekly shop, is a skill that will set you apart from the rest.
- Implement your new language stream of 'no touch' to your shopping trip and you will be able to safely guide your child and ensure you don't have to continually take things off him once he's collected them off the shelf, thus reducing the trigger for tears.
- Always be sure you've given your baby the opportunity to learn new language cues and requests at home while you have time and patience to follow through to ensure you don't confuse him.

Remember, it's all about giving your baby the opportunity to learn before asking anything of him in a more challenging environment.

The 'lie down' game

If a parent makes it home in time, nudie playtime is one of the most enjoyable one-on-one times of the day, and a wonderful way to close a busy day on a great note.

Keep this game a parent-governed line of communication. During your normal nudie playtime when you see your baby lie down say 'Awwww lie down' and lie your head on the bed. If the baby sits up, say 'Good sleeping'. Everyone should clap and cheer at this wonderful new game. You can encourage him with positive language like 'Good lying down'. Once this basic game has begun, repeat your cue, 'Okay, Mummy/Daddy lie down', and make sure the adults lie their heads on the bed and say 'Awwwwww lie down'. Pretend to sleep. Snore, and have your eyes closed (but keep him in your sights for safety reasons). Stay still for a moment then end the session with a big 'Good sleeping' and sit up. He will leap up with you and proudly clap himself. Everyone clap and cheer again.

If your baby instigates more lying down, you can join him and repeat the game, but be careful about one thing: if he jumps up, don't let him end the lying-down session after that initial start to the game. The completion to lying down should be retained as a parent-governed line of communication for sleep-training purposes, since that is the whole purpose of the game. Encourage him to lie down by either staying there sleeping, or telling him to lie down until you're ready, 'Quick lie down, wait.' He will quickly learn that when he lies down, you'll call an end to the situation and he'll wait grinning at you from her lying position. This means he's used to you governing the end of a lying-down session, and prevents confusion at sleep time.

Meal-time cue: 'bib on'

Place a bib on your baby by showing him the bib and saying, 'Bib on' with a smile on your face. Remember your inflection. This is not a punishment. If he becomes upset, remember the role you and your attitude play in helping her calm down and feel safe. Make sure you put the bib on correctly, and then define what the statement 'bib on' actually means.

If your child tends to try to fight you putting it on or tries to remove the bib, it's important you take the bib out of his grasp and repeat the statement 'Bib on' patiently and gently. Tuck the ends in under his buckles or around their sides (it should be big enough), or hold the bib in place with your hand for older children so they can't lift it or take it off. If he's protesting heavily about his bib don't even try to feed him at this point. 'Bib on, bubba' is a simple request you've made when you're governing the outcome of a situation. If he fights you about something as simple as having his bib put on, it is usually a symptom of a more significant communication problem that is contributing to meal-time dramas and stress for him. It's important your child can relax and allow you to do things for him, like put his bib on him, so that the task of spoon-feeding his is *not* where your biggest battle takes place. This means persisting until he stops trying to remove the bib, or at least can be managed more easily before you start to feed him.

'Nappy change' communication broken down into component parts

Pre-empting: 'Bella, Mummy is just getting dressed but *soon* it will be time for nappy change. Nearly time to lie down and wait for Mummy.'

Forewarning: 'Last one, Bella, then it's time for nappy change, *nearly time* to lie down, wait for Mummy.'

Stating event and expectation: 'It's time to change your nappy, let's go.' Bella looks up and you say 'Up, up' and she raises her arms. You then carry her if she is still a crawler or say 'Let's go' and gesture to her to follow you. Your toddler will grab a toy and run towards the room where the change table is and stand waiting for you. You pat the table and say, 'Lie down, wait for Mummy'. You lay her on the change table and say 'Lie down, wait for Mummy' again. She lies comfortably and babbles, chats or sings along with you while you change her nappy. As the nappy change draws to a close, you play a little game or do a little nursery rhyme much to her delight.

Defining your statement: If she moves to roll over or stand up, make the wait sign with your hand and say, 'Wait'. 'Lie down and wait for Mummy' means 'Don't even try to reposition'.

Praising: If she is lying happily and doesn't look like she's going to challenge you, praise her: 'Good lying down, Bella; 'Good waiting for Mummy, Bella.' Praise and praise good behaviour throughout.

Following through: To manage behaviour use your cues: 'Lie down', 'wait', 'legs down', 'hand out, Mummy do it!' Add nursery rhymes, small toys and songs to hold her attention.

Completion: At the end of the nappy change, when *you're* ready, get your baby up with your up cue or use the wait game. Give her a cuddle and kiss, then leave the room with a little ritual that could be closing the door or turning off the light or putting the nappy into the bin together and washing hands.

Mason, a bundle of energy

If you need more proof that getting your child to position calmly is a good idea then let me introduce Mason, a beautiful little boy who was the most physically mobile and active six month old I had ever come across in my entire career. His mother was desperate with exhaustion and had literally been everywhere to try and help her little boy sleep and eat. Both these tasks were extremely stressful for Mason and his mum and dad. As a result the entire family's future was at stake as Mason's parents' relationship was crumbling. They had been to three sleep schools, employed two private sleep consultants and visited various paediatricians and clinic sisters to seek advice and had been given a whole range of settling and feeding strategies, none of which had been successful. Mason's mum was absolutely convinced that no one could help her as all the other experts had told her that this was just the kind of baby Mason was, and it was better to adjust to that than to try to fix it. But she knew he needed to sleep and to eat.

Mason's mum told me she was frightened her little boy was hyperactive or had ADHD (though she didn't know it, it is absurd to even suggest such a thing at his age) as he was extremely active and others had suggested this to her. I wondered if positioning and really basic communication misses could be the main problem we had to deal with, so I decided to visit the family to see for myself. When I arrived I was a little taken aback by how petite Mason was. He looked the size of your average four month old and was way off the bottom of the chart for height and weight. After dozens of tests with no results he was about to be medicated with a calorie booster. More shocking to me, however, was the fact that this tiny, teeny weeny little baby boy was standing independently and was cruising furniture confidently on his own and had been doing so for nearly seven weeks. When he wasn't standing and walking around he was crawling either commando-style or on his knees double time. He was like an Energizer rabbit, but faster.

I asked his mother to pick him up and hold him and, as I suspected, he would not stay still for even a single moment despite her most valiant efforts. He stood on her hip, moved himself from one hip to the other like a little orangutan, and then spent most of the time trying to push off her with his hands and feet while she clung on desperately. He was not wanting to get down, he was just enjoying the challenge this new physical situation presented him with. I asked to observe her breastfeeding him. This was equally as frantic with a counted 23 attachments in a three-minute window. He was up and down, and sitting, then squatting, then dancing with one foot twirling beautifully or jumping, all while feeding.

His poor mother burst into tears and my jaw was literally on the floor. She was completely exhausted and clearly a little bit frightened about his excessive physicality. And this was the root cause of Mason's sleeping and eating problem. It was not some random suggestion of ADHD – which almost implies permitting the behaviour – but simple positioning and communication like asking him to 'stop, and be still please'. While this might be a shocking suggestion to a number of people, it is an absolutely vital request and boundary that should be set for some, if not most, babies. Mason needed to learn how to sit still, and be still and to relax, and to start to observe the world around him sometime *before* he acted. So his frazzled mother and father needed to learn how to set new boundaries.

We set up a new positioning plan to tackle the main issue and then a week later we planned to start a sleeping and eating program. We decided on just one sitting position on an adult's lap, and eliminated all other sitting options for him for the short term. We decided on one comfortable breastfeeding position and eliminated all other options in the short term. We decided on one hip-carrying position and eliminated all other options in the short term. We locked in simple cues for these new positions: 'sit down, wait for Mummy/Daddy', and 'lie down, wait for Mummy'. And I showed her how to define what those cues meant and how to be consistent until they achieved the results. Based on his response to my initial requests to sit still, it was going to be hard work.

I waved farewell, aware that even for me the next two days would be extremely tiring and challenging. However, within two days Mason was able to sit, to lie, to wait quietly on his parents' hips with no tears and no tantrums. He was able to eat, feed and play more effectively. He was starting to calm down. They were doing great. So it was time to start his new routine. Within two days of starting his new sleeping and eating program Mason was able to self-settle, and resettle independently (with the aid of a no-movement wrap creating a single sleeping position), eat solids in his high chair and relax and enjoy a complete unbroken breastfeed. His parents said their new baby was 'bliss and happy to boot'. The best of both worlds.

Were there tears when Mum and Dad put the new boundaries in place? Most certainly. He was furious in fact, and it took one and a half days for him to learn the new expectations of how to sit, lie and be carried in the new ways. There were lots of cranky baby moments, and lots of tears. Was it worth it? Well, his weight increased within three weeks and he was no longer required to start a calorie booster. He was full, well rested and happy. His mother came off her antidepressants within three months, and his parents repaired their tattered relationship and are still together years later. Mason still sleeps and eats beautifully and is a healthy, happy, bright little boy with a new baby brother. While he did learn some simple positioning boundaries, he always remained a vibrant and energetic little man, just in a more balanced and healthy way. I'd say that was a happy ending. Absolutely worth every moment required to correct his positioning issues.

The case of Miss Melanie and the laptop

To highlight the capacity of a mobile baby, and therefore a busy toddler, to learn and understand the simple 'no touch' language cue, I would like to share a story about a little girl and my laptop. I was fortunate enough to work with a family in Melbourne who had the most adorable little ten-month-old girl called Melanie. She was bright, inquisitive and delightful company despite her dreadful lack of sleep. Her mother and

I giggled the week away as we watched the clever and cheeky antics of this sweet little baby girl. Melanie learnt very quickly how to not touch the kitchen oven, which was at her height, and within one day was able to crawl up to the door, put her hand up without touching it and blow while looking at her mummy. This was Melanie's way of confirming the item was still definitely a no-touch zone. When her mother said 'That's right bubba, no touch', Melanie would happily go on her merry way and find something else to do.

Within three days Melanie was so effective with understanding the basic cue of 'no touch' that her mummy could put a glass of water on the coffee table and if Melanie reached to grab it, a polite 'no touch, Melanie' would result in the little girl confirming she definitely couldn't touch the item with a little raised hand and a blow. All was going beautifully and Melanie was enjoying her new communication with her mummy and me. This was until I brought out my laptop and put it on the coffee table.

Melanie's little eyes lit up at the sight of a million buttons and she immediately stood up on the couch and admired the screen from a distance. Her eyes twinkled as she toddled her way over to my legs and turned to look at the laptop. I then did the unthinkable: I asked her to 'no touch, Melanie'. She looked up at me, held her hand up to the computer and blew a few times. I confirmed it was definitely a no-touch zone, which she accepted but couldn't help but look at the screen. It was almost too tempting to resist, so she checked with me one more time by raising her hand towards the item, looking at me and blowing. I again confirmed it was a no-touch zone and gave her a little cuddle. She laid her head on my lap . . . then tried once again. With an unstoppable smile I confirmed to her that, despite her lovely cuddle, it was still a no-touch zone. Melanie accepted this and decided to stand, holding the coffee table and looking at me while I worked.

After a few minutes she asked again, only this time her hand was almost touching the monitor. I gently brushed her hand away and repeated the cue with a smile, knowing she was finding it very hard to resist. I was just about to pack away my laptop as I could see it was too tricky for her when she picked up a coaster and asked me again, only this time she used the coaster as a way of almost touching my computer. I repeated the cue as I started to pack away. Finally, in a desperate bid, Melanie threw the coaster at the computer and, having finally touched it in the most indirect way, clapped her little hands with delight.

Children are often more receptive to and more able to accept boundaries in the morning.

When you first teach your child to not touch an object she's used to being able to touch, you may need to prevent her from touching the object for a full five minutes, and occasionally longer per intervention.

Melinda and the dreaded sunhat

Melinda was a beautiful 13 month old with a lovely home play environment, including Melinda's most prized possession, a big blue sandpit in the backyard. The pit was filled with her favourite toys and she regularly gazed down from the balcony at its splendour. On the morning I arrived, Melinda's mother filled me in on all of her little bunny's sleep-time dramas and daytime difficulties, but commented that the one thing that was guaranteed to make her happy was the sandpit.

As the first morning progressed, Melinda became tired, which is normal when working to correct sleep-time problems, so we ventured down to the sandpit. I popped my hat on, her mother put her hat on, and we headed for the door.

'Where's Melinda's hat?' I asked.

Her mother laughed. 'You'll be lucky if you get within 100 yards of her with the thing.'

With that response, I instigated a new important communication boundary: 'Sheyney says hats on', and that's just that. This is when I am absolutely no-nonsense. I used my flow of communication to put the hat on but immediately she took it off. I repeated the 'hat on' cue and action all the way to the sandpit. Melinda continued to remove it. I put her hat on again and with lightning speed (which you need to have) I stopped Melinda's hands from even reaching her hat. Every time she would try, I would block her hand and repeat my cue 'hat on'. It didn't take long for Melinda to get frustrated with me.

'How long is this going to last?' her mother asked anxiously.

'Until she stops taking it off,' I confidently replied.

'We could be here a long time, Sheyne,' she gulped.

She was right. For 25 minutes her little girl absolutely battled to take her hat off, and I would not let her. I stayed calm, and either blocked her hands, or held the hat on her head while I released her hands as she tried desperately to remove it. On the rare instance that she did get it off, I would pop it back on immediately. Needless to say, she got very upset with me. She rolled over because she was kicking her feet, so I sat her up, replaced the hat, and carried on. The whole time we intermittently tried to distract her with the sandpit, but she was one determined little button. We praised her, reassured her, but stuck 100 per cent to defining the statement 'hat on'.

Could we not have just gone inside? Sure, but she would have learnt nothing, and it would have all been in vain. Melinda was definitely going to spend more time outside over the next four years of her life, particularly as she loved her sandpit so much, so leaving her hat on was a long overdue boundary that needed to be set, so I decided to work right through it until she stopped fussing and left it on.

Finally, far more tired than when she started, she picked up her spade and started to play. I adjusted her hat, praised her, and we had a lovely play. She would occasionally reach for her hat, but a simple 'hat on' would remind her, and after a brief 'waaaaah' as she dropped her hand again she would resume playing.

That afternoon, we headed out for a walk down the street and her mother and I used the PRM flow of communication to keep the established 'hat on' boundary in place, and guess what . . . instant success. No tears, no tantrums, no attempts to even touch the hat and no skin damage. Her mother sent me an e-mail when she was almost three saying, 'Melinda has never taken her hat off again, nor cared about her hat going on since that first day in the sandpit. Now, if we want to go out to the sandpit, she reminds *me* to get the hats.'

Make a decision about a certain boundary and stick to it. Your child will only need to be exposed to it once or twice to understand there is no negotiation when it comes to wearing his sun hat. His skin is far too precious to just 'give up' on!

The case of Charlie's baby-proof world

I met Charlie, a beautiful little 18 month old, when his parents were finding it more and more difficult to get him to do anything without a massive tantrum. Things hit a crescendo when he became so distressed he cried for over 24 hours straight. This is a crisis- or critical-care case, so I dropped everything and arrived on their doorstep in another Australian state just over six hours after talking to the parents on the phone. I was greeted by his crying but also by a grateful mum and dad. Both mum and dad hugged me in relief and I went to sit next to their very distant-looking baby boy.

Charlie was sitting in front of the television sobbing, a little more settled than earlier when I was on the phone, but totally tuned out. I just sat quietly next to him watching his favourite episode of *The Wiggles* and observed the environment. The whole house was bare. The TV cabinet was emptied of any adult items and filled with toys and the doors were taped closed. There were no bookcases and every single cupboard and door was sealed shut. The kitchen was blocked off with a gate, the coffee table was removed and the room was literally pared down to its bare walls, a couch, a baby seat, a television and toys. Charlie was living in a world where he never had to experience the normal request to not touch certain things. His parents, in their desire to make his life easier, had actually made it so foreign for him to need guidance that he became the ruler of his own domain.

As he got older, it became less and less possible to guide him at all until ultimately the concept of being guided by his parents became something that evoked foreign uncomfortable feelings inside him. In the end, his parents were resigned to doing whatever it took to make him happy, until suddenly their tiny little boy who desperately needed guidance was being burdened with the task of guiding his parents to raise him. This finally became too much and he was no longer able to cope, let alone guide them. This meant all three family members had no one to guide them and didn't know what to do.

That night, once Charlie was asleep, I sat down with Mum and Dad. 'What is it you're wanting from me?' I started.

'Help,' they replied. 'Help us, just tell us what to do, we just don't know anymore.' My heart broke for them.

'So what you're wanting from me is exactly what your baby is wanting from you: some guidance, the burden lifted off him, some good ideas from your pool of wisdom.' Both parents looked at me glassy-eyed.

'Yes please,' they sighed. 'Our poor little man,' his mother sobbed, 'we thought this would make him happy but he just got so stressed.'

The three of us set off on a five-day mission to turn their lives around. I gave them the ability to be the same lifeline to their son that I was to them. As confident, guiding parents with a balanced set of communication streams in a house with a normal amount of things he had access to, some of which he could touch, and some of which he couldn't touch, Charlie became happy and settled. He suddenly began to talk and participate in a huge range of normal, healthy listening tasks.

The case of Alex and the Mack truck

I met the lovely Alex when I visited his family in the south of Sydney. Alex was 11 months old and had developed a really profound fear of the sound of truck engines. This was not just your usual reaction by a baby: it was near hysteria that would often take him between one and two hours to recover from. Most people would think that while this was unfortunate, it was okay: how often does your child encounter a truck when playing at home? Sadly, though, in Alex's case the neighbour was a truck driver and he owned a giant Mack truck. Much to Alex's horror the truck would rumble into life right next to his house at all hours of the day and night.

In this scenario we needed to help Alex overcome his fear and become more relaxed about the noise made by the truck. Initially, we used the 'white noise' setting on a sound therapy spa to eliminate the noise from his environment altogether as his reaction was one of significant distress. We needed to take this measure because trying to teach him to get used to the noise when we didn't have the opportunity to give him some forewarning was clearly going to be too difficult for him, and for us. Instead, we went to the neighbour and recorded the sound of the truck on to a digital recorder and made a CD. In addition to the truck sound, we recorded a series of normal household sounds and created a loop of the six different sounds, one of which was the truck. We then made picture cards to match each sound.

On the first day we sat down with our CD and picture cards and worked through each sound. We made sure the volume was set to low and, knowing the truck was coming next, we would pause the CD, show him the picture of the truck and make the sound with our mouths. This would initially evoke a reaction of real fear in little Alex but we would stay calm and confident for him. Slowly, one loop at a time, Alex became more and more used to the fact that the truck sound was coming. After playing the game four times the first day Alex was getting better and better about hearing the sound.

We repeated this same strategy on day two and as he got more and more used to the sound loop he began to show a desire to play elsewhere and lost interest in the CD. This was a great sign for us. The next part would be easy. We simply left the CD playing and went to a new area of play. As the day progressed, we increased the volume of the CD until it was quite loud. We would carry on as usual and occasionally see him hear the truck and look up at us. As he crawled towards us, we would smile, reassure him and make the truck sound with our mouths while handing him the picture card, then offer him a toy. The truck sound would end its cycle and he would go back to what he was doing. In just two days he went from near hysteria to a whole new level of coping.

We played this CD every day for a week for between one and two hours after an initial sitting-down game. By the third day, the sound of the truck starting up was no longer something that even drew his attention. His mother and I were delighted for him and he has never had a problem with the sound of trucks since.

Safe cot environments

When checking your nursery is safe to pursue independent sleeping for your baby, you should always utilise the latest information and research available to you. The reduction in the incidence of cot death over the past 16 years since the commencement of the SIDS and Kids public education campaign has been a staggering 70 per cent. For the latest information please see their website (www.sidsandkids.org). When shopping for a cot, if the product does not have a label or information indicating it has passed the basic safety standards test as set by Standards Australia for cots (www.standards.org.au) don't purchase the product. Some other basic hints and tips include:

- always place your baby on his back to sleep
- keep his environment smoke free, meaning 100 per cent smoke free always

- don't overheat your baby with excessive bedding or headwear
- don't leave hats, bonnets or other headwear such as hooded tops on your baby while he sleeps as babies cool themselves through their heads
- when tucking in your baby, lie him down towards the bottom end of the mattress to ensure he doesn't wriggle down below tucked-in bedding and risk sleeping with his head covered
- securely tuck in all bedding so it doesn't come loose through the night
- don't use electric blankets, hot-water bottles or heated wheat bags as a means of keeping a baby under two years of age warm
- keep the cot away from any curtains or dangling curtain/blind cords as these represent a significant accidental asphyxiation risk if the child gets the cord or connectors caught around his neck
- unless you're deliberately tucking them into their beds securely, babies under two years of age should be wearing nightwear that will keep them warm rather than trying to cover them with loose blankets – sleeping bags are excellent sleepwear for the cooler months, rather than blankets
- ensure your baby does not have access to uncovered power points, or power leads coming from those points
- there should be absolutely no pillow or cushions, regardless of your child's age or whether he is sleeping or not, while he is in the cot as the risk of overheating or asphyxiation is far too great – pillows can be introduced after your child turns two and he is moved to a bed environment.

Hand-me-down/second-hand cot safety

If you've been given a cot that is older than four years, I would personally recommend you don't use it. If you have a family cot that has been passed down through the years, I usually recommend you put it in a safe place as a keepsake only and don't use it as a sleeping environment for your baby. If you've been given a cot that is not too old, you must ensure it is safe and meets current safety standards set out by Standards Australia for cots, and you must always replace any mattress with a well-fitted, standards-approved mattress. If you're setting up a cot you used with your first child, I always recommend purchasing a new well-fitted, safety-standards-approved mattress as well.

If you're unsure, the following basic common sense guides will help you:

- Cot bars are no less than 5.5 centimetres apart and no more than 8.5 centimetres apart.

- There are no broken, loose or missing elements to the cot.
- The cot mattress should be brand new and safety standards approved; if not, you will need to purchase one.
- The cot mattress fits the cot well, bearing in mind that gaps larger than 2.5 centimetres between the cot bars and the mattress represent a hazardous sleeping environment.
- Any mattress protector is well fitted and breathable – I personally resist the use of these as they overheat children and the mattresses are durable and can survive for two years easily without protectors.
- The cot paint is not toxic lead based.
- Nothing at all can catch on your baby's clothing and trap or hook him if he loses his footing.
- Nothing can catch, trap, or hurt little fingers when they explore the cot.

Hot tips for feeding

Pay attention to your child's feeding habits and positioning. As your baby get older encourage more efficient feeding, and don't allow feeds to be played out over an hour or two because of fussiness or snoozing. By eight weeks most babies are feeding effectively for about 20 minutes on each side, and they gradually become more and more efficient as they grow older. Do note, though, that some babies are far more effective than this, while others may need a little longer. If they start to fuss after a healthy amount of feeding time, simply finish the feed and wait until the next appropriate feed window. If your little one has become fussy, encouraging a longer gap between feeds by ending a feed session after a normal amount of time will encourage better feeding and less fussing at the next feed, and help change the cycle of sluggish to more effective feeds.

Full recovery routine checklist

Has your baby become profoundly overtired, indicated by:

- being unable to sleep for more than one, two or a maximum of three daytime catnaps of between ten and 30 minutes in length
- sleeping less than 12 hours in every 24 hours
- requiring excessive amounts of breastfeeding, or needing to feed for excessive lengths of time to cope with his day
- being unsettled during the night with prolonged wakings in excess of an hour at a time, regularly

- being unable to fall asleep without significant or lengthy intervention
- being unable to go back to sleep without significant or lengthy intervention
- being unable to stay asleep for more than two to three hours at a time at night
- being unable to be placed in his cot without displaying significant distress
- being extremely clingy, and you're unable to put him down
- being distressed and crying for prolonged periods during the day or night both during sleep and non-sleep times of the day, regularly
- not accepting solids or sleep without a big fight?

Have you:

- previously done control crying for more than a three-day window and had no success
- been following a 'classic' routine of two longer sleeps a day carefully, trying to allow your child to self-settle and been unsuccessful
- failed any kind of sleep training that was either designed by or managed personally by a 'professional' sleep consultant even when you stuck 100 per cent to the plan
- been unable to be helped at sleep school, and have been sent home with a 'we are sorry, we can't help you' farewell?

Has the mother of the child:

- been diagnosed with postnatal depression and is not coping terribly well
- feeling that she is not coping or not understanding her baby's needs and is feeling like a failure?

If you're experiencing a combination of some or all of the above symptoms and have a very overtired and unsettled little one with significant stress being experienced by the mother and father, then it's time to quickly repair your sleep through the use of full recovery PRM.

Appropriate foods for your baby's age

As you know, when your baby starts to eat solid foods you need to be careful about what you give him. Below are the foods you can introduce at appropriate ages, how much of them he can eat together with some warnings about foods that might cause a reaction and recommendations on what to avoid in your baby's diet.

For a six to nine month old

Fruit: apple, avocado, banana, cooked apricot, mango, peach, pear

Vegetables: carrot, cauliflower, green beans, lentils (watch in case of reaction), potato, pumpkin, sweet potato, turnip, zucchini

Protein: chicken, egg yolk (reaction watch), fish (reaction watch), lamb

Portion size: 110–170 grams (between the size of a four to six months or seven to nine months jar of bought baby food). Some may want a little more, some may want a little less.

For a ten to 12 month old, in addition to above

Fruit: dried fruit – prunes

Vegetables: Brussels sprouts, cabbage, leek, mushroom, onion, parsnip, pulse beans, rhubarb, beetroot, eggplant, garlic (small portions initially) tomato (watch for rash on face or bottom)

Protein: beef, cheese including cream cheese and ricotta (watch for dairy reaction), liver

Portion size: 130–180 grams, some may want a little more, some may want a little less.

For a 12 month old plus, in addition to above

Fruit: berries (reaction watch for strawberries), melon, plum

Vegetables: bean sprouts, cucumber, celery (once he has enough molars to chew it), lettuce

Protein: custard, regular milk, shellfish (watch for reaction – introduce from 18 months plus)

Portion size: 150–200 grams, some may want a little more, some may want a little less.

Water:

You have *no* idea how important water is from six months of age or when a baby starts to take solids. When I conduct my workshops, the last thing I tell everyone before I send them home is that I want to see their babies beautifully hydrated. I want to see glistening lips and perfect, oily-slick, beautiful big eyes. I want drool and plump hydrated little faces, arms and legs. The level of water each baby will need to achieve this varies according to how active the child is and his diet and his climate, but the most important thing to be mindful of is to just offer your baby several good sips of water often throughout the day. Even if he pushes it away, try a couple more times. Offer no water 30 minutes before breakfast, lunch or dinner for fussy eaters until the meal is completed.

Notes:

- Be mindful of foods that might cause choking. Grapes are not appropriate until around 12 months of age and then they should always be cut in half or quartered, as should berries, to avoid choking.
- No child under two years of age should have a sandwich for lunch unless he can consume a healthy portion of vegetables and iron within that sandwich in addition to at least half the bread. Bear in mind, the content of a sandwich should have a nutritional value vastly higher than the bread. Bread with a spread – Vegemite, cheese, etc. – is not a nutritionally balanced meal. As lunch is the most important meal for sleep, this meal must provide a good balance of vitamins, minerals and iron.
- As iron absorption and stores play such a crucial role in sleep, if you feel that your baby is not eating an adequate quantity of his lunch's meat source, then be sure to offer an evening meal containing meat as well. Once he is eating effectively at lunch, dinner can become predominantly vegetarian.

Warnings:

- Foods to avoid until a child's third to fifth year include honey, kiwi fruit and nut products.
- Honey is definitely not appropriate until a child is 12 months old, although I would be extremely cautious when introducing it to your little one's diet at any age.
- Avoid *all* nut-based products due to the high risk of the potentially fatal allergic reaction called 'nut anaphylaxis'. Don't cross contaminate butter containers or food items by even using a knife that has been in the peanut butter or Nutella jar. Having a nephew who almost lost his life at nine months of age to his nut allergy, I cannot stress the importance of your vigilance where this is concerned. Even a seemingly untraceable quantity of nut product can prove fatal to a child suffering this form of allergic reaction.

When things are definitely not okay

Significant clinical depression and/or clinical anxiety in a parent can be a major cause of ongoing night wakings and daytime wakings. I believe this is because children need to feel comfortable and know everything is okay for them to be able to relax enough to sleep. If one or both parents give off a signal that things are not okay, sleep disruptions become a symptom of a shaky emotional grounding during the day. In other words, parents provide the emotional solid ground that children stand on, but when that ground is not so solid, the foundation for a child's sense of security is unstable, resulting in unsettled behaviour, clinginess, and a lot of crying. Many of these children try to predict the next part of their day by creating it themselves to feel secure. This is when a child-governed line comes forward. Babies under two without a solid parent-governed line of communication become unsettled because they are overburdened by thinking they need to govern their day.

The reason I mention all this is to highlight the importance of identifying the causes of sleep problems, and to go easy on yourself and your child if you're recovering from depression. If you suffer from significant depression/anxiety it may be worth seeking assistance from a medical professional for the condition while you also gain assistance and guidance to work through your baby's sleep-time issues. You can then comfort your child, and not stress him, or alternatively, get some much-needed hands-on help with a professional like myself to implement the program for you.

It's a difficult situation because often troubling bouts of emotional stress from either one or both parents can be directly related to their own sleep deprivation. This will be resolved once the baby starts sleeping, but a vicious cycle occurs here and it means you need to be as calm and confident as possible as you correct your child's sleep-time issues before you can achieve sleep yourself. Make sure you have solid support, and have read and learnt as much as you can. Being forewarned is forearmed and this will also give you a sense of control as you predict the day and your future progress. If, however, you're not coping, look into getting someone to come in to help you until things settle down. A book is not going to be the solution for everyone, and sleep deprivation has some devastating effects on new parents.

Go easy on yourself and get some support until your baby, and then you, can recover. Know you're not alone. Many people out there, like me, are desperately trying to keep up and make a difference to your parenting journey, and never give up on finding harmony in your house.

Never underestimate the value of role playing

I met the amazing baby Joseph when he was a tiny but boisterous eight month old. He had the loveliest giant, round cloth nappies and did the best one-legged dance I had ever seen. I digress . . .

Joseph was a very unsettled sleeper. Before I met his family, his mother and father had talked to every possible person they could who dealt with sleep-time issues who avoided control crying. After all the homespun remedies and routine and settling suggestions they felt they had no other options left available to them and decided to try control crying. On their first attempt, Joseph cried for three hours, much to their horror. They were told to continue. They did. For four days. For each sleep it took an average of two to three hours to get him to go to sleep, and this didn't guarantee he'd stay asleep for more than 40 minutes. Eventually, and wisely, they stopped. Then his exhausted mother and father would take turns for hours and hours on end to rock and pat this beautiful big-nappied baby back to sleep.

One morning, Joseph's father saw me on the breakfast television program *Sunrise*, offering advice on how to get babies to sleep, and decided to give me a call. Because they had all been through so much, I knew trust needed to be re-established, especially after the control crying. On the first day, Joseph showed me just how clever he was by picking up his little toy and saying 'octopus'. It occurred to me that even at eight months Joseph was smart and just needed to be told what was going on.

We role played his new settling routine, including wrapping his blue bear, at least three times before I put him to bed for the first time. Joseph needed a firm wrap to emulate his mummy's cuddles but it took him just three minutes to put himself to sleep the first time. It took him 30 seconds to fall asleep that night. And then I was up all night with his mother, who was crying as she was concerned he had been asleep for too long. Joseph's new sleeping pattern has not faltered since, and he has just started school. He just needed to know what was happening, and what to expect.

Surface-sleep pause for resettling

When your child is learning how to go back to sleep without intervention during surface sleep, you'll need to pause and interpret his crying before deciding to attend to him or not. This process is not about watching a clock; it's about observing his sleep patterns and listening to his cries. Often, the more you fuss the more he'll fuss, so avoid going in during the first ten minutes if at all possible. If he appears upset, however, turn to 'Interpretating your child's cries' to help you determine if you should attend or not. If you do need to attend in the first ten minutes, there is a far higher likelihood that he will get off the bus and you will need to assist him until the next Sleep Bus arrives in 40 minutes' time. The length of your initial pause will increase, in the first few days of learning to go back to sleep, in the following pattern:

Day 1: wait a minimum of five minutes before interpreting his cries, deciding to attend or not, and using your new resettling routine.

Day 2: wait a minimum of six minutes before interpreting his cries, deciding to attend or not, and using your new resettling routine.
Day 3: wait a minimum of seven minutes before interpreting his cries, deciding to attend or not, and using your new resettling routine.
Day 4: wait a minimum of eight minutes before interpreting his cries, deciding to attend or not, and using your new resettling routine.
Day 5: wait a minimum of ten minutes before interpreting his cries, deciding to attend or not, and using your new resettling routine.

These times are only for when you feel you have no choice but to attend in those first ten minutes, until he's become fully conscious of his environment, or gone back to sleep.

A little history of the Sleep Bus

The Sleep Bus is a simple concept based on years of record-keeping while observing children as well as on the study I've undertaken on sleep. I first noticed the pattern I call 'the Sleep Bus' when I started working with children in daycare, but it was not until 1993/94, when I started comparing the data from my mountains and mountains of observations of different children, that I actually discovered a clear distinction in day versus night and settling versus resettling sleep patterns. I noticed that a child put to bed at a certain time comes back to surface sleep at specific times, so it is possible to predict times when a child will cry naturally during the night.

I named it 'the Sleep Bus' because of the different lengths of time it took sleep to come at night compared to the time it took during the day. I was living in London at the time and one night as I sat waiting at Trafalgar Square to get the bus home it felt like an eternity, and I was tired and freezing and desperate for the bus to arrive. So I got up to check the timetable. What I saw was a mirror image of what I was seeing and using as a prediction method to assist children to settle to sleep, or to go back to sleep, during the day and night. It was ironic to me, because the same desperate wish for the bus to come that was filling me, was just as it is after I wanted a little person to go back to sleep when they've woken during the night, but the bus only comes according to the timetable and I needed to be patient.

In 2003 I introduced the Sleep Bus to all of Australia on Seven's *Sunrise* program, and it caught on like wildfire. I am very proud to release it here completely, and believe it has the potential to change the way sleep time and wakings are ultimately managed everywhere.

The case of Jed and his train

I once travelled for an hour by car, two hours by plane, an hour by bus, four hours by train and an hour in a car again to discover the cause behind the mysterious frequent wakings of a baby who seemed to be on just the right routine. Usually I can identify what the cause of most sleep problems are fairly quickly by just chatting on the phone, but occasionally a baby like Jed turns up and no matter how much I investigate I just can't put my finger on the cause.

After I arrived, Jed's parents apologised that their house was right on the railroad tracks. Not long after a train tooted and the entire house went into a flat spin. Jed became frantic. Dad ran for Jed with great excitement, Mum ran for the door keys, and baby Jed squirmed eagerly as Mum unlocked the door. When the door was opened we all ran to the back fence. I looked on with great interest as Jed and Daddy waved to each of the 35 carriages before heading back inside.

'Does that happen every time the train goes by?' I asked in amazement.

'Yep,' Dad said proudly, 'he sure loves his trains. He's such a little boy!'

Needless to say, this was the source of the problems. Twenty-four hours a day that train rumbled by and Jed had become so used to running for the door to see it that even when he was asleep he'd hear it a mile away and panic, calling urgently to be picked up day and night. He'd become so unsettled at sleep time that we had to take drastic measures. We quickly stopped responding to the train altogether and, within two days, I was able to happily wave goodbye. The moral of the story is, 'Beware of the habits you create for your child.'

Diversity in sleep repair requirement

The parents of seven-month-old Mia asked me for assistance with Mia, who woke more than ten times a night and would only sleep in her mother's arms during the day. Despite this, Mia's average sleep requirement, calculated through a sleep diary over a seven-day period, was 15 hours, 45 minutes. I placed Mia on a high-sleep-requirement routine, placing an emphasis on communication, environmental factors such as needing to be wrapped, and routines for predictable settling, resettling and waking.

Through this management, Mia's sleep in her cot was quickly restored and within three days she could self-settle, self-resettle, stay asleep peacefully, and be content to be in her cot awake. After that her parents were very careful and consistent for three full weeks so Mia felt safe in her new routine because her sleep disruption triggers were difficult to work through. Mia had to learn how to be in her cot awake and put herself to sleep, and her parents had to learn *not* to rescue her from that normal and safe environment.

Acknowledgements

This book was only possible because of my beautiful, courageous, funny, vivacious and amazing daughter, Dasha Sofia, who fought so hard to beat the cancer she was diagnosed with at just two years of age.

So, firstly I would like to thank my darling little girl, Dasha, for showing me the true depth of love a human heart is capable of. You are my reason for being, my one and only and forever. You are the most extraordinary human being I have ever met. Thank you for trusting me as you walk your life's path, and for enduring the unimaginable so we can journey forward as a family. Thank you for ringing that bell, my precious baby girl. Mumma loves you more than you will ever truly understand.

To my husband, Diego Fernando Soto – what a ride! Thank you for our baby girl, and thank you for all you have done, and do every day, to ensure we get through even the toughest of battles and enjoy the brightest of days. I love you with all my heart, and always will!

To my amazing family for all their incredible love and support over the last 18 super-challenging months, all the prayers, tears, time, effort, determined faith in her recovery and endless love and dedication to us was unbelievable. I truly believe I have the best family in the entire universe. I love you all so deeply.

To aunty Limmy (Simmeone Hanlen), you are one outstanding human being. Not only did you stand by my side every single day while Dasha was so ill, coming to every single scan, chemotherapy day and hospital stay, you also spent your spare moments cooking, cleaning, washing, visiting, supporting and loving us. You were our literal liferaft – and you never, ever left my or Dasha's side, on even the darkest days. I cannot tell you how grateful I am. I don't know how we could have done it without you but I do know that we did it so well because of you. We love you, love you, love you! Thank you, Simmy.

To my amazing friends, Tina Cholakyan, Rebecca Tait Hecker, Melissa Mozley, Fiona Drane, Susanne Knowlings, Lynette Dibbs, Jane Groves, Tamika Yea and my mothers' group and the many other wonderful friends who got us through a year of chemotherapy treatment and have always been there to help – my thanks comes from the deepest part of my heart.

To the amazing medical and nursing teams who got us through at the San hospital, especially Dr Hanna ('Easy does it!') and to our life-saving Dr Servinch (thank you for hearing a desperate mother's cries and listening to both me and your instincts). May God always guide your work with children. Our thanks is difficult to put into words – you saved Dasha's life. To our outstanding oncology, surgical, nursing and emotional support teams at Westmead Children's Hospital – you are all incredible human beings and your knowledge, wisdom, love and enthusiasm is out of the world. I can only ever hope to achieve in my lifetime just a fraction of the support and life-saving care to families you provided us with through each day we relied so heavily on you for our miracle. Thank you seems inadequate.

To all the other amazing organisations that got us through, from Red Kite to Cure Our Kids, Neuroblastoma Australia, Capes for Kids, Geelong Crochet For Cancer, Bravery Beads, Starlight Foundation, Camp Quality, Make A Wish and many more – thank you!

To the incredible support I have received from Allen & Unwin (I knew you were my dream publishers for a reason), especially Louise Thurtell – your integrity, heart and patience has been so wonderful. Thank you also to my editor Michelle Swainson.

To my amazing clients over the years, and to all my *Dream Baby Guide* graduates who taught me how to compile this second book – for your trust, dedication to the philosophy and ongoing dedication to the care of other families as you pay the wisdom forward – as well as to my own during our time of need, your kindness has been inspiring, and I am so proud. Thank you.

To my angel nephew, Caleb. You are always with us, never forgotten. Thank you.

Most importantly, to God, thank you for hearing our cries, and answering our prayers. Without my faith, I would have crumbled. Please God, be with us always, and bless all the precious children of this world. I love you.

Index